Children with Neurological Disorders: Book 1

Neurologically Handicapped Children:
Treatment and Management

Children with Neurological Disorders: Book 1

Neurologically Handicapped Children:
Treatment and Management

EDITED BY

NEIL GORDON
MD FRCP
Consultant Paediatric Neurologist,
Booth Hall Children's Hospital,
Manchester

AND

IAN McKINLAY
BSc DCH FRCP
Consultant Paediatric Neurologist,
Booth Hall Children's Hospital,
Manchester

FOREWORD BY

PROFESSOR SIR PETER TIZARD
Emeritus Professor of Paediatrics,
Oxford

BLACKWELL SCIENTIFIC PUBLICATIONS
OXFORD LONDON EDINBURGH
BOSTON PALO ALTO MELBOURNE

© 1986 by
Blackwell Scientific Publications
Editorial offices:
Osney Mead, Oxford, OX2 oEL
8 John Street, London, WC1N 2ES
23 Ainslie Place, Edinburgh, EH3 6AJ
52 Beacon Street, Boston
    Massachusetts 02108, USA
667 Lytton Avenue, Palo Alto
    California 94301, USA
107 Barry Street, Carlton
    Victoria 3053, Australia

First published 1986

Set by Setrite Ltd, Hong Kong
and printed and bound by
William Clowes Ltd,
Beccles and London

DISTRIBUTORS

USA
    Year Book Medical Publishers
    35 East Wacker Drive
    Chicago, Illinois 60601

Canada
    The C.V. Mosby Company
    5240 Finch Avenue East,
    Scarborough
    Ontario M1B 2X4

Australia
    Blackwell Scientific Publications
    (Australia) Pty Ltd
    107 Barry Street
    Carlton, Victoria 3053

British Library
Cataloguing in Publication Data

Children with neurological disorders
Bk. 1, Neurologically handicapped
children: treatment and management
7. Pediatric neurology
I. Gordon, Neil   II. McKinlay, Ian
618.92′8046 Rf486
ISBN 0-632-00827-X
        0-632-01593-4 (PBK)

Contents

v

Contributors

Jean Aicardi, *Clinique de Génétique Médicale et I.N.S.E.R.M. (U12) Hôpital des Enfants Malades, Paris, France*

Jean-Jacques Chevrie, *Clinique de Génétique Médicale et I.N.S.E.R.M. (U12) Hôpital des Enfants Malades, Paris, France*

Ena Davies LCST, *National Advisor, Blissymbolics Communications Resource Centre, South Glamorgan Institute of Higher Education, Cardiff*

Christopher Dodd FRCS, DO, *Consultant Ophthalmologist, Manchester Royal Eye Hospital, Manchester*

Dian Donnai MRCP, DCH, *Consultant in Medical Genetics, St Mary's Hospital, Manchester*

Charles Galasko MB, ChM, MSc, FRCS, *Professor of Orthopaedic Surgery, Royal Manchester Children's Hospital, Manchester*

Neil Gordon MD (Ed), FRCP, FRCP (Ed), *Consultant Paediatric Neurologist, Booth Hall Children's Hospital, Manchester*

John Holland, *Principal Clinical Psychologist, Chichester Health Authority*

Alan Huntington BA, *Honorary Senior Research Associate, Department of Audiology, University of Manchester*

Jean Huntington MA, *Senior Lecturer in Education of the Deaf, Department of Audiology, University of Manchester*

Audrey Leatherbarrow BEd, DASE, CertEd, *Head of Department, Assessment Unit Booth Hall Children's Hospital, Manchester*

Ian McKinlay BSc, DCH, FRCP, *Consultant Paediatric Neurologist, Booth Hall Children's Hospital, Manchester*

George Marshall OBE, *Formerly Headmaster, Exhall Grange School, Coventry*

Robert Minns, *Senior Lecturer, University of Edinburgh, Department of Child Life & Health; Consultant Paediatric Neurologist, Royal Hospital for Sick Children, Edinburgh*

Ingemar Olow MD, PhD h.c., *Medical Director, Bracke Ostergard Habilitation Centre, Göteborg, Sweden*

Nigel Ring MA, MSc, *Formerly Technical Director of the Rehabilitation Engineering Unit, Chailey Heritage, Lewes, Sussex*

Lewis Rosenbloom FRCP, DCH, *Consultant Paediatrician, Alder Hey Children's Hospital, Liverpool*

John Stephenson MA, FRCP, DCH, *Consultant in Paediatric Neurology and Physician with responsibility for the EEG unit, Royal Hospital for Sick Children, Glasgow*

Maurice Super MD, MSc, FRCP, DCH, *Consultant Clinical Geneticist, Royal Manchester Children's Hospital*

David Taylor MD, FRCPsych, *Professor of Child and Adolescent Psychiatry, Royal Manchester Children's Hospital*

Ian Taylor MD, DPH, FRCP, *Ellis Llwyd Jones Professor of Audiology and Education of the Deaf, Department of Audiology, University of Manchester*

David Thursfield DPH, MRCPsych *Consultant Child and Adolescent Psychiatrist, Royal Preston Hospital, Fulwood, Preston, Lancashire*

Foreword

Professor Sir Peter Tizard
Emeritus Professor of Paediatrics, Oxford

At least a quarter of all children seen by paediatricians in their out-patient clinics are suffering from chronic (i.e. long lasting) disorders of the nervous system (brain, spinal cord or peripheral nerves). The com-monest of these conditions are emotional and behavioural disorders, learning difficulties, mental retardation, fits and cerebral palsy; less com-mon are defects of vision or hearing of neurological origin, spina bifida and degenerative disease of the brain or nerves and there is a multitude of rare conditions requiring expert diagnosis.

The editors of this book are both consultant paediatric neurologists in Manchester where the senior (Dr Neil Gordon), starting nearly thirty years ago, built up the first comprehensive service for paediatric neurol-ogy in this country—at least outside London.

This book is unusual for several reasons. Drs Gordon and McKinlay have made an admirable selection of contributors, half of whom are from Manchester, the remainder being specialists from other parts of the United Kingdom or continental Europe, and they have evidently given these authors their reins! Each chapter is a lengthy, authoritative and up-to-date essay on every aspect of the condition under review.

Next, the book is not only addressed to doctors—especially to paedia-tricians, neurologists and psychiatrists—but also to members of the several groups of non-medical professional workers, who play such important roles in the lives of handicapped children—therapists, psychologists, social workers and teachers. But the individuals most obviously involved in the care of handicapped children are, of course, their parents and this is a book that could be read and understood by intelligent men and women whose occupations have no connection with medical matters. What it will teach them is how complex are these disorders and how seriously studied by the experts, how much *is* known about them and how much can be done to help a handicapped child to lead a normal life, even when curative treatment is not available.

The third unusual feature of this book is the amount of space devoted by the editors in their personal contributions and by many of the invited authors to discussion of doctor/patient and doctor/parent relationships, to the exchange of mutual understanding—the doctor learning the practical and emotional problems imposed by a handicapped child on his family (and vice versa), the parent learning the medical background to the condition, its causation (when known) and the possibilities of treatment in its widest sense.

Finally, I must draw attention to the kindness and informed concern for their child patients and their families shown by the editors and many of the authors. They do not only refer to concepts which, I am glad to say, have become commonplace in British paediatrics in recent years, but show their awareness of the practical measures by which their good intentions may be achieved.

It is a pleasure and a privilege to have been asked to contribute a foreword to this work.

Introduction

Ian McKinlay & Neil Gordon

Neurology has been described as 'the unspeakable in pursuit of the untreatable'. As it becomes a less remote speciality and as communication with families has grown, neurologists are becoming less formidable. Also the main purpose of their 'pursuit' is not the search for obscure diseases ('interesting cases'). While many common neurological disorders are not at present curable, there are possibilities for explaining them to the family. Consequences for the child and family may be limited by treating symptoms, organizing educational opportunities, facilitating care and promoting acceptance of the family's predicament. Although efforts to help the disabled person may sometimes produce small changes, the benefit to the family as a whole in terms of prevention of secondary illness and distress justify a thorough service. This aspect has perhaps been misunderstood by doctors or others who feel uncomfortable with disabled people and are not frequently involved in their care. Confidence in the treatment and management of neurologically sick or handicapped children derives partly from familiarity and partly from a structured approach (the same is true of surgery).

This book, and its companion volume (*Neurologically Sick Children: Treatment and Management*), seek to clarify the role of the doctor and the contribution of medicine within a wider service. They also acknowledge the place of other experts within that service. The first book deals with long-term management of chronic disorders and aims to convey the philosophy evolved by paediatric neurology departments. The second book is more specifically about the management of acute or complex disorders. The opportunity is also taken to describe the contribution made to treatment and management by the computerized tomography brain scan.

It is logical to include any condition that affects the central and peripheral nervous system under the rubric of paediatric neurology. This encompasses all the problems related to mental retardation and to specific learning disorders particularly of language, those due to motor disabilities such as cerebral palsy, all the varied aspects of the management of epilepsy in childhood, as well as the rarer neurological diseases, for example, metabolic disorders, defects of muscle chemistry, infections, hereditary conditions and neoplasms. There are strong arguments for increasing the resources devoted to this speciality, especially in terms of teaching and research, although most of the medical commitment must be provided by paediatricians, family doctors and community child health services.

The growth of paediatric neurology: the last 25 years

There have been considerable developments in community and child health services for disabled children in the last 25 years. Technical advances have seen the development of chromosome testing, computerized tomography, peripatetic EEG, metabolic screening of neonates, and greatly enhanced biochemical investigation including serum drug levels. Attitudes to handicap and disability have also been changing. For 15 years all mentally handicapped British children have had the right to receive education; schools have replaced the health authorities' junior training centres. Local sports centres and holiday schemes increasingly offer facilities for handicapped people, and local authorities are becoming more aware of problems of access, care, mobility, further education, occupation and leisure. In many parts of Britain, admission of mentally handicapped children to long stay hospitals has ceased, though a proportion of these children do need alternative accommodation to their family home. It has become commonplace to see handicapped children with their parents or guardians in shopping precincts, holiday resorts and cinemas. Certain public attitudes to handicap are still a problem, however, and will not change as quickly; the funding of services remains precarious, and parents may still be embarrassed when they ask for allowances or services. Indeed, the effect on families with a handicapped child of the new policies of community care has been little studied. But there is no doubt that there have been improvements in the predicament of handicapped or disabled children and their families.

The present position

Handicapped children, including those who are mentally handicapped, now usually receive initial specialist medical advice from a paediatrician with a developmental interest, rather than a psychiatrist with an interest in mental handicap. The reason for the handicap will be investigated and will be successfully found in two-thirds of the children. If the problem is complex either diagnostically or therapeutically, many paediatricians will involve a paediatric neurologist, if one is available, for further discussion and advice. The neurologist commonly makes a contribution, often involving the genetics service, over a short period of time and then refers the child back to the paediatrician for continuing care. As the child grows, the neurologist is often asked for a second opinion about treatment and management. This may be in a local shared clinic (paediatrics/neurology) often held monthly. These clinics maintain good links between local and teaching centres and reduce travelling for parents. (In Manchester each consultant paediatric neurologist holds one such clinic each week on average.) Problem patients may be seen on the ward during such visits also.

Combined clinics are also carried out by paediatric neurologists and paediatricians with community doctors, for example in special schools near the teaching centre. This allows the neurologist to meet school doctors, teachers, community nurses and therapists, as well as the parents. The improved briefing so obtained helps in the consultation with the child, and also minimizes conflict between school and hospital.

Neurological paediatrics is having an impact in treatment as well as diagnosis. Drug treatment for epilepsy is more easily monitored and has been simplified. Of the 54 mentally handicapped schoolchildren with epilepsy in Salford near one of our hospitals, half receive one drug only and a few have been withdrawn from all drugs (which had proved ineffective). It is exceptional for drugs to be prescribed for behavioural problems if a service is available for behavioural advice and social work or nursing support.

Therapists, social workers, teachers, childrens' nurses (in hospital and community) and psychologists have become much more involved with handicapped children and have been developing expertise that is making life easier for their families. At one time the doctor was liable to be offered the results of pent-up frustration, anger and distress caused by handicap in families at their wits' end. There is now more to offer and there are more people to share the problems with. That has potential for confusion and duplication of effort, but if the work is well co-ordinated and led the service is enriched.

Becoming an adult

The changing situation for children is beginning to affect adult services, which are much less prepared (in the sense of facilities and professional education) to continue the paediatric style of management. Children with chronic neurological handicaps who have been regularly reviewed throughout childhood find a great change when they grow up and request help. Specialist appointments tend to be on an *ad hoc* basis only; the family doctor may or may not have expertise in advising handicapped people and the community health services are often much more developed for schoolchildren than for adults. The proposals to close large mental handicap hospitals is prompting review of these services in a way that may be beneficial to those living at home also. There is a case for establishing posts in clinical community medicine throughout the country to ensure that the service is co-ordinated and, by occasional reviews of handicapped adults, that individuals are receiving that service. There is also a case for establishing consultant posts with special interest in neurological rehabilitation to co-ordinate the hospital services. Such health and rehabilitation services could be based in resource centres that are an adult extension of the concept of child development centres. At present, some units for the young chronic disabled, the brain injured and the paraplegic have been equivocal in their response to young adults with cerebral palsy, mental handicap or spina bifida. (Handicapped people can have quite strong prejudices about people with other handicaps—perhaps because when they were younger they were told 'Well, at least you're not mentally handicapped', 'You don't have epilepsy', etc.) In-patient planning will be needed for some handicapped adults when they become ill. For most, some extra nursing cover will enable treatment to proceed within existing services. However, when disturbed handicapped people become ill (e.g. disturbed from psychosis or epilepsy), it is doubtful whether they would be best served by those services in their present form.

Accommodation for disabled or mentally handicapped adults is at present limited in availability and scope. Those with multiple care needs, difficult behaviour or criminal records are often excluded from hostels or sheltered housing schemes. As parents age, fall ill, tire or expand their working responsibilities, requests for accommodation will increase.

Although imaginative schemes for employment, further education and occupation of disabled or handicapped adults exist, there is still a great deal of boring or unsuitable activity in overcrowded or inappropriate accommodation. In times of mass unemployment and controlled public spending, change is likely to be slow unless enlightened self-funded schemes emerge at a local level.

Development of paediatric neurology: the next 25 years

If paediatric neurology is to remain an integral part of paediatrics, as it surely must do, a wider knowledge of all that can be accomplished in this field is essential. The need for specialized training in neurology is recognized, but the time and opportunity for teaching and research, with rare exceptions, is not. The aim of these books is to indicate to those working in general services how extensive and varied the therapeutics of neurology can be; and also to provide a stimulus for future research of treatment and management techniques.

These books aim to present 'the state of the art' of treatment and management for children with neurological disorders. It is to be hoped that the transformation of the last 25 years will be repeated in the next 25 years, both for children and especially for young adults.

Further reading

Anderson, E.M. (1973) *The Disabled Schoolchild*. Methuen, London.

Anderson, E.M., Clarke, L. & Spain, B. (1982) *Disability in Adolescence*. Methuen, London.

Baird, H.W. & Gordon, F.C. (1983) Neurological evaluation of infants and children. *Clinics in developmental Medicine*, **84/85**. S.I.M.P., Heinemann, London.

Cunningham, C.C. (1979) Parent counselling. In *Tredgold's Mental Retardation* (ed. M. Craft), 12th edn. Ballicre Tindall, London

Downey, J.A. & Low, N.L. (1982) *The Child with Disabling Illness: Principles of Rehabilitation*, 2nd edn. Raven Press, New York.

Drillien, C. & Drummond, M. (1983) Development screening and the child with special needs. *Clinics in Developmental Medicine*, **86**. S.I.M.P., Heinemann, London.

Farnham Diggory, S. (1978) *Learning Disabilities*. Fontana/Open Books, London.

Francis Williams, J. (1974) *Children with Specific Learning Difficulties*, 2nd edn. Pergamon Press, Oxford.

Gordon, N.S. & McKinlay, I. (1986) *Neurologically Sick Children: Management and Treatment (Children with Neurological Disorders*, Book 2). Blackwell Scientific Publications, Oxford.

Hall, D.M.B. (1984) *The Child with a Handicap*. Blackwell Scientific Publications, Oxford.

McCarthy, G.T. (1984) *The Physically Handicapped Child. An Interdisciplinary Approach to Management*. Faber & Faber, London.

Raine, D.N. (1977) *Medico-Social Management of Inherited Metabolic Disease*. MTP Press, Lancaster.

Scheiner, A.P. & Abrams, I.F. (1980) *The Practical Management of the Developmentally Disabled Child*. Raven Press, New York.

Thomson, G.H., Rubin, I.L. & Bilenher, R.M., eds (1984) *Comprehensive Management of Cerebral Palsy*. Grune and Stratton, New York.

Williams, P. & Shoultz, B. (1982) *We Can Speak for Ourselves. Self Advocacy by Mentally Handicapped People* (Human Horizon Series) Souvenir Press, London.

Woods, G.E. (1983) *Handicapped Children in the Community: Medical Aspects for Educationists*. Wright, Bristol.

Chapter 1
The Sick Child's Predicament

David Taylor

'Whole sight, or all the rest is desolation'
John Fowles: Daniel Martin

Introduction

When the group of doctors that became the British Paediatric Neurology
Association met in Manchester in 1971, I took time to visit the Whitworth
Gallery and I saw Epstein's *The Sick Child* for the first time. The model
was his daughter Peggy, aged 10, who was at home and unable to play
because of an eye infection. So Epstein immortalized her. Not all sicknesses have so positive an outcome. It depends in part upon the nature of
the sickness, whether the sickness represents the battle (as it might be
with a cancer or an infection) or is merely the instrument of surrender
(as in the unique metabolic familial recessives). Even then, people are
capable of being ennobled by their manner of coping as well as being
brought low by their failure to cope.

Mostly these are just potential fates, for when sickness strikes it is
usually trivial and leads to nothing but triviality. For this reason doctors,
inundated by sickness of little import, are prone to be seduced into
attempting to trivialize even serious, prolonged and potentially lethal
disorders. A vehicle much favoured for the process of trivialization is high
technology. By rivetting our attention to the disorder of part function, we
hope to be excused our lack of attention to the whole. Frequent success
intermittently reinforces the power of this way of functioning. But equally,
failure is inevitable. The result has been the progressive decline in the
status of medicine despite its successes.

There are additional problems for child neurologists. Children are
'temporary non-persons' sociologically speaking, and the mentally handicapped, those with chronic brain disease and the mentally ill, likewise not
being entirely responsible, are excused social obligations at the price of
not ever being considered quite as people (Locker, 1981). Children's
doctors and doctors of the mentally ill and handicapped have themselves

I

been diminished by association, so that they too occupy a partial non-status. But since serious chronic sickness is not only found amongst groups, such as the young, the elderly and the diminished, whose person status is reduced, it may be that most doctors will soon be accorded a negative regard, along with their patients, by the majority of the fit people aged between 15 and 65.

Reinforcing the public's disregard for medicine has been its failure to meet needs that are not contingent upon high technology but are constituted in what have been dismissed as 'problems of living'. It seems to me that dealing with 'problems of living' at every level represents the highest aspiration of medical practitioners.

A previous essay, originally entitled 'On refreshing the parts that anticonvulsants cannot reach' (Taylor, 1981), was a reminder that there is more to therapeutics than pharmacology, because there is more to sickness than disease and illness. It is immediately apparent that there is a need to agree what these words mean. The dictionaries are not helpful, they are as confused as we have been. I have had to suggest constraints on the use made of these terms and provide a set of considerations that might be used when attempting to differentiate the various components of a sickness (Taylor, 1982). Disease relates to physical realities, evidence of which is accessible to the sense organs. Disease is about things. Illness is the declaration of a sickness in a social context; it is an account, an enactment of a subjective experience. But it can be a behaviour, a role. Illness is about processes. Predicament derives in part from its *Oxford English Dictionary* definition, 'a state of being, condition, situation, or position especially one which is unpleasant, trying, or dangerous'. It encompasses people's psychosocial interconnections, their social ramifications, the sense in which they are understood. Predicaments are about how people are.

In developing the theme of the sick child's predicament I shall first distinguish predicaments from environments. Then I shall consider how predicaments antecedent to sickness might exert their effect. I shall outline how a predicament is discerned and I shall describe some dangerous and some excruciating predicaments. Then I shall discuss the predicament of sickness and finally the hospital as a predicament.

Environments and predicaments

There are hazardous environments, inhospitable terrains, uncomfortable climates. Man can, and does, create his own deserts. A good example was given by Carter (1981) recently. He quotes Thomas Ansell, the Medical Officer of Health for Poplar, giving evidence to a House of Lords Committee in 1862:

> There are four factories and distilleries dealing with the refuse of gas, commonly called naphtha; seventeen manure works for making manure, chiefly from fish, decaying organic matter and night soil; there are ten works connected with the boiling of bones and other animal matter, including a candle factory and a soap factory; there are five varnish makers; there are eleven manufacturing chemists manufacturing various articles such as vitriol and muriatic acid including one smelter of antimony; there is one set of coke ovens and one gas works.

Our understanding of the depredations caused by these environments is a product of bioscience. They speak directly to our dearly won and valued rational expertise. Lead and sulphur in our air; bacteria and isotopes in our milk; smoke, asbestos and silica in our lungs; darkness in our skies. Each is a lesson in elementary chemistry and physiology. Each leads to testable hypotheses. The agents are perceptible and preventable. But there are more subtle vectors.

John B. Calhoun (1973) experimented, albeit with mice, to determine the effects of producing a perfect environment. His memorable paper, entitled 'Death squared: the explosive growth and demise of a mouse population', opens thus: 'I shall largely speak of mice, but my thoughts are on man, on healing, on life and its evolution. Threatening life and evolution are the two deaths, death of the spirit and death of the body.'

Calhoun raised mice, starting with four identical disease-free pairs, in a perfect environment, protected from emigration, resource shortage, inclement weather, foul atmosphere, free from predation. His 'universe' could have supported 3840 mice for nesting sites; 6144 for water supply; and 9500 for food. After an initial pause, its population grew rapidly at first, plateaued, reached a maximum of 2200, declined and *all* the mice died of old age.

He learned that mice have a social organization, and that his paradise was not constituted in accordance with the spirit of that organization. Key social roles became blocked by adults of post-reproductive age. Without appropriate places in the organization in which to learn appropriate sex behaviours, fertile mice were deprived of reproductive opportunities. They did not fight or become sexually deviant. They became drones or 'beautiful ones' capable of nothing but congregating together, eating, sleeping and preening themselves. In the phase of social disorganization,

young mice were prematurely rejected by their mothers so they too failed
to learn the social behaviours necessary for reproductive survival. A
perfect environment proved to be an insupportable predicament. It did
not take the intangible, social needs of mice into consideration. Social
behaviour proved not to be just some superficial nicety. However intangible, it was a fundamental fact of biology.

The social behaviour of children is, similarly, a fundamental fact of
biology. It is dependent upon adequate functioning of the central nervous
system. The level of organization at which it depends upon CNS function
is 'higher' than that which is normally examined by neurologists. It is an
obvious truth that many children who are apparently neurologically sound
are functioning in a grossly deficient manner at that level of organization.
That level is still largely beyond reach of the routines of bioscientific
enquiry. The prospect of a useful marriage between neurometrics (Baird
et al., 1981) and psychometrics, together with positron emission tomography and its developments, offers hope for the future. However, the fact
remains that certain deficiencies in performance will result from environmental rather than from structural deficiencies. These vectors, such as
inappropriate social organization, are intangible and difficult to objectify.

How we label these intangibles varies. We can call them social factors,
the spirit, the imagination. What Calhoun rediscovered by experiment
with mice, Sir James Frazer knew as a matter of social history of man. In
The Golden Bough under 'Tabooed things' he writes: 'The danger is not
less real because it is imaginary; the imagination acts upon a man as really
as does gravitation, and may kill him as certainly as a dose of prussic
acid.'

There are deleterious human environments not constituted in accordance with our social needs. They are just as poisonous in their way as the
air of Poplar in 1862. They are complicated by being translated through
human interpretation, reaction and social behaviour. The classic example
is high-rise flats. But John Lennon, who had ample choice, chose to live
in one till a bullet stopped his song. What caused his death? He died of
his wounds, or of another's mad imagination, or of the major endemic
sickness of New York City, or of his fame. The causal sequences are
more difficult to untangle. Which are the agents, which the vectors, which
the enabling conditions? I see a marked discontinuity between these
complex factors and what we usually mean by 'the environment' and I
prefer to call them Predicaments.

Because they are intangible it is more difficult to understand how
predicaments act in harmful ways than it is to understand the effects of

environmental agents. Gilbert Ryle pointed to this philosophical problem of psychosomatics, indicating that there was no way in which immaterial mind could alter organic structure. But many of us are shy of crediting somatic effects to extraneous causes without the intervention of physically tangible agencies. Yet evidence increasingly suggests it (Schmale, 1959; Ader & Cohen, 1975; Cobb, 1976; Rowland, 1977; Barltrop *et al.*, 1977).

Ryle, of course, was arguing against mind being immaterial. If perceptions lead to states of being, cerebral states, rather than states of mind, and if certain brain states lead to less efficient homeostasis and alter the deployment of defence mechanisms, then predicaments which lead to those states will have as much aetiological force as *Legionella* in the shower water (Stein *et al.*, 1976; Haggerty, 1980; Kashani *et al.*, 1981). It would also make sense of psychological healing, techniques such as re-affirming self-esteem, reviving of spirits, the inspiration of hope, which have been part of the therapeutic equipment of doctors for centuries.

Though we have far more therapeutic equipment nowadays, there is a price to pay for ignoring or diminishing the personal aspects of sickness. It is no part of my argument to deride or belittle the triumphs of bio-science and biotechnology. The statistics of the Royal Manchester Children's Hospital and Booth Hall Children's Hospital 50 years ago in 1931 reveal that most of the sicknesses then given as causes of death have been eliminated, or are better explained. But others assert themselves and death, disability and diminishment still powerfully obtain. The very success of bioscience highlights its failures. The failures lead to criticism, which in turn lead to negative attitudes which reduce medicine's resources.

There are critics within and outside medicine, constructive and destructive. Ivan Illich (1975) attacks the whole technological tinkering basis of medical practice; its presumption, he predicts, will lead to nemesis. More recently, Ian Kennedy (1981) unmasked medicine to explore what he saw as its authoritarianism, its carelessness, its dubious ethics, and its power. In the book *The Aquarian Conspiracy*, which documents wide-ranging changes in the climate of social attitudes, a chapter is given to 'Healing ourselves' and it documents 'what happens when consumers begin to withdraw legitimacy from an authoritarian institution' (Ferguson, 1981).

The withdrawal of legitimacy means that we can no longer presume that we will be left alone to make whatever clinical decisions seem most appropriate in our eyes. Our clinical decisions, our expenditure and our needs are no longer entirely ours to make, to dispense, to provide for.

According to Jonathan Miller (1978) medical authority has been accorded in three ways: *ex officio*, symbolized by granting the title Doctor to Bachelors of Medicine; by charisma, symbolized in personal reputes, foibles, quirks; and through rational expertise, demonstrable knowledge, symbolized in registration and control and Institutes of Learning.

As legitimization is withdrawn, our *ex officio* status is reduced; charisma is latterly not much revered; and our rational expertise is being questioned. Oxygen, Thalidomide, vaccine damage, the mounting price and frequency of suits for negligence; wardships to prevent hysterectomy in a handicapped girl, to permit surgery on a Down's syndrome boy; the Arthur trial; each of these corporate social acts reflects an aspect of public disillusionment with medicine as it is. From within medicine Tudor Hart (1981) tells us we are training the wrong sort of person to be the wrong sort of doctor. Thomas McKeown's Rock Carling volume (1976) is dedicated to the premise that individually delivered biotechnology compares poorly for effectiveness with public health measures. George Engel (1977) and others have been striving to reintroduce the person into the equations of medicine. The silent critics are the astonishing growth of private practice and 'alternative medicine'.

I abstract from all this that medicine is failing at the personal level, and the interpersonal level. The ready solutions provided by bioscience seductively draw us past the person towards the complaint. We are not oriented towards intimacy because many of the solutions we can offer do not require it. Some doctors feel, as Szaz (1972) does, that if the sickness is not biotechnical it is not medical. But who else is supposed to explain that to patients?

In paediatric neurology many of the more impressive and recondite disorders from which neurologists derive their repute are spectacularly biotechnical but have no specific cure. Most of the wide range of minor dysfunctions which make up the bulk of practice give rise to complaints that respond to reassurance and quite general measures.

Even so, we ask 'How are you?' but we do not care to know how people are. We want to know how the disease or the illness is getting on.

Discerning the predicament antecedent to sickness

In his introduction to the American *Basic Handbook of Child Psychiatry*, Justin D. Call (1979) writes: 'The infant is as much a person as is the adult. As growth proceeds, the individual is not only what has emerged, he is a person with a history. Without this history he is an enigma both to himself and to everyone about him'.

History taking is the key to the predicament, but a special type of history taking. What we are seeking is context. A traditional medical history is aimed at determining whether the account being given accords with the technical specifications of a disease. Such social detail as is examined is an extension of the biotechnical, to determine the feasibility of genetic or infective agents being relevant. It is not regarded as a means of making the acquaintance of a patient.

One useful contribution of psychiatrists has been that they set up their interviews in a way which produces historical information from patient and family, but which also generates enactments of how they habitually function and the feelings which they attach to their complaints. Medical consultations seem to us to be geared deliberately to avoid such events, which if they do break through are seen as troublesome intrusions.

It is no wonder that we have a limited understanding of the psychosocial antecedents of sickness and personal vulnerability. I want to know *why* some children are prone to virulent disorders following infectious mononucleosis. Having discovered that measles is a cause of encephalitis, what is it that allows occasional children to suffer measles encephalitis? Why do some children who had prolonged severe febrile seizures not suffer from temporal lobe epilepsy later? The history could be the vehicle through which the antecedents of sickness are explored. Not just the story of the sickness but the story of how it might have come about. It is the opportunity to explore the child's place in its social structure, to examine the traditions of the family, to understand their concept of explanations.

To deepen our knowledge of the predicament means deriving information from which we can make inferences. First, what sorts of attachments and supports have been available, and have these changed? This requires an assessment of the real structure of the family. Is the apparent father, the father? Is he actually present? Does he provide the support which this presumes? Is mother a 'good enough' mother? Is she a 'well enough' mother?

Second, what value is accorded this child, and has that value system been changed? The intrusion of a new baby, a foster child, or a change in parents' interests or preoccupations will be relevant.

Third, does the child have the capacities to meet the demands being made of it? Developmental delay, failure to achieve an expected performance, to conform, to fulfil an affectional need, are the bases of some failures.

Fourth, have there been real changes which reduce 'frequent registrations of consistency', those acts and experiences that diminish the affirmation of social roles, alter social habits, reduce available options?

Totman in his *Social Causes of Illness* (1979) portrays the person at high risk for developing a wide range of disorders: 'He emerges in the throes of significant social change which for one reason or another leaves him socially paralysed—unable to relate to his changed situation in a meaningful and effective manner'.

Life events research, though necessarily constrained by limited formulae for what is and what is not considered meaningful, nevertheless provides general support for this conception of the predicament antecedent to sickness.

Dangerous predicaments

It is simply a mistake to believe that medical biotechnology holds the key to the bulk of child sickness. In the United States in 1970, for example, the death rate for children aged 1–4 was 84.5 per 100,000. A third of these deaths were due to accidents. In the age group 5–15, accidents were responsible for half the deaths (Vaughan *et al.*, 1979). The liability to accident is not random across social groupings, but unduly affects the poorer social groups. The size of the problem and the carnage produced was shown in Adelstein's (1975) figures for England and Wales. Between 1961 and 1971 there were 705,029 injuries and 9219 deaths by accident. Social class is a crude summary of predicament but its effect on child mortality statistics was evident enough to become a matter of national enquiry (Black, 1980).

Being illegitimate is dangerous. In Salford in 1931 one in five illegitimate babies died in the first year of life; twice the rate for the legitimate born. But in Chamberlain & Simpson's book (1979) on the British Births' Study there is a study of deaths in the first year of life. Sudden Infant Death accounted for 35, congenital malformations 40, and all the rest 35. SID occurred in one in every 700 babies in classes 1–4 and one in 262 in class 5, 'other' and 'unsupported'. The ancient association between 'nosos' and 'penia' which at times has seen illness and poverty equated still reasserts itself above all our technology.

Excruciating predicaments

The language of human distress is very limited. At times the body speaks for what the tongue cannot utter.

CASE   A 13-year-old pallid, affectless youth has been off school for a year since he entered secondary education. He has established a habit of chronic vomiting. He is the illegitimate only child of an only child of ageing grandparents. Grandfather is sick and unemployed, grandmother is also at home where her daughter takes in work. The boy has been told that his father died before his mother could marry him. He might wonder why there is no objective evidence of his ever existing; photographs, artefacts or relatives. The family is largely house-bound, enshrouded with lies and deceit. He has been hospitalized for several periods, including one of 16 weeks on a paediatric ward.

CASE Seen on a neurological ward, her presenting complaint was that she walked on a lateral malleolus of her foot but with her foot so internally rotated that the toes pointed backwards. Many tests had been undergone to investigate the possible physical basis of this complaint and an orthopaedic fixation of the foot was planned by the parents. This solitary 'symptom' was the last residue of a sickness of nearly 4 years' duration. This phase, some 3 years old, owed its origins to an episode of hyperventilation and tetany on a coach with 36 classmates which was met on the motorway at 1.00 a.m. by police and ambulancemen and which, followed by 'marked somnolence' the next morning, was investigated as 'encephalitis'. Although the doctors were certain that the coma was entirely fictitious, by the time they had concluded this the child and her parents had been convinced, by the extent and assiduousness of the investigations, that the child was the victim of a mysterious disease.

CASE A wildly overactive 5-year-old boy regressed in his speech at 3 and now rarely utters and looks autistic. His mother has no siblings, no relatives, and her father died in her infancy. At the time of the regression in the boy's speech, her mother died, her disastrous lover left her, and her equally disastrous husband briefly attempted a reconciliation after a prolonged absence. Mother now muddles by in a depressive dream state, scarcely coping with his female co-twin and an older sister, who are said to remain imperturbably normal. Mother had been unable to breastfeed this voracious nine pounder while she fed his delightful twin sister for 6 months.

CASE An 18-year-old attractive girl has suffered numerous wildly dramatic fits in the office where she works. This is the latest in a series of sicknessess of mysterious provenance which suddenly beset her at the menarche. Emotional distress is denied. She is the illegitimate child of an illegitimate mother, who is the daughter of her adoptive mother's sister. She had sensed these facts from a family tree which she found in a Bible which she glimpsed in her youth in her grandmother's house. She might be forgiven some concern when the menarche faced her with the reality of her own femininity.

CASE A 9-year-old boy was admitted to a psychiatric unit having relinquished all voluntary behaviours. He did not speak, move or eat. He lay in a heap glowering between his fingers with which he covered his face. He had suffered glandular fever, which when it recurred months later was thought to be leukaemia. Extreme solicitude was withdrawn when this proved not to be the case. It took weeks to realize that his regression had a deliberate quality to it. While on a 3-hour ambulance drive to see a specialist, he developed retention of urine caused by his antidepressant drugs. The last words he had spoken, months before admission, had been to his father when he was about to be catheterized, 'Don't let them do that dad'.

The predicament of being sick

A new predicament is established by falling sick. Occasional episodes of minor illness allow periods of rest, quiet, private warmth and closeness, the delicious regressions towards dependency, the opportunity to retrace and rehearse some developmental stages. This idyll is likely to be curtailed in conditions of damp, overcrowding, and where mother feels she ought to be at work.

I sense that people's tolerance of the threat of illness has decreased with reduced incidence of threatening illness and a falling death rate. The improbability of early death or a life of handicap actually heightens its unfairness. Perhaps too the prejudices are built not on current statistics, but on those of our own or even our parents' childhoods. Fifty years ago at the Royal Manchester Children's Hospital there were 2716 admissions and 151 deaths. In 1980 there were 83 deaths in 8416 admissions. A significant decrease despite the aggregation of mortally sick children in that hospital. Equivalent figures at Booth Hall Children's Hospital show a precipitous decline from 486 in 1931 to 29 deaths in 1980. There is a marked relative increase in known cancer deaths and from degenerations of the central nervous system.

Sickness, as well as recruiting protective reactions, is also a nuisance and a threat. A sick child may experience ambivalent attitudes. We have still to allow that sickness leading to hospitalization will be alarming. However, the hospitalization of children to cover brief episodes of relatively minor illness seems to be on the increase. In the British Birth Study, 20% of children had been admitted by the age of 3½. In the study of Davie *et al.* (1972), 45% of children had been admitted by the age of 7. The figures suggest that domestic overcrowding, large sibships and a working mother do indeed increase the tendency to admit a sick child. Paediatricians call these 'social admissions', in the sense that they would have felt it safer to let the child stay at home if that seemed more competent. The policy might be supported by the dramatic reduction in death rates, or it might just increase the probability of repeated admissions for children from disadvantaged homes, the group whom Rutter (1976) showed to be the most psychologically vulnerable to them. It is worth recalling that the original purpose of 'incubation' was the belief that sleeping overnight in the Temple increased the potency of its magic.

The hospital as a predicament

There is no need for a further review of hospitalism. The works of Spitz & Spence and Bowlby & Robertson are commentaries on a scene now, I am sure, outdated. I only draw attention to the similarity of the phases of protest, despair and detachment which these workers outlined in the reaction of children to traumatic separation, and the work of Engel & Schmale (1972). They claim to have distinguished a 'giving-up'–'given-up' reaction in adults: an experience of hopelessness and incompetence to cope, which is associated with increased vulnerability to disease and death. It is discernible in species other than man, but I know of no empirical work with children. Are there perhaps times when hospitalization becomes counter-productive? Might it foster the very sickness of which we would be rid?

Admitting a child to hospital produces three of the violations of social functioning which Totman (1979) concluded were conducive to producing psychosomatic disorder:
- An abrupt change in a person's social environment so that familiar rules are inapplicable.
- Severance from a reference group.
- A change which requires new rules.

Do hospitals function in ways that tend to limit the trauma of the resultant predicament?

Sociological research summarized in *Beyond Separation* by Hall & Stacey (1979) suggests that, in the hospitals they visited at least, there is a long way to go before the suggestions of the Platt and subsequent Committees are adequately implemented. The regular practice of giving parents rooms to stay in remains largely an option, or a plea, or a possibility, rather than a strong widespread expectation.

Margaret Stacey makes seven useful points in her conclusions about 'the organisation of the hospital'. She does not refer to the way in which hospitals are planned, or the fearsome constraints imposed by antique plant.

If we seriously believe that children and parents in hospital deserve to be related to as well as treated, then we shall have to provide for the possibility. We shall have to decide whose job it is to relate to them, to provide surrogates for inadequate care, models of caring.

Consider child abuse. The management of the whole situation has fallen to the lot of the paediatrician. Not just the care of the abused child's injuries, but the provision of asylum, nurture, and such repair as is possible of the infant's capacity to trust. Many paediatricians use the caring relationship that they establish with the child, to establish a working therapeutic relationship with the parents. They recognize that the injuries were a function of a predicament and they work to alter that predicament, albeit sometimes through legal process. Yet, where the excruciating predicament falls short of abuse, where the illness speaks up, or disease supervenes, there is sometimes less enthusiasm to involve parents in therapy. I suppose it is the awesome implications of the practice of socially-oriented medicine that keeps us determined to exploit to the maximum the possibilities of bioscience.

Conclusion

The concept of predicament is offered as an understandable and historically available alternative to unconscious process in assessing children's difficulties. For health professionals who are not psychiatrists, the implication of unconscious process is that it is deep structures which are inaccessible except to the experts which are important in the mental well being of children. On the basis of this belief their commonsense judgements are suspended. I hope I have shown, through the impact of the vignettes presented above, that there is likely to be a broad measure of agreement as to the sorts of distress that the other might be experiencing once their predicament is exposed. The science of predicaments is in its infancy, but its language is the ordinary speech of people involved in health care as they describe their patients' plights to one another. The scientific propriety of 'accounts' is increasing and has had a variety of usages (Dingwall, 1976; Harre, 1979; Totman, 1979).

Even a psychiatry that accepts the idea of the unconscious recognizes that the only access to it is the patient's account of any given situation or experience. The therapist works on this account hoping for reconciliation. A fuller account of functioning within families, a family's manifestation of their predicament, is provided by 'family therapy'. But this ordinary action of listening with attention and respect to the unfolding of the predicament of others is in danger of being obfuscated and mystified by the process of professionalism.

This essay has been a plea that significant time should be spent by doctors in evoking and listening to detailed history. This aspect of modern medicine is seriously underplayed because it is undervalued as compared to empirical findings and test results. But diagnosis is not limited to finding diseases; sickness is not only the story of a disease. Diagnosis must extend into the patient's context. If the context is misconstrued or misunderstood, even acts of good faith may be seen by patients as dangerous intrusions. There will be loss of faith, poor adherence to regimes, anger with the limitations of practice, and a litigious approach to medical failure.

Consider the surgeons' operating time. Hours of effort, on the part of a team of people supported by complex technology, are expended in the hope of benefit. It might well prove economical of time if, after screening, a great deal of time was spent by physicians coming to a comprehensive diagnosis that includes the patient's predicament.

The psychological aspects of medical practice that matter most are not those which emerge painfully over years or months of probing. They are more likely to be mundane, self-apparent and readily available in the forefront of the minds of people who are only too anxious to unburden themselves if they are only given a chance to do so.

References

Adelstein, A.M. (1975) National statistics. In *Paediatrics in the Environment* (ed. D. Barltrop), pp. 57−67. (Fellowship in Postgraduate Medicine) London.

Ader, R. & Cohen, N. (1975) Behaviourally conditioned immunosuppression. *Psychosomatic Medicine*, **37**, 333−334.

Baird, H.W., John, F.R., Ahn, H. & Maisel, E. (1981) Neurometric evaluation of epileptic children who do well and poorly in school. *Electroencephalography and clinical Neurophysiology*, **48**, 683−693.

Bartrop, R.W., Luckhurst, E., Lazarus, L., Kiloh, L.G. & Penny, R. (1977) Depressed lymphocyte function after bereavement. *Lancet*, **i**, 834−836.

Black, D.K. (1980) *Inequalities in Health*. DHSS, London.

Calhoun, J.B. (1973) Death squared: the explosive growth and demise of a mouse population. *Proceedings of the Royal Society of Medicine*, **66**, 80−88.

Call, J.D. (1979) Introduction. In *Basic Handbook of Child Psychiatry* (ed. J. Noshpitz), Vol. 1, pp. 3−10. Basic Books Inc., New York.

Carter, J.J. (1981) Vitiated air: a Victorian villain? *Journal of the Royal Society of Medicine*, **74**, 914−919.

Chamberlain, R.N. & Simpson, R.N. (1979) *The Prevalence of Illness in Childhood*. (Fellowship of Postgraduate Medicine) Pitman, London.

Cobb, S. (1976) Social support as a moderator of life stress. *Psychosomatic Medicine*, **38**, 300−315.

Davie, R., Butler, N. & Goldstein, H. (1972) *From Birth to Seven. A Report of the National Child Development Study*. Longmans, London.

Dingwall, R. (1976) *Aspects of Illness*. Martin Robertson, Oxford.

Engel, G. (1977) The need for a new medical model; a challenge for biomedicine. *Science*, **196**, 129–136.

Engel, G. & Schmale, A.H. (1972) *Conservation-withdrawal, a primary regulatory process for organismal homeostasis*. Ciba Symposium 8, Elsevier, Amsterdam.

Ferguson, M. (1981) Healing ourselves. In *The Aquarian Conspiracy*, pp. 241–277. Tarcher/St. Martins, London.

Haggerty, R.J. (1980) Life stress, illness and social supports. *Developmental Medicine and Child Neurology*, **22**, 391–400.

Hall, D. & Stacey, M. (1979) *Beyond Separation*. Routledge and Kegan Paul, London.

Harre, R. (1979) *Social Being*. Basil Blackwell, Oxford.

Hart, J.T. (1981) A new kind of doctor. *Journal of the Royal Society of Medicine*, **74**, 871–883.

Illich, I. (1975) *Medical Nemesis*. Calder and Boyars, London.

Kashan i, J., Hodges, K., Simonds, J. & Hilderbrand, E. (1981) Life events and hospitalisation of children: a comparison with a general population. *British Journal of Psychiatry*, **139**, 221–225.

Kennedy, I. (1981) *The Unmasking of Medicine: Based on the B.B.C. Reith Lectures*. Allen and Unwin, London.

Locker, D. (1981) *Symptoms and Illness: the Cognitive Organisation of Disorder*. Tavistock, London.

McKeown, T. (1976) *The Role of Medicine: Dream, Mirage, or Nemesis?* (The Rock Carling Fellowship) The Nuffield Provincial Hospital Trust, London.

Miller, J. (1978) *The Body in Question*. Jonathan Cape, London.

Rowland, K.F. (1977) Environmental events predicting death for the elderly. *Psychological Bulletin*, **84**, 349–372.

Rutter, M. (1976) Parent–child separation: psychological effect on the children. In *Early Experience* (eds A.M. Clarke and A.D.B. Clarke). Blackwell Scientific, Oxford.

Schmale, A.H. (1959) Relationships of separation depression to disease. *Psychosomatic Medicine*, **20**, 259–277.

Stein, M., Schiavi, R.C. & Camerino, M. (1976) Influence of brain and behaviour on the immune system. *Science*, **191**, 435–440.

Szaz, T. (1972) *The Myth of Mental Illness*. Paladin Books, St. Albans.

Taylor, D.C. (1981) Epilepsy: a model of sickness. In *Psychopharmacology of Anticonvulsants* (ed. M. Sandler), pp. 129–135. Oxford University Press, Oxford.

Taylor, D.C. (1982) The components of sickness: disease, illness and predicament. In *One Child* (eds C. Ounsted and J. Apley). Heinemann, London.

Totman, R. (1979) *Social Causes of Illness*. Souvenir Press, London.

Vaughan, V.C., McKay, R.J. & Behrman, R.E. (1979) *Nelson Textbook of Paediatrics*. W.B. Saunders, Philadelphia.

Chapter 2
Genetic Counselling in the Management of Children with Neurological Disease

Maurice Super & Dian Donnai

Introduction

'Could any further children we have be similarly affected?' This is one of the first questions which parents may ask when faced with an abnormal child. The timing of genetic counselling requires care. Soon after the diagnosis has been made, a rejection phase may occur, with the parents wanting second opinions and their thoughts fixed on prognosis and treatment possibilities. These can seriously affect their view of recurrence risks. Unfortunately, an exact aetiological diagnosis and prognosis are not always possible, especially in infancy in various forms of mental handicap. Providing clear answers on which reproductive decisions may be based can be very difficult.

The counselling exercise differs from the traditional doctor–patient relationship in that it tries to be non-directive. One objective is to provide the family with the facts on which to base their own rational decisions. Whilst the family doctor, paediatrician or paediatric neurologist are providing supportive care, the geneticist, to increase the insight of the family, may have to explain in detail the known range of a particular disorder. Where no curative treatment exists, the best that we have to offer for the future may be an accurate assessment of the recurrence risk, and in a few conditions prenatal diagnostic tests and selective abortion of affected pregnancies. To ensure that the various roles do not become too divorced, combined clinics, e.g. of paediatric neurologist and geneticist, work well for some of us.

The genetic counsellor needs to give an idea of the burden of the condition. This is assessed in terms of pain, mental or physical handicap, abnormalities of excretion, operations, admissions to hospital, life-span, financial implications for the family, and the possible effect on the other children and the marriage.

We make much use of the specially trained genetics health visitor, who visits the family at home to gather some of the background information and give some idea of what to expect at the clinic visit. She sits in during this, observing the couple's reactions and supporting them, and follows up with a home visit when their retention of information is checked and their further queries answered or brought to our attention. Often she will provide support when further pregnancies are planned or during them, especially if antenatal diagnostic procedures are undertaken. There are deep moral and religious issues involved. People of varying ethnic backgrounds may have different views or accept handicap more philosophically than others. Preferable to employing interpreters when these are needed would be trained counsellors and health visitors of the same background. Unfortunately, this is not always possible and a great deal of effort may still leave poor mutual understanding.

Diagnosis

The essence of accurate counselling is the diagnosis. Since the brain can only respond in a limited number of ways to insult, genetic and acquired brain damage may present with exactly the same signs. There are several genetic mechanisms underlying neurological dysfunction, including chromosome imbalance, abnormal genes either arising by new mutation or inherited, and polygenic disorders such as neural tube defects. All can

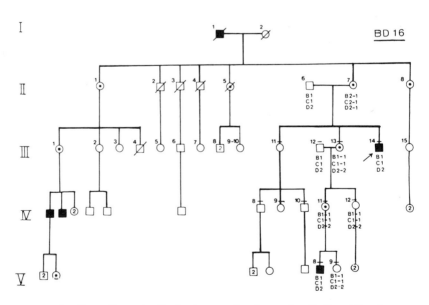

Fig. 2.1. A family pedigree for Becker's muscular dystrophy. B, C and D refer to DNA polymorphisms.

interfere with the formation and function of the brain and neuromuscular system.

There is no substitute for a careful family, pregnancy and disease history and a meticulous physical examination both of the patient *and his or her parents*. Apart from the obvious clinical relevance, we have been struck with how often this parental examination has psychotherapeutic advantages (one of the editors of this book described it as having 'an almost symbolic power'). The formal family pedigree may provide direct help in making the diagnosis. An example (Fig. 2.1) is shown where spinal muscular atrophy (see later) had been diagnosed, and the pedigree, supporting an X-linked recessive disorder, allowed the correct diagnosis of Becker's muscular dystrophy to be made, with confirmation of carrier status in some female relatives and a new diagnosis in the 10-year-old boy shown. Physical examination includes a specific search for dysmorphic features, with detailed measurements including those of the face, hands and feet, and comparison with normal ranges. Deformations and malformations should be identified (see Smith, 1982). Sometimes, investigations that may not have been otherwise clinically relevant, e.g. CT brain scan, may allow a more accurate assessment of the genetic risk. Structural brain abnormality is often not genetic in origin.

When history and examination do not provide an answer as to whether a disorder is more likely to be genetic or acquired, one may sometimes be in a position to give empiric counselling based on observations in similarly affected families. Some common examples from the published literature follow (Table 2.1). In all of them the load is considerable. Markers of the

Table 2.1. Empiric risk of some neurological disorders

Condition	Arithmetical risk
Idiopathic microcephaly (with no abnormal neurological signs)	1 in 8 (male or female)
Idiopathic ataxic cerebral palsy	1 in 8
Idiopathic athetoid cerebral palsy	1 in 8
Idiopathic symmetrical spasticity	1 in 8
Aqueduct stenosis	1 in 8 (in brothers)
Cerebral malformation on CT brain scan	1 in 100
Male with IQ 30–50, no abnormal neurological signs	1 in 5 (in brothers)
Infantile spasms (after exclusion of tuberous sclerosis)	1 in 100

genetic forms of these conditions would be invaluable in separating them from the non-genetic.

Clinical conditions

Examples are given below of clinical conditions with neuromuscular features, some where the aetiology is known and some where it is not, bringing out certain features in the history and examination that will enable accurate genetic counselling to be given.

Chromosome abnormalities

The presence of extra or missing chromosome material interferes with growth and development before and after birth.

The most common autosomal chromosome abnormality causes Down's syndrome, usually associated with trisomy 21, though occasionally with unbalanced translocation or mosaicism. The geneticist is often asked how the condition arose and how handicapped the child will be. It is helpful to show parents of any child with a chromosome disorder the karyotype and to explain how this is obtained. They may also require a simple explanation of egg and sperm formation and conception.

The geneticist should inform the parents that the extra chromosome in Down's syndrome could have arisen from either of them. Despite the association with advanced maternal age, in as many as 25%, the non-disjunction is of paternal origin. Unless he has a special interest in Down's syndrome, the geneticist is not too specific about developmental potential, but he can provide some information about the range within the syndrome and encourage the parents to discuss with the paediatrician the various developmental tests that are done in infancy and childhood.

Part of the investigative work on a dysmorphic child with developmental retardation is chromosome analysis, and occasionally a child will be discovered to have duplicated or deleted chromosome material. This situation may have arisen *de novo* in the child or may result from a balanced translocation state in either parent. The most common balanced translocation involves chromosomes 14 and 21. Where the parent is found to be a carrier, e.g. 45XX (or XY) t(14,21), careful explanation is necessary and the couple need to be reassured that the translocation will have no effect on the carrier's health, though chromosomally unbalanced conceptions may occur in future. The possible viable offspring when such a translocation exists are 46XX (or XY), 45XXt(14,21) or 46XXt(14,21), the last being translocation Down's syndrome. The whole concept of prenatal diagnosis and termination of affected foetuses should be discussed. Some parents may decide that they would like to embark on another pregnancy and take advantage of prenatal tests; other parents when faced with this possibility may decide not to increase their family. If a balanced translocation within one member of a family is identified, there may be other family members also at risk of carrying it and thus of having handicapped children. Either through the family or through the General Practitioner, such people should be contacted and a simple explanation of the situation given to them. Those who wish to pursue investigations would then have blood lymphocyte chromosome analysis to determine whether they are or are not carriers.

Sex chromosome abnormalities. Klinefelter syndrome (47XXY) is common (1 in 600 males born) but is seldom diagnosed in childhood. Long-term follow up of children diagnosed by newborn screening has shown that there may be delay in the onset of speech. Intelligence is generally normal or slightly reduced. At puberty there may be psychiatric problems, the incidence of which is reduced by testosterone therapy. In some other chromosome abnormalities there may be autistic behaviour (e.g. XYY and fragile X syndromes: see below). Chromosome analysis should be undertaken whenever such symptoms are unexplained.

As technical advances in cytogenetics occur, some conditions not known previously to be due to an abnormality are discovered to be associated with minute chromosome changes. The recognized triad of aniridia, mental retardation and Wilm's tumour is now known to be associated with a minute deletion in the short arm of chromosome 11. The Prader-Willi syndrome of hypotonia especially in infancy, truncal obesity, hypogenitalism and mental retardation, with characteristic face and hand features, is associated in at least 10% of cases with an abnormality of the long arm of chromosome 15.

The fragile X (Renpenning's) syndrome. It has been recognized for some time that mental retardation without obvious physical abnormality is more common in boys than girls. Martin & Bell (1943) first suggested that X-linked genes should be considered in the aetiology of non-specific mental retardation. In 1969, Lubs noted the presence of a marker X chromosome in affected males belonging to a pedigree where mental retardation was segregating as an X-linked recessive characteristic. In 1977, Sutherland showed that this marker was a fragile site occurring at band q27 of the X chromosome. It was found that culture conditions were critical to demonstrate it: blood needs to be cultured in a medium deficient in thiamine and folic acid, and the fragile site is demonstrable only in a proportion of an affected boy's cells and in an even lower proportion in carrier women. Mental retardation is more marked in affected males (IQ 30–50); carrier females may have moderate retardation. Delay in the onset of speech or autistic behaviour has been associated with the fragile X syndrome (Fig. 2.2).

Mendelian disorders

There may be heterogeneity within a particular diagnostic category. For example, many disorders such as sensori-neural deafness and retinitis pigmentosa can be inherited in any of the three main mendelian ways: autosomal dominant, autosomal recessive and X-linked recessive. The family pedigree and clinical presentation may allow confident counselling. In disorders like spinal muscular atrophy most are autosomal recessive, but the rare varieties presenting late in childhood or adulthood include significant numbers of autosomal dominants which may have arisen by mutation or inheritance. The dominant and recessive forms are clinically indistinguishable.

Autosomal dominant disorders

Some dominant disorders are notoriously variable in their clinical expression. Before a mutation is presumed to have occurred and a low recurrence risk given to apparently normal parents of an affected child, detailed physical examination of both of them and full family pedigree are needed. Specifically, stigmata of disorders such as neurofibromatosis and tuberous sclerosis should be sought in the parents of children with neurological disease. Freckling in the axilla is pathognomonic of neurofibro-

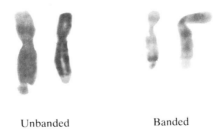

Unbanded   Banded

Fig. 2.2. Fragile X chromosome. This is often more easily seen in unbanded preparations.

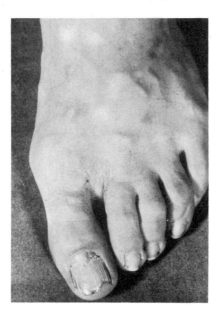

Fig. 2.3. Ungual fibromas seen in patients with tuberous sclerosis.

matosis and the subject may have no other signs of the condition. One mother with this finding asked for genetic advice after an astrocytoma had been discovered in her 2-year-old son. As yet this boy has no skin lesions (these may appear up to the age of 10 in neurofibromatosis).

Hypopigmented patches, best seen in blue or ultra-violet light, and ungual fibromas typical of tuberous sclerosis should be searched for in the parents and child in any case of idiopathic mental handicap or fits. (Figure 2.3 shows a photograph of ungual fibromas.) These cutaneous stigmata may be the only signs of the condition.

Myotonic dystrophy is again very variable in its clinical expression. Classically it presents in the third, fourth or fifth decade of life with weakness and wasting of muscles, myotonia of grip and other non-muscular signs, such as frontal baldness, cataracts and endocrine disturbances. However, it has been recognized that sometimes the offspring of affected women (but not affected men) can be severely affected at birth. Indeed, when presented with a child with hypotonia in the new-born period, it is important to examine the mother to see whether she has any signs of myotonic dystrophy. This should include slit-lamp examination of the lenses and electromyography. Amongst women with myotonic dystrophy there is a high rate of pregnancy and labour complications. Their offspring have a high perinatal mortality and morbidity and the children who survive are often retarded in mental and motor development, though not necessarily to equal degrees. Some show limb deformities. A typical presentation in a family follows.

CASE A new-born full-term male presented with hypotonia, talipes, poor suck and swallow, after a pregnancy complicated by polyhydramnios. His mother suffered a postpartum haemorrhage after his birth. A previous sibling had similar problems and died of a respiratory infection at 12 weeks of age. The mother denied any muscular symptoms or family history, but detailed examination of her revealed a degree of dysphonia, an horizontal smile, inability to bury her eye-lashes and slightly impaired relaxation of grip. Pedigree data included a maternal grandmother with cataracts and a maternal uncle with a weak grip and 'joint stiffness'. The baby required tube feeding for some weeks. His mental and motor development has been slow, and at the age of 3 years he has marked facial weakness, strabismus and very little speech development (Fig. 2.4)

Autosomal recessive disorders

It has been estimated that individuals are heterozygous for the equivalent of three to five abnormal genes. Most people marry a partner who has different abnormal genes to themselves but homozygous offspring occur more frequently if the couple are consanguineous or if they come from

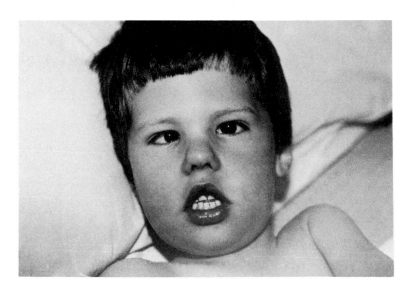

Fig. 2.4. Boy, aged 3, with myotonic dystrophy.

isolated or other inbred communities. Many of the inborn errors of metabolism are inherited in a recessive fashion where precise biochemical diagnosis can be made both of the affected child and of carrier parents or other relatives. About 50 inborn errors of metabolism are amenable to prenatal diagnosis by specialized laboratories. Many have no available treatment, but a few, for example phenylketonuria, can be prevented from causing handicap by appropriate dietary manipulations. A mother with phenylketonuria (PKU) may give birth to a child with a combination of microcephaly with mental handicap, congenital heart disease and cleft palate, all presumably the results of the effects of phenylketones on the developing embryo and foetus. The mother of any microcephalic infant should be checked for this condition. If she takes a special, low phenyl-alanine diet, before and during a future pregnancy, such a child may be mentally and physically normal, though there may still be some risk of handicap. With generations of children diagnosed as having PKU by new-born screening now growing up, one will be faced increasingly with the need to monitor such pregnancies and their outcome in affected women.

Autosomal recessive conditions have a 1 in 4 risk of recurring within a family and a couple's decision whether to proceed with another preg-nancy may depend on the availability and ease of treatment (e.g. dietary) and the availability of prenatal diagnostic tests, as well as the duration of survival of the untreated child.

Many mental retardation-malformation syndromes are inherited in an autosomal recessive fashion. The problem with most of these is that the basic defect is not known so that most are diagnosed purely on their clinical presentation, for example, the well-described though fairly rare Smith-Lemli-Opitz syndrome. Meticulous attention must be paid to previous reports of the syndrome and a child must not be assigned to a particular diagnostic category without good evidence, since labels are difficult to shed and the ensuing genetic risk of 1 in 4 may be unfairly prohibitive. If genetic markers were available for such conditions, their diagnosis would obviously be much easier and counselling based on the diagnosis much more confident.

X-Linked recessive disorders

Duchenne muscular dystrophy is the commonest X-linked neuromuscular disorder. At least 50% of affected boys show mild global retardation mainly with motor delay, and this may be the presenting feature. The mean age at diagnosis is 5 years, by which time a second affected boy may have been born. A creatine phospho-kinase (CPK) estimation should be part of the investigation of any boy with delay in walking or running, especially if not walking by 18 months of age, or when mild mental handicap is suspected.

As in other X-linked recessive disorders, biological factors may reduce the usefulness of tests or markers. With only one X chromosome active in the somatic cell of the female (Lyon hypothesis) a normal test result does not necessarily exclude carrier status of a female relative. In Duchenne muscular dystrophy, CPK levels are abnormal in only 70% of obligate heterozygotes, e.g. women with two affected sons or an affected brother and son. The accuracy of the risk estimates to females in a family with one isolated case of Duchenne muscular dystrophy are increased by having CPK estimated in a specialized reference laboratory on all the first-degree female relatives of the mother. These results are incorporated in Bayesian calculations which take account of the number of unaffected brothers and sons of the mother.

It is important to remember that a normal CPK result does not prove that the female is not a carrier. Although one in three new family cases of Duchenne muscular dystrophy arises by new mutation, it would be very wrong to presume mutation on the basis of such normal results. New recombinant DNA technology gives the hope that very soon it will be possible to demonstrate the presence of an abnormal gene in the cell, whether or not it is being expressed. Then one will be able to diagnose the carrier state or new mutation with certainty and accurate prenatal diagnosis will then become possible. There is, sadly, less certainty that our increased knowledge of the gene will lead to effective treatment. These comments, whilst made in some detail about Duchenne muscular dystrophy, should apply in time to many genetic disorders.

Multifactorial disorders

Most common birth defects do not have a mendelian or identifiable chromosomal basis, but many have an increased recurrence risk which is considered to indicate a considerable genetic component, termed polygenic or multifactorial. Generally, the additive effect of a number of genetic loci, together with environmental factors, are believed to be operating. Genetic counselling for such disorders lacks the precision of a mendelian disorder and only empiric risks can be given. Neural tube defect is the commonest multifactorial disorder in the United Kingdom. There are regional differences in recurrence rate. In the north-west of England a couple who have had one child with a neural tube defect have a one in 20 chance of such an occurrence in the future, and a couple who have had two affected children have a 1 in 8 risk. In the past, all that one could offer the couple was prenatal diagnosis by serum alphafetoprotein measurement, ultrasound scanning and amniocentesis to measure the levels of amniotic fluid alphafetoprotein (and more recently gel electrophoresis to detect acetylcholinesterase). Observations in the past suggested low vitamin levels in women delivered of children with neural tube defect. In a recent collaborative study, such women were given a multivitamin preparation with folic acid and iron—Pregnavite Forte F (Smithells *et al.*, 1980)—for at least 1 month before and for 2 months after conception. The results of this study appear encouraging in that the observed recurrence risk in the treated group was significantly lower than amongst the controls who had the same recurrence as expected from large earlier studies. An MRC study is under way in an attempt to define exactly which vitamin is responsible for the reduced incidence.

Specific syndromes of unknown or uncertain aetiology and with a low recurrence risk
The Sturge-Weber, Rubinstein-Taybi, Williams, Prader Willi and Cornelia de Lange syndromes are all well-defined and generally occur sporadically in families. *Before giving a low recurrence risk, one must be sure of the diagnosis.* Even when this is certain there are occasional families in whom there have been recurrences.

General aspects of genetic counselling

Regardless of the main reason for referral for counselling, the wish of most parents is for healthy future children. A certain amount of general advice may be given. A medical and gynaecological check-up before a new pregnancy is a good idea. Ideally, the mother should have ceased oral contraception at least 3 months prior to conception and should be known to be immune to rubella. She might need dietary advice and she should not smoke (Sidle, 1982) or take alcohol (National Council of Women, 1980; Wright *et al.*, 1983; Edwards, 1983). She should avoid unnecessary medication, at least in the first 3 months of pregnancy. She is made aware of serum alphafetoprotein screening and ultrasound in the prenatal diagnosis of neural tube defects. The couple are asked to make contact with the clinical genetics team during any future pregnancy so that colleagues may be alerted to earlier problems and provided with gathered information.

One objective of genetic counselling is the reduction of genetic disease. Even when the recurrence risk for a seriously handicapping disorder is high, authoritative counselling has a role to play in the peace of mind and mental health of the family. To quote Fraser (1974):

> Genetic counselling is a communication process which deals with the human problems associated with the occurrence, or risk of occurrence, of a genetic disorder in a family. The process involves an attempt by one or more appropriately trained persons to help the individual or family (1) comprehend the medical facts, including the diagnosis, probably the course of the disorder and the available management; (2) appreciate the way heredity contributes to the disorder, and the risk of recurrence in specified relatives; (3) understand the options for dealing with the risk of recurrence; (4) choose the course of action which seems appropriate to them in view of their risk and the family goals, and act in accordance with that decision; and (5) make the best possible adjustment to the disorder in an affected family member and/or to the risk of recurrence of that disorder.

References and further reading

Edwards, G. (1983) Alcohol and advice to the pregnant woman. *British Medical Journal*, **286**, 247–248.

Emery, A.E.H. (1979) *Elements of Medical Genetics*, 5th edn. Churchill Livingstone, Edinburgh.

Fraser, F.C. (1974) Genetic counselling. *American Journal of Human Genetics*, **26**, 636–659.

Kessler, S., ed. (1979) *Genetic Counselling Psychological Dimensions*. Academic Press, New York.

Lubs, H.A.A. (1969) A marker X chromosome. *American Journal of Human Genetics*, **26**, 636–659.

McKusick, V.A. (1983) *Mendelian Inheritance in Man*, 6th edn. Johns Hopkins University Press, Baltimore.

Martin, R.H. & Bell, J. (1943) A pedigree of mental defect showing X linkage. *Journal of Neurology and Psychiatry*, **6**, 154–157.

National Council of Women (1980) *The Fetal Alcohol Syndrome*. National Council of Women, London.

Sidle, N. (1982) *Smoking in Pregnancy—a Review*. Hera Unit, The Spastic Society, London.

Smith, D.W. (1982) *Recognisable Patterns of Human Malformation*, 3rd edn. W.B. Saunders, Philadelphia.

Smithells, R W , Sheppard, S. & Schorah, C.J. (1980) Possible prevention of neural tube defects by periconceptual vitamin supplementation. *Lancet*, **I**, 339–340.

Sutherland, G.R. (1977) Marker X chromosome and mental retardation. *New England Journal of Medicine*, **296**, 1415.

Wright, J.T., Toplis, P.J. & Waterson, J. (1983) Alcohol and the fetus. *British Journal of Hospital Medicine*, **29**, 260–266.

Chapter 3
Mentally Handicapped Children

Ian McKinlay & John Holland

Those who are involved in the treatment and management of mentally handicapped children need to understand each other's roles as they work within, and compete for, limited resources. The last 25 years have seen considerable expansion in understanding within paediatrics, paediatric neurology and related specialities of the causes of mental handicap and the treatment of its consequences. Genetic counselling has become much more accurate and accessible. As the 'medical model' of long-stay hospital care for children has become obsolete, a new 'medical model' is evolving. There has also been considerable expansion of knowledge and resources for community care and education of mentally handicapped children. Where the disciplines co-operate best, the service will improve most. This chapter discusses current medical and behavioural contributions for mentally handicapped children and their families

Health services

Health services offer prevention, identification and treatment of mental handicap and its consequences. Preventive measures include health education (peri-conceptional health), maintenance of a good diet, and avoidance of drugs, irradiation and alcohol in pregnancy, rubella immunization (Weatherall, 1982), genetic counselling and monitoring of obstetric and perinatal medicine. Identification may be possible at birth (e.g. for children with Down's syndrome), but more usually occurs as the result of increasing concern about delayed development. Treatment is possible for epilepsies, with simplified treatment and monitoring of drug levels, visual and hearing losses, physical deformities, dental, psychiatric and general physical disorders.

Doctors who are involved in regular treatment of mentally handicapped people develop particular expertise in looking for health associations with particular diagnoses. For example, people with Down's syndrome are prone to congenital heart disease and to development of progressive deafness, hypothyroidism, presenile dementia (Olson & Shaw, 1969; Gath, 1981) and leukaemia (Smith & Berg, 1976). Tuberous scler-

27

osis is associated with infantile spasms and other serious epilepsies, bone cysts and osteomalacia with fractures in those being treated for epilepsy, hamartomas and gliomas (Hunt, 1983). Those with congenital infections commonly suffer severe hearing and/or visual loss and/or heart disease.

For those who suffer from epilepsy or behaviour disorder there has been a tendency to try to treat these by too many drugs in too large doses. Handicapped people have difficulty in indicating side-effects and in questioning the effectiveness of treatment. Some handicapped people become much more active, communicative and able to learn when their treatment is reduced or stopped (Taylor & McKinlay, 1984). To maintain a balanced diet to prevent anaemia or constipation and promote growth may require dietetic advice for children with feeding difficulties or fussiness.

The health of mentally handicapped children in general differs from that of the general childhood population both in the frequency with which individual health problems occur and in the frequency with which different health problems coexist. The majority of mentally handicapped children have eye defects (Bankes, 1974; Millis, 1981) or other visual disabilities. One-third suffer from epilepsies (Neuhauser, 1977) and one-fifth suffer from cerebral palsies (Blomquist, 1982). Hearing deficits, respiratory tract infections and physical deformities are very common. Disproportionate communication deficits from language and articulation disorders are found. Gastro-intestinal disorders such as vomiting, oesophagitis, constipation or diarrhoea are common, incontinence is rife, respiratory difficulties are frequent and psychiatric illness is excessive. Several such associated disadvantages commonly coexist in individual children requiring a team approach to minimize their effects (Robinson, 1973).

New patterns of the organization of health care for mentally handicapped children are evolving (Fogelman, 1983). In time, this will come to influence the health services for mentally handicapped adults also (Richardson *et al.*, 1979). The rehabilitation services for physically and mentally handicapped children are based in child development centres linked to local paediatric services. There is a strong case for developing adult rehabilitation services, linked to adult medical, neurological and psychiatric services in a local area, perhaps based in a health resources centre analagous to the child development centre. Life expectancy for handicapped people has increased considerably in recent years (Kirman, 1980; Carter & Jancar, 1983). This, added to the closure of the institutions and the expectations raised by the services for children, will bring pressure to bear for improved adult facilities. There is much to be done, and reason to suspect that 'community care' may conceal community neglect (Bax, 1967; Williams, 1969; Harris *et al.*, 1971; *British Medical Journal*, 1979; Chamberlain, 1981, 1984; Gloag, 1983; Tripp, 1984).

CASE   A young man of 18 was referred to an experienced paediatric clinical psychologist because of outbursts of aggressive behaviour and irritability. He had broken the arm of a member of staff in his training centre, but hours later he saw the staff member's arm in plaster, expressed concern and appeared to have no recollection of the cause of the injury. The psychologist thought a medical opinion should be sought and raised a question about psychomotor epilepsy. This was not confirmed after investigation by a paediatric neurologist, but a history of a mentally handicapped brother and several other mentally handicapped male relatives was obtained. They were shown to have a fragile X chromosome in the laboratory. Eight females in the extended family were at risk of carrying the abnormal chromosome with a 1 in 2 risk of mental handicap in their sons and of a carrier status in their daughters. The man (and his brother who had similar episodes) benefitted from a low dose of chlorpromazine. Genetic counselling was very helpful to the family. Treatment with folic acid is being considered.

The first part of this chapter outlines the potential area of medical expertise, directed towards questions parents ask or would like to ask if they could put them into words (Taylor, 1982). It is sometimes frightening for them to ask because they know the answers could upset them. Yet many of the oblique pressures put on those who deal with handicap derive from suppression of such questions. The second part of the chapter concentrates on developments in behavioural management and precision teaching techniques. Above all, parents seek information and appropriate skills.

Is there something wrong?

Children may be referred to doctors or nurses because parents or professionals are concerned about their development. There may be disagreement about the significance of the child's behaviour. Parents may worry about a child inappropriately because of their limited knowledge of child development. Professionals may worry inappropriately about a child who is normal for a particular family. It is important for parents to know that the doctor has listened to their story. Secondly, the doctor gains by being seen by the parents to engage *with* the child as well as to talk *about* the child. Difficulty in distinguishing behaviour that is within the normal range from deviant behaviour may derive from a lack of professional expertise (e.g. delegation to a junior doctor) or lack of concentration (e.g. when pressed for time in a hectic clinic). It may also derive from an ambiguity within the child—the child of uncertain development whose prognosis would be uncertain to any expert.

CASE A 3-year-old child has just been discharged from the clinic after a year's follow-up but no investigations. When first referred at the age of 2 he had been able to roll over for three months and had just pulled himself up to stand for the first time. The child was attentive and understood speech though he uttered none. He was hypotonic but otherwise physically normal. His parents knew of relatives with delayed motor development and did not share the concern of the referring professional. The child had been improving, had no physical features suggestive of a condition requiring medical treatment or of unequivocal neurological abnormality, and the parents were not seeking genetic counselling as they had completed their family. There was no pressure to investigate. General advice was given by the physiotherapist and the child began to attend a playgroup. After a year he could name colours, count up to 10, form fairly complex phrases and sentences, and there were (good-humoured) complaints from the family about the boy's fearless climbing, jumping off cupboards and tendency to rush around the house.

Children who turn out to be severely handicapped may seem to behave normally in early infancy (Aylward *et al.*, 1978). Conversely, it is not unknown for parents of children who turn out to be quite normal to have become involved in their local spastics society or mental handicap organization at the time their child's 'handicap' is being investigated medically. Even when the child is found to be normal later on, he may not be perceived as normal because of the earlier experience (see also Hagberg & Lundberg, 1969; Nelson & Ellenberg, 1982; Chaplais & Macfarlane, 1984).

Though mental handicap or developmental delay may be present in the child, this may not be the reason for the parents' consultation. They may have come for help with a feeding or sleeping problem, irritability, seizures or constipation in the child. Some doctors may be excited by having spotted a few features suggestive of a syndrome but should not forget what prompted the referral.

Parents of children who turn out to be mentally handicapped will often say 'Why didn't they tell us earlier?' Certainly, if a child is known to be mentally handicapped this should be discussed with the parents. Before that stage, if parents want, the professionals may share their *own* uncertainty (which is *common*) and organize suitable advice or support during the uncertain period. Playgroups for children with doubtful development, offering informal or structured advice, allow parents to meet other families in the same situation. This fosters the realization that failure to reach a diagnosis is not because the doctor is not clever enough or trying hard enough, but because the situation cannot be resolved yet. If colleagues who are in more regular contact with the family are kept informed, such as the family doctor and health visitor, conflicting professional advice can be minimized and the family may be dissuaded from seeking multiple medical consultations. Though opinions offered in specialist clinics have some power, it would be remarkable if these were remembered accurately and completely and could, unaided, sustain a family for the months until the next clinic appointment. Sending parents a copy of the written paediatric report to the family doctor and copies of assessment reports can both inform the family and restrain gossip in the reports (Jolly, 1984).

If the mother is pregnant again or if the child is to be placed for adoption, there is added pressure to investigate. For example, if a boy presents with non-specific motor delay and delayed speech and language, there are strong reasons for checking serum creatine kinase to exclude Duchenne dystrophy from the family's point of view. When the child is for adoption, the interests of the boy and the prospective family conflict, and there is a need for discussion before tests are carried out. If the parents are anxious to add to the family but the mother is not pregnant, they may be advised to delay until the child's diagnosis is clearer.

There is an obligation to detect remediable factors in a child's developmental delay, however. Thus ophthalmological, orthoptic and audiological services, medical social workers and other health professionals need to be considered and their involvement will often be welcomed.

What is wrong?

If a child's developmental delay is likely to persist, this should be discussed with both parents together (Cunningham, 1979) or with a parent's friend or relation present to give support. The child should be immediately accessible. It is unwise and unkind to give one parent bad news and expect this to be passed on by that parent to the other. If both parents hear the same explanation, they have no need to dispute the information between themselves, are more likely to be mutually supportive and can be involved with the child's habilitation together from the start. Not all the information is understood or even agreed at the first counselling session and other sessions may be needed. It can be helpful, with parents' consent, to include the medical social worker or a nurse in the first interview so that a home visit can be arranged to discuss the interview with both parents. It may be that the mother will be more involved in daily caring for the young handicapped child, but the parents should be advised to plan to share domestic responsibility. When parents both have interests and friends outside the home they are more likely to find the personal resources to care for the child and for each other. It has not always been so:

> A wise son maketh a glad father but a foolish son is the heaviness of his mother (Proverbs 10.1).

Formal assessment, with due allowances for ethnic factors, temperamental variability or any physical impairments, complements the history by relating observed behaviour to established norms. It is not a process that should lead to a catalogue of flaws but to a detailed contemporary knowledge of the child's assets and limitations. This provides a clearer definition of the type of handicap(s) the child faces. If a child is uniformly delayed with a developmental attainment of half the average standard for his age or less, he may be described as mentally handicapped. But it is prudent to make sure that vision and hearing are normal and that the child does not have a severe motor disorder (e.g. athetoid cerebral palsy). Ignorance of cultural factors and language barriers can lead to incorrect assessment. Severe psychosocial deprivation can present as apparent mental handicap. Specific disorders of language development should also be considered.

There are many children who are less severely or less uniformly delayed. They may have normal motor ability but severe delay in understanding language. Or there may be a mixture of language and motor immaturity in a child who nonetheless performs within the average range for some types of play and self-care. They partly perform as if mentally handicapped and partly as normal children. Though it is increasingly common for such children to be described as having 'learning difficulties', this is not easy to communicate with granny, the man on the bus or the next door neighbour who may be more familiar with such terms as: 'a bit backward', 'brain-damaged', 'slow' or 'late developer'. Terminology is a problem.

Someone in the early years, this is often a doctor, needs to collect the assessment information and interpret it to the parents. The confusion between mental handicap and mental illness may need to be discussed. For children with cerebral palsy the term 'spastic' can be upsetting. It is commonplace for teenagers to call each other 'spastic' or 'mental' as forms of abuse. Hearing such words used only a few years later to describe their own children may provoke confusion or anger in parents (see also Fraser, 1980; Sensky, 1982).

Why is the child handicapped?

By no means all pregnancies are planned but, even when they are, parents are taking a biological risk, though the degree of risk may not be known. Parents do not know which conditions they may be carrying but they hope to prove themselves reproductively competent. There may also be pressure from grandparents to confirm this. If a child turns out to be handicapped, part of the parental distress derives from the thought that they may be biologically responsible.

Thoughts also turn to the time of conception (e.g. 'just after I came off the pill'), health in pregnancy ('I had a lot of sickness'), possible drug intake, including attempts to induce abortion, smoking, alcohol consumption, sexual activity, accidents, continuing to work till late pregnancy, or making a lot of house alterations till the last minute. They wonder if the doctors or midwives missed something or made mistakes during the delivery. Could the mother have passed on some infection which harmed the baby or has the child caught something after birth? The parents will also wonder whether the handicaps are part of the child's make-up or the result of mistakes in their parenting.

The answers to these questions and to the genetic implications of a handicapped child emerge from thorough biological investigation. They are fundamental and parents who may seem demanding in other ways may not have had them answered. This major opportunity for a medical/ scientific contribution can be used very therapeutically too, in establishing a basis of trust.

CASE A severely mentally handicapped girl with frequent seizures had been going to school within another authority but funded by her local authority. When the girl was 13 the local authority tried to withdraw the transport and offered a local school. The mother, previously quiet, became furious. 'They caused her handicap; they can pay' was her opinion. This prompted the first active review of the diagnosis for 10 years. The perinatal history—to which mother had attributed the handicap—had been fairly unremarkable. The child's prominent mandible, cheery manner in spite of multiple myoclonic fits and severe handicap, jerky movements and continuous seizure discharge on EEG suggested Angelman's syndrome. This led to useful discussion with the family who had never managed to ask many questions before. With increased confidence they questioned the girl's need for medication (which was withdrawn with beneficial results) and participated more in a joint programme with the school.

CASE   A very small severely mentally handicapped 12-year-old girl had been placed in a hostel 10 years previously after being abandoned in hospital. Her father had served 5 years in prison for murdering a sibling and the family was hostile to all authority. The girl was referred because she had been screaming. It was found that she had oesophagitis which was relieved by antacids. She was also found to carry a partial trisomy. This properly explained her handicap, which had previously been attributed to concealed non-accidental injury or perinatal hypoglycaemia. Her family was pursued. It was found that her father and two sisters carried a balanced translocation. This interaction led to renewed family involvement and the girl began to make regular home visits.

CASE   In the same hostel a 9-year-old girl with average agility but no language was referred because of faecal soiling and hyperactivity. In the course of investigation of the cause of her handicap it was found that she, her mother, mentally handicapped brother, and uncle all suffered from dystrophia myotonica. Her mother, who was quite disabled but who had never been diagnosed or referred to a specialist, benefitted from treatment with phenytoin. Genetic counselling was possible for the healthy sister who had previously decided to have no children. The handicapped girl's problems responded to a behavioural programme.

Although doctors should be strenuous in their efforts to find a biological explanation, families seek another type of explanation. There are ancient moral interpretations:

> *Delicta maiorum immeritus lues* (Horace, *Odes* III.6.1)
> ['Though guiltless you must expiate your fathers' sins']

Be sure your sins will find you out (Numbers 32.32).

The marriage or pregnancy may have been disapproved of by the extended family. The conception may have been unplanned and unwanted. The parents may have been in dispute or feel guilty about their behaviour during the pregnancy. Pregnancy may have followed treatment for prolonged infertility. The child may not be legitimate; abortion may have been attempted. In these circumstances the handicapped child may seem to be a punishment. Whatever doctors may think about such beliefs or superstitions, they should be aware that some families, including some from other cultures, may regard them as more important than the biological explanations.

What does the future hold?

Discussing the prognosis is part of the counselling role of the doctor, who needs to know the variability of the condition diagnosed. Parents may say they want to know the worst; all the possibilities they may have to face. This presents the doctor with difficult decisions, counselling people they do not know well. If parents understand the sickness and its implications, they and their children seem to do better. It is worth the time and organization to explain what is known. Some parents will benefit from reading books or articles about their child's condition. Many learn a more mature philosophy of life; that caring and sharing are more important than status and higher income, that health and happy times are to be treasured, and that suffering is a widely shared part of the human predicament. They enjoy their handicapped children and realise that all children generate pleasure and problems.

One example of potential difficulty is discussion of the possibility of epilepsy. About a third of severely mentally handicapped children will develop epilepsy (i.e. more than 60 times more likely than in people who are not mentally handicapped). Seizures are frightening to parents who often think the child is dying in the first major seizure. The anticipation of epilepsy is also frightening and some parents may be reluctant to leave the child if they know of the possibility of seizures. Given that two thirds of the children will not experience epilepsy, is it right to discuss the possibility with all parents? The support available to parents will affect this decision (e.g. whether it is possible for the doctor or a well-informed social worker or nurse to follow up the initial interview by further discussions until parental anxiety is put into perspective). Involvement in parent support groups will often help.

Medical knowledge will influence the information given to the parents about epilepsy. Virtually all children with Sturge–Weber syndrome and the great majority of those with tuberous sclerosis (80%) will suffer from epilepsies. Relatively few (about 2%) of those with Down's syndrome will do so. The better the doctor knows the family and the more information the doctor has about the child's condition, the easier it is to offer appropriate advice.

Discussion of the prognosis of the mentally handicapped autistic child of 3 or 4 years who does not appear to understand any speech and utters very little sound is difficult. It is true that some of these children develop surprising practical or artistic skill, and a few learn to speak or communicate in other ways, better than would have been predicted. But most will never learn to communicate well or even to relate satisfactorily to close relatives, especially if the child is of low IQ, has seizures or an abnormal gait. They are more demanding and less rewarding than most to care for through to adult life. The child with severe cerebral palsy as well as profound mental handicap may also show very little progress in spite of immense input. The parents often become dispirited, may demand even more therapy or criticize the school. Once more, the quality of the support services will influence the amount of information given early on. A realistic prognosis, adequately discussed with a suitably supported family, may prevent excessive expenditure of time and money in unrealistic remedial efforts and may allow development of a better family life.

There are children such as those with the Prader—Willi or Renpenning syndromes who appear to be severely mentally handicapped in infancy but turn out to be mildly handicapped after a few years. Children with athetoid cerebral palsy are commonly thought to be severely mentally handicapped in the first 2 years, yet they may show evidence of average intelligence later. A few are of above average intelligence.

CASE   A boy aged 12 was referred because further surgery was being contemplated for deformity. He attended a school for severely mentally handicapped children and was in their special care unit. At the age of 18 months he had attained a DQ of 25 on the Griffiths test. The parents were advised that the child was severely handicapped, but they did not find that easy to accept as the boy seemed alert. Both parents received psychiatric help and eventually became resigned to accept the expert opinions. Though severely incapacitated, the boy was obviously attentive at the time of admission and had a good sense of humour. On the Columbia test using eye-pointing he achieved a quotient in the 60 to 70 range. Within 2 weeks he had learned to play draughts (checkers) and was learning to read, so he was transferred to a school for physically handicapped children. He found it difficult to learn to concentrate but has made substantial progress.

Counselling of the families of handicapped children is an activity for experienced people. The doctor is a source of specialized biological information which can help families understand the nature of their child's condition and the causes of that condition. Doctors consulted early on about the child's delayed development may initiate more broadly based assessment and management advice by referral to colleagues. Though time spent with the doctor is influential, it is brief, and the key worker (or 'named person') to whom the parents should later refer will usually not be the doctor. The parents or key worker will commonly require specific medical advice from time to time. This does not mean that the doctor is the central figure from the family's point of view eventually.

Treatment of the neonate thought to be severely handicapped

There is a popular belief that most handicapped children would not survive if it were not for medical intervention. When neonatal paediatrics was a new speciality, more handicapped children lived than would have been the case previously because of the survival of sick neonates whose treatment had been only partially effective. However, the great majority of mentally handicapped children suffer their brain lesions in early pregnancy (Hagberg, 1975; Fryers & Mackay, 1979; Crawfurd, 1982; Hagberg & Kyllerman, 1983), and perinatal care only has a small effect on the prevalence of handicap.

Nonetheless, some difficult issues arise when children who are very likely to be handicapped become ill or show malformations that need surgical treatment in the perinatal period. Uncertainty about legal implications, wide differences of opinion between individual doctors, nurses, parents and families, social workers and others involved with the children professionally, sensational press treatment of individual children's experiences and the lack of a clear public concensus add to the pressure on those trying to decide on the management of individual children. Robertson & Fost (1976) suggested the establishment either of clearer criteria for infants who can be allowed to die, or of an improved decision-making process, with a preference for the latter. When an anonymous children's physician discussed sedation of severely defective newborn babies (*Lancet*, 1979b), this provoked considerable but divergent correspondence. Sedation was described as 'surely warranted in the case of an infant with Down's syndrome and duodenal atresia for whom no operative treatment is intended' in a later anonymous leading article (*British Medical Journal*, 1981). Both stressed the need for openness with parents and sharing of decisions between colleagues. During this period in Britain, a decision was made by a social services department to overrule an agreement between parents and doctors to withhold surgery from a Down's syndrome child with duodenal atresia. The child was taken into care for the purposes of obtaining surgery and was subsequently returned to the care of the parents who had sustained heavy legal fees in the meantime. A paediatrician was tried and acquitted of murder following care of a multiply malformed infant with Down's syndrome which included use of chloral hydrate and dihydrocodeine.

A British public opinion poll carried out at that time by Market and Opinion Research International (MORI) asked if a doctor who, with parental consent, 'sees to it' that a severely handicapped baby dies should be found guilty of murder. Seven per cent said 'Yes' and 83% said 'No'. The same organization asked 2062 British respondents aged 15 or over whether it should be arranged for a severely handicapped newborn baby (A) to die by the withholding of food or necessary medical treatment, or

(B) to be looked after in a home or hospital for the handicapped or by foster parents. The replies were: 'A' 37%, 'B' 45%, 'Undecided' 13%, and 5% gave other replies (*Lancet*, 1982). Living with ambiguity is a common medical experience and does not preclude a process of ethically sound decision-making at either extreme of the lifespan of the affected individual (British Paediatric Association, 1981; President's Commission for the Study of Ethical Problems in Medicine, 1983).

The competence of informed parents to reach a decision with their baby's doctor should be respected. Such decisions are not extremely urgent and an instant decision should not be expected. The doctor will be wise to share clinical judgement and assessment of the prognosis with an experienced colleague or colleagues, whether or not the parents request a second opinion. The presence of a nurse or social worker during interviews with the parents may be helpful, if the parents agree, as this may allow further informed discussion prior to a further interview with the doctor. The immediate postnatal period is a difficult time for such decision-making, and the avoidance of bias on the part of the doctor, though intended, may not be easy to achieve. These are unavoidable factors, however. Recent wider discussion is to be welcomed by doctors and parents. Clarification of what *should* be done as opposed to what *could* be done (Goodall, 1984) will evolve best through such open negotiation.

What can be done to help?

Medical treatment
There are general conditions which are treated by the family doctor. Common examples include otitis media, chest infections or constipation. Irritability in relation to mealtimes may be the result of colicky pains in the constipated child. Oesophageal regurgitation is underdiagnosed (Cadman *et al.*, 1978; Byrne *et al.*, 1983) but responds well to appropriate positioning, food consistency and antacids between meals. An enthusiastic family doctor, knowing the handicapped child, could be in the best position to interpret symptoms presented by other family members. However, many such doctors are not especially interested, so specialized community child health and hospital doctors will continue to have a role.

Specialist advice will be helpful for treatment of the common visual or hearing impairments and of seizures. The epilepsies of mentally handicapped children can be difficult to treat, and at times it has to be recognized that drugs have failed or even worsened the situation. Too often, the desperate attempt to improve epilepsy leads to the child taking large doses of several drugs without benefit. Especially if the diet is poor, they are at risk of developing deficiency of folic acid and vitamin D. The drugs may lead to deterioration of behaviour (barbiturates, valproate), gingival hyperplasia and hirsutism (phenytoin), excessive weight gain or alopecia (valproate), excessive salivation and increased chest infection (benzodiazepines), or nightmares (carbamazepine). These may be too high a price to pay. ACTH has a role for infantile spasms (40 U/day decreasing over 4 weeks) and should be considered for other refractory seizure disorders. The ketogenic diet has a definite place for refractory epilepsies, especially myoclonus. Rectal diazepam solution for prolonged or serial seizures may be a satisfactory alternative to continuous oral medication. Advice on first aid and general management are as important as the drugs. In a recent unpublished survey of drugs for epilepsy in mentally handicapped children in Salford (54/154 children were affected), the most commonly used drugs were sodium valproate and carbamazepine. Half were on a single drug and over 5% with fits no longer took drugs.

Physical deformities are common in mentally handicapped children. About 20% of mentally handicapped children also have a degree of cerebral palsy. Their physical deformities are generally best dealt with by physiotherapy. At times the possibility of surgery is raised. A regular working relationship between a physician, a particular orthopaedic specialist and the physiotherapist will offer the best prospect of a wise decision. Not all surgery is beneficial for deformity in the long run, and the experience of admission can be hazardous for an immature child. Serial plastering techniques can be beneficial for a tight tendo Achillis but need to be applied and supervised by an experienced person. More needs to be learned about the indications for tendo Achillis lengthening—sometimes a success, sometimes harmful. Scoliosis can develop during school years, and in adolescence especially. In the Salford study, 58 out of 154 mentally handicapped children had a scoliosis, and a similar number had deformities of the feet, often needing special or adapted footwear and advice from chiropody services. Amongst severely handicapped children who move very little, scoliosis occurs in intelligent children with intermediate spinal muscular atrophy as well as mentally handicapped children with marked spasticity (Fulford & Brown, 1976), and there is a long-recognized risk of developing a windswept postural deformity leading eventually to gross distortion. This is probably preventable by regular changes of posture and promotion of physical activity; even passively if active movement is difficult, but the effort required is considerable.

There has been much discussion recently about the management of the subluxating or dislocated hip in multiply handicapped children. On the one hand, even expert physiotherapy supervision may not prevent dislocation and the hip may become painful in early adult life. On the other hand, effective surgery (e.g. Girdlestone's arthroplasty) is quite a major procedure and may not have a permanent effect. If parents are to be encouraged to agree to such surgery for a child who does not appear to be distressed, they will need more evidence about the natural clinical history than is available at present. However, difficulty in positioning a child comfortably and problems with hygiene in the groin may justify an early operation.

Another specific area of potential medical involvement is the treatment of behaviour disorders, including sleep disorders, self-injury and 'hyperactivity' (Corbett, 1972; Rutter, 1972; Forrest & Ogunreni, 1974; Corbett & Campbell 1981). Doctors, asked to help in the management of handicapped children who are restless, aggressive, destructive, self-mutilating or not sleeping, have tended to prescribe drugs rather than consider a broader approach. Some of these behaviours have emerged because of the inadequacy of available resources to give the child an interesting day or to relieve the family when necessary. Drugs have been used as a 'chemical straight-jacket', especially in institutional care. However, aversion therapy can still be useful; there are psychotic mentally handicapped children and adolescents who benefit from major tranquillizers, e.g. phenothiazines or butyrophenones. Drugs can also be used in a short-term way to reinforce a behavioural programme, e.g. trying to establish a regular sleeping habit. An interesting recent approach has been to use B blockers, e.g. propanolol, to modify the systemic effects of anxiety for a short period while other adjustments are being made. However, long-term tranquillizers or sleeping pills, e.g. nitrazepam or promethazine, often have no sustained effect. Cyproterone acetate, a testosterone antagonist, is occasionally useful for adolescent boys with unacceptable sexual behaviour.

Rather than responding to a request for help with prescriptions, the doctor should first consider whether the presenting behaviour is appropriate for the child's developmental age or outside normal experience. Normal immature behaviour is unlikely to respond to drugs. Secondly, it is worth considering whether a different approach would resolve the issue, e.g. regular short-term care, behaviour modification, a sheepskin on the mattress of the child who wakes at night or a lock on the door for a child who wanders at night. Thirdly, colleagues who are regularly involved with the family may be able to contribute useful information or advice. It may be that one parent is not sharing the care sufficiently and the other is being worn out. If drug treatment is used, its purpose needs to be explained and its effect needs to be monitored carefully.

Contraception, sterilization and sexual counselling

Sexuality of handicapped people evokes strong reactions from the general population and from parents. The elements underlying this include: the need to discuss sexuality which many still find embarrassing, the persistent infantilization of handicapped people, unjustified fear of associated violence by males (Gebhard *et al.*, 1965), exploitation or promiscuity of females, and concern about eugenic issues (Reed & Reed, 1965). Mentally handicapped people may be more liable to engage in sexual activity, such as masturbation, in public, but as a group their levels of sexual activity and fertility are reduced (Gebhard, 1973; Hall, 1975), not least through lack of unobserved opportunities. It is not long since girls who had illegitimate babies and who were rejected by their families could be described as moral defectives and sent to the same institutions as the mentally handicapped.

Discussion of handicapped people's sexuality may need to be facilitated by medical input or by teachers, social workers and psychologists in a planned way (Stewart, 1978; Dorner, 1980). Handicapped people will often have opinions and questions to discuss, given the opportunity (Bancroft, 1983). Some parents criticize this (suspecting that it is putting ideas into the heads of their children) if they are not involved in planning how to approach the issue. When the child or adolescent causes embarrassment by public masturbation, advice may be given about acceptable contexts for behaviour, reinforced by a behavioural programme as required.

There are several methods of fertility control available to the general population and no single method is universally acceptable. Similarly, no single policy is applicable to handicapped people. The individual's circumstances need to be taken into account at the time of referral, in terms of the prognosis and in the light of genetic implications. Attitudes of the family are also important but these can come into conflict with those of social service agencies.

CASE A severely mentally handicapped girl, a member of a large sibship, one of whom was moderately handicapped, left school and began to attend an adult special care unit. Her care was shared between her mother and a short-stay public facility. On one of her last visits to the child development centre she appeared to be unwell and was admitted for investigation. She was found to be severely anaemic and 20 weeks pregnant. Intensive enquiry failed to identify the father but a 15-year-old brother was among those implicated. The girl's (divorced) father requested termination of the pregnancy and sterilization. Her mother requested continuing obstetric care, no sterilization and custody of the baby, handicapped or not, though this meant continuing the care circumstances in which the girl became pregnant. After detailed discussion within and without the local services, it was decided to take the girl into care, to treat her anaemia, continue her pregnancy, sterilize her after delivery by caesarean section under general anaesthetic, to allow the grandmother to look after the new baby (whose development is uncertain), and to maintain the girl in public care after delivery with supervised home visits to maintain links. There was persisting disagreement between professional and family views about the sterilization.

CASE A woman with Down's syndrome, who was capable of independence, married and had six children, three of whom had Down's syndrome. She rejected amniocentesis on the grounds that she would not contemplate termination of pregnancy for a condition she had herself.

The parents of severely handicapped, mobile adolescents, cared for at home, often request sterilization (*Lancet*, 1979a; *British Medical Journal*, 1980; Wolff & Zarfas, 1982), and may continue to request it after discussion of alternatives with their family doctor, child development centre physician, family planning service and gynaecologist. It is likely to be considered especially for girls who are incapable of parenthood and unable to manage other forms of contraception reliably, or who carry a genetic disorder. If the young person is wholly or partly in the care of the social services, their views will also be expressed. Where uncertainty persists, the matter should be referred to an ethical committee or, as a last resort, to the courts, who may be asked to make a ruling with independent representation for the mentally handicapped person. Should there be uncertainty about the ultimate prognosis, it would be wise to oppose sterilization.

In the Wolff & Zarfas (1982) study, over 70% of parents of mentally handicapped young people favoured sterilization, even if the young people were capable of sustaining a marriage or when the parents were Catholic. However, there are religious and moral parental objections to sterilization, or even contraception, which need to be taken into account for adolescents or older handicapped people when parents have sole care. It may be held that intervention in natural fertility contravenes religious teaching or promotes promiscuity. Advocacy of any alternative view on behalf of these young handicapped adults is only considered in exceptional circumstances. Parental views do not preclude unwanted pregnancies, however, and such can prove exceedingly traumatic for all concerned.

One method of sterilization used for handicapped girls is hysterectomy (Wheeless, 1975). Though this carries the risks of general anaesthesia and surgical interference, it does remove the need to cope with periods without inducing a premature menopause. Hysterectomy is also considered for very handicapped incontinent girls in whom hygiene can be a difficult problem (Vining & Freeman, 1978). Continuous contraceptive medication is an alternative, but can lead to disease of the endometrium, breast discomfort and weight gain (Savage, 1978).

Sterilization or medical modification of sexual behaviour of mentally handicapped men has not received much attention (*Lancet*, 1979a). In the Wolff & Zarfas (1982) study, parents of mentally handicapped men were as anxious as parents of mentally handicapped women that sterilization should be carried out, but such parents are not usually asked. If a mentally handicapped man is married or has a stable sexual relationship, and it is thought that the couple could not cope with parenthood, a vasectomy is safer and simpler than female sterilization. Another problem may be that a mentally handicapped man is promiscuous and prone to take advantage of mentally handicapped girls who do not reciprocate sexual interest but cannot prevent it, though they may or may not resist. Vasectomy will prevent conception but not assault. Castration is probably not justifiable. Medication either in the form of sedation or use of cyproterone acetate (Davies, 1975; Dein, 1975) may affect the personality and needs continuous supervision, but is at least reversible.

Sterilization of mentally handicapped people unable to give informed consent is illegal in the United Kingdom and is only carried out after wide discussion which may include medical defence organizations. However, Batshaw & Perret (1981) reported from the United States that at the time of their writing 16 States had compulsory sterilization laws especially for mentally handicapped institutional residents prior to release. This, and the issues for people living at home, are reviewed by Haavik & Menninger (1981). Discussion on this subject has taken increasing account of the capacity for friendship, love, marriage and sexuality of handicapped people (Mattinson, 1975; Craft & Craft, 1978, 1979). This trend will undoubtedly continue as others ask handicapped people about themselves (Madge & Fossam, 1982; Anderson *et al.*, 1982) and as self advocacy is encouraged (Williams & Shoultz, 1982). Marriage for handicapped people is still prohibited by law in some places but the laws are increasingly unenforced (Edgerton, 1979). The confused and unsatisfactory state of the law reflects the lack of a clear public opinion in a climate of changing circumstances for mentally handicapped people.

There is a case for a long-term prospective study of practice in fertility regulation amongst handicapped people, including self advocacy as far as practicable (Madge & Fossam, 1982; Anderson *et al.*, 1982; Edgerton, 1979; Williams & Shoultz, 1982).

Dental care

There is a need for a comprehensive preventive dentistry approach in the home, school and health services, yet this is often poorly co-ordinated (Nowah, 1976). As Miller (1965) pointed out, the overall problem created by the child's handicap may leave the parents and/or guardians apathetic about dental needs. Yet most dental disease can be prevented and early treatment may make subsequent, more elaborate, treatment unnecessary. The congenital or acquired causes of mental handicap may lead directly to associated dental disease. Initial routine involvement of dental health services should follow from the early diagnosis of handicap. This may be through hospital or specialist community services. A good diet, use of fluoride (*British Medical Journal*, 1972) and removal of plaque, especially by brushing the teeth, are habits to establish early. Avoidance of excess intake of sucrose in drinks or frequent snacks and foods of suitable texture are recommended (Rosenstein & Rosenberg, 1964).

Later assessment, perhaps in several sessions, may be attempted through local services. The school dental service may be able to examine the children in a familiar setting and achieve good co-operation. (This has also been the experience of adult training centres.)

If instrumental treatment is required, handicapped children often require premedication to reduce anxiety and restlessness prior to the use of local analgesia or nitrous oxide and oxygen. For older children the addition of intravenous diazepam to the above may achieve sufficient relaxation and amnesia to obviate a full general anaesthetic (Rosenberg, 1982). Ketamine is a possible alternative but should be avoided in people with hydrocephalus because of its tendency to raise intracranial pressure. Some children may show signs of disturbance during recovery. If general anaesthesia is required, as it often is for treatment of younger handicapped children, the agents used are generally anti-convulsant. However, there needs to be collaboration between dentist and doctor concerning medication prior to anaesthetics being given.

Physiotherapy may be recommended before and after anaesthetics in handicapped children prone to chest infections. Care in the use of benzodiazepines for such children is suggested because of their tendency to provoke excessive salivation and bronchorrhoea.

Orthodontic advice will often be indicated. Malocclusion is common amongst many groups of mentally handicapped children (Koster & Rosenstein, 1978), for example those with Down's syndrome, craniofacial abnormalities or cleft lip and palate. Any child wearing a Milwaukee brace may experience pressure on the mandible and teeth, and may require an adapted appliance. Periodontal disease may relate to inadequate dental hygiene or to side-effects of treatment (phenytoin or sodium valproate). It is the commonest pathological condition of mentally handicapped people.

Damage of teeth through attrition, abrasion or trauma is more likely in people with cerebral palsy, epilepsy or self-mutilation. There is an increased need to assess such people's need for restorative dentistry. Handicapped children with poor motor control may find it easier to use a thickened rubber handle to hold their toothbrushes or may prefer to use battery operated brushes. Those with over-sensitive mouths may prefer to avoid toothpaste and to brush their teeth using water only, because they may drool excessively or fear choking if toothpaste is used.

Care of the teeth of handicapped people requires an early start, good organization and experienced practitioners more than special techniques. Excellent results can be obtained.

A family approach

Families of newly diagnosed mentally handicapped children usually know little of therapies, social work, available allowances, special education or concepts of shared care (Tizard & Grad, 1961; Ballard, 1978; Featherstone, 1981; Phelp & Duckworth, 1982). There is much to be said for letting them know what is available and how they can gain access to those they think appropriate. They will usually meet the different members of the team during the initial assessments and develop an understanding of what each has to offer (Mackay, 1976). As helping agencies have developed, there has been a risk of overwhelming families by an intrusive team, rather than allowing them the opportunity to find solutions appropriate to their own family. Services may be directed towards the handicapped child only, rather than considering the family as a whole and their social handicap (Carr, 1970; *British Medical Journal*, 1972; MacKeith, 1973; Gath, 1973; Solomons, 1978; Judson & Burden, 1980). Families have not had much say in how services should be developed but receive what the experts have planned. The development and use of self-help groups for families should be encouraged (e.g. Hunton, 1980).

The availability of information about services varies greatly. In some areas, small booklets or pamphlets have been produced which give clear details of all the relevant information, together with names, addresses and telephone numbers of the key people to contact. Another approach has been to hold a series of local meetings (perhaps at the local child development centre or school) at which various specialists outline the role they play in the management and treatment of handicapped children. Such meetings, as well as providing opportunities for parents with similar problems to get to know each other, also allow time for general questions to be asked which may be difficult to discuss fully in a busy clinic setting.

There are families who, sometimes for cultural reasons, are very accepting of handicap. As one father said, 'Some children are clever and some are not but that's OK': he could not understand why his son had been referred and was quite content to accept him with an unexplained IQ of 60 though his other children were within the average range. Other families, perhaps for social or cultural reasons, tend to ignore the child and deprive him of potentially beneficial advice, compounding the disability. They want a cure or nothing. Allowances may not be spent for the child's benefit. It may help to be more directive with some parents and to agree simple goals for the child with a high prospect of success. This may motivate further involvement. Occasionally, the handicapped child may be so neglected or abused (Solomons, 1979) or inhibited within the family that alternative care or residential schooling is required. There is also a risk of over-concentration on the handicapped child to the detriment of siblings (Bentovin, 1972a, b; Grossman, 1972; Simeansson & McHale, 1981) or the marriage (Hanid & Harvey, 1978).

There is no doubt that services for mentally handicapped children in the United Kingdom have improved considerably in recent years. All children can go to school. Assessment and remediation have become more sophisticated. Long term care in large institutions has become obsolete and resources for community services are increasing. The mentally handicapped school leaver, however, does not have comparable opportunities available. This must be the next priority if the energy that has gone into helping mentally handicapped children and their families is not to be wasted.

Who cares for the expert?

Though work within the services for handicapped children is intellectually demanding and potentially rewarding, the interactions are often stressful. Doctors may be anxious from the outset, as the family commonly blames 'Medicine' for their predicament. It is not easy to work with distressed people when solutions are partial and resources are limited. The best professional efforts may be unsuccessful and the consumer cannot be expected to be grateful. It helps to work within a democratic team who can be mutually supportive. If members trust each other, know what they can and cannot expect from each other and work at effective communication, then organizational tensions can be limited. Each team member needs to achieve personal development from life outside work if a personal contribution is to be sustained. It would be ironic if the humanity of the consumers were to be increasingly respected at a cost of professional 'burn-out'. In-service education for team members is also an essential source of renewal. This is discussed in relation to intensive care medical work (Walker, 1982; Valman, 1982; Parente, 1982; Pritchard, 1982; Asthury, 1982), but similar problems also affect those working in services for the handicapped.

Behavioural treatment

One particular approach which has shown itself to be an effective way of providing parents with practical help is the behavioural approach, which aims to analyse behaviour in terms of its environmental contingencies and subsequently to develop practical intervention strategies. It has been common to consider this approach solely in terms of a set of behaviour-modifying techniques that are applied to particular problems, the so-called 'cookbook' approach. However, it is important to recognize that appropriate intervention for any particular skill deficit or behaviour problem can only be on the basis of a careful analysis of the behaviour in question. A behavioural analysis should consist of a number of steps: observation and data collection, interpretation, intervention, and assessment of the effects of the intervention. Interested readers are referred to Tennant *et al.*, (1981) for a more detailed review of this approach.

Observation and data collection

Collecting detailed information about a particular skill deficit or behaviour problem is the important first step which is so often overlooked when faced with the need to intervene to solve a pressing clinical problem.

However, such information provides a firm base upon which intervention may be built, and can be collected from parents, diary records or by making careful and systematic observations in the settings in which the behaviour occurs. Increasingly, emphasis is being placed upon the importance of collecting data in the situation where the problem occurs, because such observation makes it possible to look not only at the behaviour of the child but also at the behaviour of those who interact with him. This latter information may be especially needed if it becomes important to develop an intervention plan that specifies changes in the behaviour of the parent.

Interpretation

On the basis of the information collected, it may then be possible to plan a teaching or behaviour programme. Whilst oversimplistic as a framework for the analysis of complex behaviour, it may be useful to interpret the available information within an A–B–C framework.

Table 3.1 illustrates important relationships between the behaviour (B) and its consequences (C) on the one hand, and the antecedents (A) and the behaviour (B) on the other. For example, if the consequences of a particular behaviour are viewed by the individual as positive, then there is an increased likelihood of the behaviour recurring in the future. The consequences influence the *future probability* of the behaviour. Similarly, if the consequences are viewed by the individual as negative then there will be a decreased likelihood of the behaviour recurring in the future. So an intervention programme may be devised which looks towards altering the existing contingent relationships between the behaviour and its consequences.

A particular place or person may become associated with particular patterns of reinforcing or punishing consequences. The handicapped child will learn to recognize these settings and behave accordingly. The child's behaviour may be different in different circumstances. It is clear that many problem behaviours occur in settings where individuals, materials

Table 3.1. The behavioural model

A	B	C
The antecedents set the occasion for	the behaviour to occur	the future probability of which is influenced by the consequences

or activities that engage the interest of the child are not available. Intervention programmes may be devised that try to alter the setting in which the behaviour occurs.

Intervention

Following an analysis of the problem it should then prove possible to draw up an initial specific intervention plan. It is important to identify the particular objective in explicit terms and not to use imprecise terms such as 'socializes more', 'responds appropriately' or 'does more for himself'. Recording information and specifying aims clearly, such as 'playing with one other child for 10 minutes, twice a day', 'makes eye contact on request', or 'puts on a pullover without help', establishes a baseline and allows the next step to be planned. In general terms it is possible to identify two main types of intervention. Firstly, those procedures designed to *increase* the child's behavioural repertoire, and secondly, those procedures designed to *decrease* the child's behavioural repertoire.

Increasing behaviours

One of the most widely used procedures for increasing the behavioural repertoire of a child is *positive reinforcement.* The administration of a positive reinforcer, consequent upon a particular behaviour, increases the probability that the particular behaviour will occur again in the future. Children have personal preferences for different types of reinforcement, which include music (Walmsley *et al.*, 1981), light, water (Martin, 1981), vibration, hugs, praise, tickles, small pieces of fruit, raisins, small sips of drink, and stars, as well as sweets. It will be important to establish which of these is most effective for a particular child by observation of the child's response.

During the early stages of an intervention designed to develop a new skill, the child should be reinforced every time the particular skill occurs. This helps to motivate the child to acquire the skill. As the skill becomes learned and established, it may be possible slowly to fade the use of reinforcers. In many teaching programmes it is necessary to show the child exactly how to carry out the particular task (Aronson & Folkstone, 1977; Wilson, 1980) and it can be useful to employ a *prompting procedure.* This involves providing either physical or verbal help to encourage the child to learn the required task. At the outset, it may be necessary for the person teaching the skill to guide the child physically and/or verbally through all the steps involved. However, as the child begins to learn the required actions, it will then be possible to fade the use of prompts leaving the child to carry out the skill independently.

Such a procedure can, for example, teach a child to use a spoon. The parent starts by placing his or her hand over the child's hand to prompt the appropriate actions. These include (i) grasping the spoon appropriately, (ii) putting the spoon into the bowl, (iii) loading it, (iv) raising it to mouth, (v) putting the spoon and food into mouth, (vi) closing mouth, (vii) withdrawing spoon, (viii) returning spoon to the dish and (ix) reloading. Prompting the development of skills in the this way also provides opportunities to reinforce appropriate behaviour more readily.

Decreasing behaviours

One way of reducing the frequency of a particular behaviour is by the use of an *extinction procedure*. This is based upon the notion that the removal of reinforcing consequences will lead to a decrease in the behaviour in the future. However, whilst such a procedure may, in the long run, produce a decrease in the frequency, duration or intensity of a particular behaviour, in the short run it will often lead to an increase in the behaviour before its eventual decrease. The age-old advice of 'just ignore him and he'll stop doing it' must be tempered by the knowledge that in the short term it is likely to have the opposite effect. Many extinction procedures are abandoned for this reason and it is important that when parents are given advice on the implementation of such a procedure to deal with a particular behaviour problem they are told about both the short-term and the long-term effects.

An alternative which involves the removal of reinforcing consequences is a *time-out procedure*. More correctly this should be known as time-out from positive reinforcement and can, if used consistently and correctly, provide parents with an effective way of dealing with specific behaviour problems. It is, however, rarely possible to provide parents with enough information in a clinic setting, as it is important both to demonstrate and to observe the parents using the procedure to ensure that it is carried out correctly. Thus, (i) following the occurrence of a particular behaviour problem, the child is asked by the parent in a clear, unambiguous way to stop. (ii) The child is then given enough time to comply and his appropriate behaviour is suitably reinforced. (iii) If he does not comply, a second clear command is given, accompanied (iv) this time by a warning that if he does not stop he will be put into time-out. As before, (v) the child is given enough time to comply and his appropriate behaviour is again suitably reinforced. However, if there is again no compliance, (vi) nothing further is said, no attempt is made to scold or admonish, but (vii) the child is put directly into time-out.

It is possible to use a bedroom or the corner of a room as a time-out area, into which the child is placed, facing the wall, with the parent standing behind the child holding his arms if necessary. Following a specified time period (between 2 and 10 minutes depending on the age of the child) he is then allowed out and encouraged to engage in alternative more appropriate activities. Placing a child into time-out can often be accompanied by crying, screaming, kicking and temper tantrums and it is important not to release the child until he is calm and quiet. Subsequently, the child will often resume the inappropriate behaviour, in which case it will again be important to carry out the time-out procedure. One of the disadvantages of procedures designed to decrease the frequency of particular behaviours, however, is that they provide the child with little indication of the range of more appropriate activities in which he might engage. Very often, undesirable behaviour fulfils important functions for the child. The child may gain something he wants, e.g. attention. For this reason it may be important also to try to develop more appropriate skills and activities which may fulfil a similar function. Ask the question: 'If he wasn't doing that, what would I want him to be doing instead?' The answer may provide ideas for an intervention plan which also aims to develop more appropriate activity. This approach to problem behaviour aims not only to be corrective, i.e. concerned with removing or decreasing difficult behaviour, but also constructive, i.e. concerned with the development of more appropriate activities which may have a similar functional significance to the child.

Assessment of the effects of the intervention
Once an intervention has been designed and used, it is important to see if it works. Such monitoring may provide information which will subsequently lead to alterations in the intervention. It is useful to keep records of progress in the form of a diary or a graph, so that even small changes do not go unnoticed. Such records may be particularly important, for example, when considering teaching programmes for children with severe learning difficulties where the rate of progress may be extremely slow.

The role of parents in the education of their handicapped children, especially in the formative pre-school years, has been increasingly recognized. No matter how many professionals are involved, parents have the most contact with their children. This had led to the development of a wide range of approaches designed to involve parents as partners and provide them with the additional advice they need to help overcome the learning difficulties of their handicapped children. These approaches have included books (Cunningham & Sloper, 1978; Carr, 1980), manuals (Baker *et al.*, 1976), workshops (Holland & Hattersley, 1980) and structured home advisory services (Revill & Blunden, 1979; Holland, 1981).

One particular approach which is widely used is the Portage Project approach (Shearer & Shearer, 1972). This goal-oriented, home-based teaching service aims to involve parents in the education of their children, and it has been shown that the service can be delivered effectively by existing personnel, such as health visitors, after only a relatively short period of training. Furthermore, the service has been enthusiastically received by parents and is able to help them teach their children even if the children are severely handicapped. The project materials are designed to help the parent and the person acting as a home adviser to produce an individual plan for each child and to provide teaching in a carefully structured way at a rate that suits the learning speed of the child. They include a developmental checklist, which provides an opportunity to assess the child's present level of competence in the areas of motor, self-help, language, socialization and cognitive skill, and a set of curriculum cards which provide teaching ideas.

Once the parent and the home advisor have decided on an appropriate task for the child, it will invariably be necessary to break the teaching down into a number of small steps which can be taught to the child in a week by week sequence. Following this, the home advisor will demonstrate to the parent the teaching for the coming week and will then supervise the parent carrying out the programme. Finally, the home advisor will plan an activity chart which, as well as providing a written description of the task to be taught and how to teach it, also provides space for the parents to record progress during the coming week. Usually the parent will work with the child in a structured way for a short period of time each day, and record the outcome on the graph. At the start of the next home visit, the home advisor will review progress over the past week and adapt the next teaching step accordingly.

It is important to evaluate which approach or combination of approaches suits which particular family. Though many approaches have been developed, few controlled experimental studies have been undertaken. However, Heifitz (1977) sought to evaluate a number of different approaches to parent training. The study involved 160 families from different social class backgrounds, all of whom had a handicapped child ranging in age from 3 to 14 years old, from mild to profound in terms of learning difficulties. For the course of the 20-week study, the families were randomly assigned to one of five different conditions.

1 Manuals only. This group received a series of instructional manuals which covered general teaching strategies as well as offering specific guidance in the areas of self-help: speech, language and behaviour problem management.

2 Manuals plus telephone calls. This group, in addition to receiving the instructional manuals, also received eight, twice-weekly telephone consultations.

3 Manuals plus groups. This group, in addition to receiving the instructional manuals, also took part in nine, twice-weekly group meetings.

4 Manuals plus groups and visits. This group, in addition to receiving the instructional manuals, took part in nine, twice-weekly group meetings and received six home visits.

5 Control: waiting list. This control group received training at a later date.

The results of this study showed that the increases in the children's self-help skills and *mothers'* knowledge of teaching principles were greater for the trained families than for the control families. More surprising, though, was the fact that there were no differences between the different training conditions, i.e. successive increments of professional assistance did not lead to greater gains in self-help skills on the part of the children. For this reason, it was suggested that the manuals-only condition was the most cost-effective approach. However, in considering the efforts that were made to reduce behaviour problems, it became clear that parents were unlikely to carry out such interventions without having an opportunity for discussion. For this reason, those families in the conditions that involved groups produced most efforts in behaviour problem management. Interestingly, the conditions involving groups produced most change in *fathers'* knowledge of teaching principles. At the end of the experimental study, parents were also asked to rate how confident they felt as teachers of their own children. Their responses showed that the parents in the manuals-alone condition reported feeling less confident than parents taught by other means, despite the objective evidence of their teaching expertise and effectiveness.

Baker *et al.* (1980) completed a follow-up study 14 months later, which was designed to assess the maintenance of the childrens' gains and the parents' knowledge of teaching principles. It was clear that the initial gains in skill and knowledge had been maintained and that 44% of the families were still engaged in teaching that could be described as useful or very useful. However, it was also noted that most of the teaching was now 'incidental', i.e. incorporated into the family's daily routine and carried out as the occasion arose, rather than formal where a regular teaching period was set aside each day. Parents were also asked to state which of the training conditions they might have preferred if they had been given a free choice, and all rated the manuals plus groups and visits condition first, while the manuals-alone condition was rated last. When asked about what they saw as the major obstacles that prevented them from carrying out further teaching, parents listed these as the amount of time available for carrying out the teaching, the severity of the learning difficulties which made observable progress slow, their own perceived inabilities as teachers, and their need for outside support and encouragement.

Further research is needed to establish the benefits of different approaches to parent guidance, but a number of observations may indicate a good service that aims to meet the needs of different families. Advice and guidance by means of lectures and written material may be most suited to those parents who are familiar with assimilating information in this way. Other parents may not find it easy to translate courses on general teaching principles into specific intervention procedures, and so may benefit from more direct action-oriented advice and guidance. Yet other parents may prefer a combination of the above approaches, whereby they receive guidance on specific intervention methods but also have an opportunity to discuss further the theoretical issues underlying specific suggestions. It is important not to undermine the parents' own problem-solving capabilities nor to reduce their role to that of an assistant to the professional, but to increase their confidence and competence in dealing with their own children. For this reason, service delivery structures are developed which can be flexible and responsive to a family's changing needs. While it may be necessary to provide parents with initial advice on a regular basis, reducing the consultations as their competence develops, it is possible to overwhelm a family with suggestions for intensive structured teaching that are unrealistic and may only set the family up to fail. It may be more realistic to provide general advice about using opportunities that may occur for incidental teaching, complementing this with more structured teaching sessions in appropriate day-care facilities. Advice to families needs to be planned on an individual basis and methods need to be reviewed regularly.

Summary

The coincidence of appropriate medical services, skilled teaching and parent-counselling services, well-informed parent self-help groups, and suitable short- and long-term care facilities, ideally in a local domestic setting or in a hostel organized on a family group basis, offer mentally handicapped children and their families a service which was impossible a generation ago.

References

Anderson, E.M. & Clarke, L., in collaboration with Spain, B. (1982) *Disability in Adolescence*. Methuen, London.

Astbury, J. & Yu, V.Y.H. (1982) Determinants of stress for staff in a neonatal intensive care unit. *Archives of Disease in Childhood*, **57**, 108–111.

Aylward, G.P., Layzara, A., Meyer, J. (1978) Behavioural and neurological characteristics of a hydranencephalic infant. *Developmental Medicine and Child Neurology*, **20**, 221–217.

Baker, B., Brightman, A., Heifitz, L. & Murphy, D. (1976) *Step to Independence Series*. Campaign, Research Press.

Baker, B.L., Heifitz, L.J. & Murphy, D.M. (1980) Behavioural training for parents of mentally retarded children: one year follow up. *American Journal of Mental Deficiency*, **85**, 31–38.

Ballard, R. (1978) Help for coping with the unthinkable. *Developmental Medicine and Child Neurology*, **20**, 517–521.

Bancroft, J. (1983) *Human Sexuality and its Problems*, pp. 362–369. Churchill Livingstone, Edinburgh.

Bankes, J.L.K. (1974) Eye defects of mentally handicapped children. *British Medical Journal*, **2**, 533–535.

Batshaw, M.L. & Perret, Y.M. (1981) *Children with Handicaps. A Medical Primer*, p. 356. Paul H. Brookes, Baltimore.

Bax, M. (1967) Medical aspects of the care of handicapped adolescents. *Developmental Medicine and Child Neurology*, **9**, 776–779.

Bentovim, A. (1972a) Emotional disturbances of handicapped pre-school children and their families—attitudes to the child. *British Medical Journal*, **3**, 579–581.

Bentovim, A. (1972b) Handicapped pre-school children and their families—effects on the child's early emotional development. *British Medical Journal*, **3**, 634–637.

Blomquist, H.K. (1982) Mental retardation in children. An epidemiological and etiological study of mentally retarded children born 1959–1970 in a northern Swedish county. *Umea University Medical Dissertations*, New Series No. 76, University of Umea, Sweden.

British Medical Journal (1972) Handicapped children and family stress. **1**, 329–330.

British Medical Journal (1979) Are they being served. **1**, 147–148.

British Medical Journal (1980) Sterilisation of mentally retarded minors. **281**, 1025–1026.

British Medical Journal (1981) Withholding treatment in infancy. **282**, 925–926.

British Paediatric Association (1981) Management of handicapped babies. *British Medical Journal*, **282**, 1001.

Byrne, W.J., Campbell, M., Ashcroft, E., Seibert, J.J. & Euler, A.R. (1983)

A diagnostic approach to vomiting in severely retarded patients. *American Journal of Diseases of Children*, **137**, 259–262.

Cadman, D., Richards, J. & Feldman, W. (1978) Gastroesophageal reflux in severely retarded children. *Developmental Medicine and Child Neurology*, **20**, 95–98.

Carr, J. (1970) Mongolism: telling the parents. *Developmental Medicine and Child Neurology*, **12**, 213–221.

Carr, J. (1980) *Helping your Handicapped Child*. Penguin, Harmondsworth.

Carter, G. & Jancar, J. (1983) Mortality in the mentally handicapped: a 50 year survey at the Stoke Park group of hospitals (1930–1980). *Journal of Mental Deficiency Research*, **27**, 143–156.

Chamberlain, M.A. (1981) The handicapped school leaver. *Archives of Disease in Childhood*, **56**, 737–738.

Chamberlain, M.A. (1984) Work for the disabled. *British Medical Journal*, **289**, 639–640.

Chaplais, J. De Z. & Macfarlane, J.A. (1984) A review of 404 'late walkers'. *Archives of Disease in Childhood*, **59**, 512–516.

Corbett, J.A. (1972) Behavioural and drug treatment of children with severe mental handicap. *British Journal of Hospital Medicine*, **8**, 141–144.

Corbett, J.A. & Campbell, H.J. (1981) Causes of severe self-injurious behaviour. In *Frontiers of Knowledge in Mental Retardation* (ed. P. Mittler). University Park Press, Baltimore.

Craft, A. & Craft, M. (1979) *Handicapped Married Couples*. Routledge and Kegan Paul, London.

Craft, M. & Craft, A. (1978) *Sex and the Mentally Handicapped*. Routledge and Kegan Paul, London.

Crawfurd, M. d'A. (1982) Severe mental handicap: pathogenesis, treatment and prevention. *British Medical Journal*, **285**, 762–766.

Cunningham, C.C. (1979) Parent counselling. In *Tredgold's Mental Retardation*, 12th edn (ed. M. Craft). Balliere Tindall, London.

Cunningham, C. & Sloper, P. (1978) *Helping your Handicapped Baby*. Souvenir Press, London.

Davies, T.S. (1975) Collaborative clinical experience with cyproterone acetate. *Journal of Internal Medicine Research*, **3**, 16.

Dein, E. (1975) Clinical problems in cyproterone acetate therapy. *Journal of Internal Medicine Research*, **3**, 13.

Dorner, S. (1980) Sexuality and sex education for the handicapped teenager. *Journal of Maternal and Child Health*, **5**, 356–360.

Edgerton, R. (1979) *Mental Retardation*. Fontana/Open Books, London.

Featherstone, H. (1981) *A Difference in the Family*. Harper and Row, New York.

Fogelman, K., ed. (1983) *Growing up in Great Britain*. (National Children's Bureau) Macmillan, London.

Forrest, A.D. & Ogunreni, O.O. (1974) The prevalence of psychiatric illness in a hospital for the mentally handicapped. *Health Bulletin*, **32**, 199–202.

Fraser, B.C. (1980) The meaning of handicap in children. *Child: Care, Health and Development*, **6**, 83–91.

Fryers, T. & Mackay, R.I. (1979) The epidemiology of severe mental handicap. *Early Human Development*, **3**, 277–294.

Fulford, G.E. & Brown, J.K. (1976) Position as a cause of deformity in children with cerebral palsy. *Developmental Medicine and Child Neurology*, **18**, 305–314.

Gath, A. (1973) The effects of mental handicap on the family. *British Journal of Hospital Medicine*, **8**, 147–150.

Gath, A. (1981) Cerebral degeneration in Down's syndrome. *Developmental Medicine and Child Neurology*, **23**, 814−817.

Gebhard, P.H. (1973) Sexual behaviour of the mentally retarded. In *Human Sexuality and the Mentally Retarded* (eds. F.F. de la Cruz and G.D. La Vech), pp. 29−49. Brunner-Mazel, New York.

Gebhard, P., Gagnon, J., Pomeroy, N. & Christenson, C. (1965) *Sex Offenders*. Harper and Row, New York.

Gillon, R. (1986) Acts and omissions, killing and letting die. *British Medical Journal*, **292**, 126−127.

Gloag, D. (1983) Caring for the young disabled. *British Medical Journal*, **286**, 1376.

Goodall, J. (1984) Balancing options in neonatal care. *Archives of Disease in Childhood*, **59**, 88−89.

Grossman, F. (1972) *Brothers and Sisters of Retarded Children: an Exploratory Study*. Syracuse University Press, New York.

Haavik, S.F. & Menninger, K.A. (1981) *Sexuality, Law and the Developmentally Disabled Person: Legal and Clinical Aspects of Marriage, Parenthood and Sterilisation*. Paul H. Brookes, Baltimore.

Hagberg, B. (1975) Pre-, peri- and postnatal prevention of major neuropaediatric handicaps. *Neuropadiatrie*, **6**, 331−338.

Hagberg, B. & Kyllerman, M. (1983) Epidemiology of mental retardation—a Swedish survey. *Brain and Development*, **5**, 441−449.

Hagberg, B. & Lundberg, A. (1969) Dissociated motor development simulating cerebral palsy. *Neuropadiatrie*, **1**, 187−199.

Hall J.E. (1975) Sexuality and the mentally retarded. In *Human Sexuality. A Health Practitioner's Texts* (ed. R. Green), pp. 181−195. William and Wilkins, Baltimore.

Hanid, T.K. & Harvey, D.R. (1978) Marital stress in families with a sick or handicapped child. *Journal of Maternal and Child Health*, **3**, 30−32.

Harris, A., Cox, E. & Smith, C.R.W. (1971) *Handicapped and Impaired in Great Britain*, Part 1. HMSO, London.

Heifitz, L.J. (1977) Behavioural training for parents of retarded children: alternative formats based on instructional manuals. *American Journal of Mental Deficiency*, **82**, 194−203.

Holland, J. (1981) The Lancaster portage project: a home based service for developmentally delayed young children and their families. *Health Visitor*, **54**, 486−488.

Holland, J. & Hattersley, J. (1980) Parent support groups for the families of mentally handicapped children. *Child: Care, Health and Development*, **6**, 167−173.

Hunt, A. (1983) Tuberous sclerosis: survey of 97 cases. *Developmental Medicine and Child Neurology*, **25**, 346−357.

Hunton, M. (1980) Caring for babies with Down's syndrome. *Journal of Maternal and Child Health*, **5**, 296−302.

Jolly, H. (1984) Have parents the right to see their children's medical reports? *Archives of Disease in Childhood*, **59**, 601−602.

Judson, S.L. & Burden, R.L. (1980) Towards a tailored measure of parental attitudes: an approach to the evaluation of one aspect of intervention projects with parents of handicapped children. *Child: Care, Health and Development*, **6**, 47−55.

Kirman, B. (1980) Growing up with Down's syndrome. *British Journal of Hospital Medicine*, **23**, 385−388.

Koster, S. & Rosenstein, S.N. (1978) Orthodontics in cerebral palsy. In *Dentistry in Cerebral Palsy and Related Handicapping Conditions* (ed. S.N. Rosenstein), pp. 95−110. Charles C. Thomas, Springfield.

Lancet (1979a) Sterilisation of the mentally handicapped: working group in current medical/ethical problems. **ii**, 685—686.

Lancet (1979b) Non-treatment of defective newborn babies. **ii**, 1123—1124.

Lancet (1982) Public opinion and severe mental handicap. **i**, 811.

Mackay, R.I. (1976) *Mental Handicap in Child Health Practice*. Butterworths, London.

MacKeith, R. (1973) The feelings and behaviour of parents of handicapped children. *Developmental Medicine and Child Neurology*, **15**, 524—527.

Madge, N. & Fossam, M. (1982) *Ask the Children*. Batsford, London.

Mattinson, J. (1975) *Marriage and Mental Handicap*, 2nd edn. Tavistock, London.

Miller, S.L. (1965) Dental care for the mentally retarded—a challenge to the profession. *Journal of Public Health Dentistry*, **25**, 3.

Millis, E. (1981) The eye in Down's syndrome. *Journal of Maternal and Child Health*, **6**, 184—189.

Nelson, K.B. & Ellenberg, J.H. (1982) Children who 'outgrew' cerebral palsy. *Pediatrics*, **69**, 529—536.

Neuhauser, G. (1977) The spectrum of cerebral palsy in mentally retarded patients. *Neuropaediatrics*, **8**, Suppl., 547.

Nowah, A.J., ed. (1976) *Dentistry for the Handicapped Patient*. C.V. Mosby, St Louis.

Parente, A.S. (1982) Psychological pressures in a neonatal I.T.U. *British Journal of Hospital Medicine*, **27**, 266—268.

Phelp, M. & Duckworth, D. (1982) *Children with Disabilities and their Families: a Review of Research*. NFER—Nelson Publishing, Windsor.

President's Commission for the Study of Ethical Problems in Medicine (1983) *Deciding to Forego Life-Sustaining Treatment. A Report on the Ethical, Medical and Legal Issues in Treatment Decisions*. Government Printing Office, Washington.

Pritchard, M. (1982) Psychological pressures in a renal unit. *British Journal of Hospital Medicine*, **27**, 512—516.

Reed, R.W. & Reed, S.C. (1965) *Mental Retardation: A Family Study*. W.B. Saunders, Philadelphia.

Revill, S. & Blunden, R. (1979) A home training service for pre-school developmentally handicapped children. *Behaviour Research and Therapy*, **17**, 207—214.

Richardson, S.A., Katz, M., Koller, H., McLaren, J. & Rubinstein, R. (1979) Some characteristics of a population of mentally retarded young adults in a British city. A basis for estimating some service needs. *Journal of Mental Deficiency Research*, **23**, 275—285.

Robertson, J.A. & Fost, N. (1976) Passive euthanasia of defective newborn infants: legal considerations. *Journal of Pediatrics*, **88**, 883—889.

Robinson, R.O. (1973) The frequency of other handicaps in children with cerebral palsy. *Developmental Medicine and Child Neurology*, **15**, 305—312.

Rosenberg, A. (1982) Dentistry for the handicapped. In *The Child with Disabling Illness: Principles of Rehabilitation* (eds J.A. Downey and N.L. Low). Raven Press, New York.

Rosenstein, S.N. & Rosenberg, A. (1964) Management of extensive restorative problems and tooth guidance following rampant caries in the young child. *New York State Journal of Dentistry*, **30**, 434—437.

Rutter, M.L. (1972) Psychiatric disorder and intellectual impairment in childhood. *British Journal of Hospital Medicine*, **8**, 137—140.

Savage, W. (1978) The use of Depo-Provira in East London. *Fertility and Contraception*, **2**, 41—47.

Sensky, T. (1982) Family stigma in congenital physical handicap. *British Medical Journal*, **285**, 1033—1035.

Shearer, M. & Shearer, D. (1972) The Portage project: a model for early childhood education. *Exceptional Children*, **36**, 210–217.

Simeansson, R. & McHale, S. (1981) Review. Research on handicapped children: sibling relationships. *Child: Care, Health and Development*, **7**, 153–171.

Smith, G.F. & Berg, J.M. (1976) *Down's Anomaly*. Churchill Livingstone, Edinburgh.

Solomons, G. (1978) Talking to parents of disabled children. *Developmental Medicine and Child Neurology*, **20**, 419–420.

Solomons, G. (1979) Child abuse and developmental disabilities. *Developmental Medicine and Child Neurology*, **21**, 101–108.

Stewart, W.F.R. (1978) Sexual fulfilment for the handicapped. *British Journal of Hospital Medicine*, **20**, 676–680.

Taylor, D.C. (1982) Counselling the parents of handicapped children. *British Medical Journal*, **284**, 1027–1028.

Taylor, D.C. & McKinlay, I.A. (1984) When not to treat epilepsy with drugs. *Developmental Medicine and Child Neurology*, **26**, 823–827.

Tennant, L., Cullen, C. & Hattersley, J. (1981) Applied behaviour analysis: intervention with retarded people. In *Applications of Conditioning Theory* (ed. G. Davey). Methuen, London.

Tizard, J. & Grad, J.C. (1961) *The Mentally Handicapped and their Families*. Oxford University Press, Oxford.

Tripp, J.H. (1984) *Unmet Needs of Handicapped Young Adults*. Children's Research Fund, Liverpool.

Valman, B. (1982) Staff strain. ABC of 1 to 7. *British Medical Journal*, **284**, 1025.

Vining, E.P.G. & Freeman, J.M. (1978) Sterilisation and the retarded female: is advocacy depriving individuals of their rights? *Paediatrics*, **62**, 850–853.

Walker, C.H.M. (1982) Neonatal intensive care and stress. *Archives of Disease in Childhood*, **57**, 85–88.

Weatherall, J.A.C. (1982) A review of some effects of recent medical practices in reducing the numbers of children born with congenital abnormalities. *Health Trends*, **14**, 85–88.

Wheeless, C.R. (1975) Abdominal hysterectomy for surgical sterilisation in the mentally retarded. *American Journal of Obstetrics and Gynecology*, **122**, 872.

Williams, I.A. (1969) Management of the adolescent with cerebral palsy. *Lancet*, **ii**, 1126–1129.

Williams, P. & Shoultz, B. (1982) *We Can Speak for Ourselves*. Souvenir Press, London.

Wolff, L. & Zarfas, D.E. (1982) Parents' attitudes towards sterilisation of their mentally handicapped children. *American Journal of Mental Deficiency*, **87**, 122–129.

Chapter 4
Children with Cerebral Palsy

Ingemar Olow

Cerebral palsy (CP) comprises a conglomerate of different non-progressive motor handicap syndromes, grouped together because they involve similar disorders of development and learning activities. The concept implies, however, a very mixed aetiology and pathogenesis.

The incidence of CP varies between different countries, the rate usually being around 2.0 per 1000 live births. In some European countries, for instance in Sweden, the rate of CP today is 1.5 per 1000. Two-thirds of all cases of CP can be referred pathogenetically to the perinatal period, often to multifactorial events. The potential negative effects of modern neonatal care on the panorama of handicap must be continuously evaluated. During the 1970s, the incidence of cerebral palsy did not decrease in the same way as in the previous decade; rather there was a slight increase, but not of severely multihandicapped children. Because of the concomitant decrease in perinatal mortality, a considerable net 'gain' in the number of lives saved without cerebral palsy has been achieved. Hagberg and his colleagues (1982) have calculated that in Sweden from 1971 to 1975 the improved prognosis of neonates as compared with 15 years previously had led to the additional survival of 2100 children, of whom 55 (2.6%) are handicapped.

Classification

The classification of cerebral palsy syndromes can be based on clinical (or neurological) signs or from the pathological point of view (Table 4.1). The incidence of different CP syndromes and the distribution of causes is seen in Tables 4.2 and 4.3.

Many of the children with CP also have additional handicaps which have to be taken into consideration in the management of the child. It is important to try to diagnose these complications as early as possible, as handling them in a proper way can be of immense importance for the child's further development. Visual disturbances and convulsions are mostly seen in the 'spastic syndromes', while impairment of hearing and

Table 4.1. Clinical and pathogenetic classification systems for cerebral palsy syndromes in Sweden (Hagberg *et al.*, 1978)

Neurological classification

Spastic
  Hemiplegic
  Tetraplegic
  Diplegic*

Ataxic
  Diplegic*
  Congenital (simple)

Dyskinetic
  Mainly choreo-athetotic†
  Mainly dystonic†

Pathogenetic classification

Prenatal group
  Clear prenatal CNS malformations
  SGA‡ (< −2 SD)
  Identical CP syndrome in sibling ⎫
  Consanguinity in parents   ⎬ + Normal peri- and
  Obvious abnormalities during pregnancy ⎭   postnatal history

Perinatal group
  Obvious complications during delivery and/or first week of life
  Birthweight < 2500 g. AGA§ and normal pre- and postnatal history

Postnatal group
  Defined causes (8 days to 2 years of age)

Untraceable group
  Birthweight > 2500 g. AGA§ and normal pre-, peri- and postnatal history

---

*Overlapping; counted together in statistical calculations.
†Counted together in statistical calculations.
‡Small for gestational age.
§Appropriate for gestational age.

speech difficulties are more often found in the dystonic forms. Thirty to 40% of all children with CP are also mentally retarded; the distribution of intellectual capacity in the different syndromes is seen in Table 4.4. It is also well known that the CP child more often has perceptual disorders than non-handicapped children.

Early diagnosis

It is important to remember that, after a complicated delivery—perhaps

Table 4.2. Incidence of CP syndromes during the four periods 1954−58, 1959−62, 1963−66, 1967−70

		Inc. per 1000 live births				
		54−58	59−62	63−66	67−70	$P \leqslant$
Spastic syndromes	Hemiplegia	0.79	0.54	0.64	0.55	
	Tetraplegia	0.14	0.08	0.01	0.07	
	Diplegia					
	Atax. diplegia	1.03	0.87	0.59	0.41	0.0005
Ataxic syndromes						
	Cong. ataxia	0.07	0.11	0.14	0.16	
Dyskinetic syndromes		0.21	0.29	0.29	0.15	0.05
Total CP		2.24	1.89	1.67	1.34	0.005
Sp/at diplegic	B.w. > 2500 g	0.31	0.33	0.27	0.21	
syndromes	B.w. ≤ 2500 g	0.72	0.55	0.32	0.20	0.0005
Number of cases		65	172	182	141	

Total number of cases = 560.
Sp/at = spastic/ataxic.
B.w. = body weight.

Table 4.3. The distribution of causes in the different CP syndromes

		Untraceable (%)	Prenatal (%)	Perinatal (%)	Postnatal (%)
Hemiplegia	$n = 200$	30	23	41	6
Tetraplegia	$n = 19$	10	42	37	11
Sp. diplegia	$n = 186$	15	25	57	3
At. diplegia	$n = 31$	13	45	39	3
Cong. ataxia	$n = 44$	41	25	18	16
Athetosis	$n = 20$	10	5	85	0
Dystonic forms	$n = 60$	2	26	65	7
Total CP	$n = 560$	21	25	48	6

with idiopathic respiratory distress syndrome and convulsions during the first few days of life—the next 2 to 4 months can be without any symptoms of brain damage. This is the 'silent period', often so confusing for parents, and for many doctors.

It has often been claimed that early diagnosis, leading to early 'treatment' and habilitation, places the CP child and the family in a better situation than when the diagnosis is delayed—even if it is not possible to offer actual 'cure'. Consequently, it may be important to have special services for so-called 'children at risk', that is for children who during

Table 4.4 The distribution of intellectual capacity in the different CP syndromes

		IQ < 70 (%)	IQ ≥ 70 (%)
Hemiplegia	n = 200	15	85
Tetraplegia	n = 19	100	0
Sp. diplegia	n = 186	31	69
At. diplegia	n = 31	29	71
Cong. ataxia	n = 44	48	52
Athetosis	n = 20	5	95
Dystonic forms	n = 60	62	38
Total CP	n = 560	31	69

pregnancy, delivery or the first weeks of life have been exposed to harmful events that we know can lead to future handicap *and* have shown neurological abnormalities at this time. The size of the group of children at risk is a question of how wide your limits are. A figure of around 10% of all children is often accepted.

In this way it is supposed that 50–75% of children with CP can be identified early, most of them between 6 and 9 months of age, especially if the follow-up is performed by an experienced neuropaediatrician. But the 'follow-up' needs to go on for at least the first 2 years of life in order to identify signs of a neurological handicap (Nelson & Ellenberg, 1982).

If the history and the development of the child suggest other neurological explanations, further investigations will have to be done, such as EEG (electro-encephalography) and CT scanning. Progression of neurological symptoms later in childhood is always suspicious of an alternative diagnosis to cerebral palsy, though physical deterioration during times of growth can occur in people with cerebral palsy. There is also the possibility of adverse effects from psychiatric disorders or medication.

Early management

Of all the children presenting with delayed motor development, only a small minority have cerebral palsy. However anxious we may be to tell parents the truth as we see it, premature clinical decisions are undesirable. Amongst the alternatives are social deprivation, genetically determined delayed motor development often associated with hypotonia and bottom shuffling, global developmental delay and neuromuscular conditions. Apart from those with an alternative diagnosis, there are two or three children in every hundred who show delayed motor development of uncertain cause and with an uncertain prognosis. Sometimes their families will be concerned (e.g. 'He's not walking at 18 months') and some will not ('Some children are slower starters, aren't they?').

If parents are concerned, review and further discussion will be necessary, and as time passes some parents seek further help. For selected families, general physiotherapy advice or attendance at a playgroup can fulfil this, both giving ideas for play for the child and the opportunity for meeting other parents of children in a similar position. Such services should be local rather than based in distant specialist centres. Home visitors have some advantages; the visitor will tend to offer more realistic advice and the families do not have to make an expedition. However, home visitors can only see a few children each day and the families do not meet other families so readily. Also, as multidisciplinary teams have developed, there has been a risk of invasion of family privacy. There is a tendency to introduce services in response to demand without monitoring them or comparing the efficiency and acceptability of alternative organizational methods. For children whose development is doubtful, home visiting should generally be limited to those (such as health visitors in the United Kingdom) who would be expected to come into the home. Then advice can be sought by the visitor and family from other experts. It is certainly possible to be helpful to families without being committed to a diagnosis. Most children with unexplained delay in motor development turn out to be neurologically normal, though some have learning problems.

When a child's handicap is diagnosed, this changes the situation for the whole family. All hopes and expectations are suddenly dashed. The first reaction will very often be desperation, alarm and insecurity. Even if parents have heard of handicapped children, they have hardly ever thought of the possibility of having a handicapped child themselves. The almost constant question to the midwife or obstetrician, 'Is the child all right?', shows a certain uneasiness but is often rhetorical. Even if the parents have been concerned that the child could be damaged, they are seldom prepared for the confirmation of handicap in their child. It should be arranged that both parents and the child are present when the diagnosis is given. Fathers may find it harder to become involved with their children through not having experienced pregnancy, and can become detached from a handicapped child.

Very often the diagnosis of CP cannot be made for a few months and the family with a 'child at risk' has to be advised in a special way, with delicacy and understanding, meeting the same experienced doctor and other members of the team, such as social worker and physiotherapist. They must be given all the time they want and need for discussion.

When the diagnosis is certain, the parents have to be informed together, in detail, about all that is known at that time of the degree of the handicap and how the problems may be managed. The possibilities for treatment must also be explained, who is going to give it and where. The physiotherapists, trained in early treatment and handling, must be introduced to the parents if they do not already know each other.

It is important to start physiotherapy as soon as the diagnosis of 'cerebral palsy' is given. Even if there is no known method that can 'cure' a child with cerebral palsy, early stimulation of motor functions is of great value for the child's development during the first years of life. It also gives the parents a better understanding of the child's problems and how to cope with them. At least children should be given experience of different postures and given every incentive to move by the means that are most effective for the child. Parents may be encouraged to play with the child physically from the start.

It is important to be honest in your information, to tell the parents what you know—but also what you do not know. At an early age it is difficult even for experienced doctors to give an exact prognosis. Even if this first information will be very upsetting, it is better in the long term to tell the truth in a straightforward way and with plenty of time for discussion. This gives a sense of security to the parents and prevents them from consulting too many people. Changing from unit to unit and from one doctor to another may waste valuable weeks or months and may mean that important assessments and early training will not be carried out at the right time.

So the very first information and guidance to the parents is most important. How to give it and what to say has to be very selective, depending on (among other factors) the type and degree of handicap, the circumstances of the family and the parents' first reaction; and of course, this first information has to be followed up very shortly and then repeatedly during the next few months. Fathers tend to find it harder to express their distress. It can help if a social worker or nurse is present at early interviews and then visits the home to discuss the information given. In this way questioning can be made easier.

We know from experience that the parents, perhaps most often the mother, can have a sense of guilt about what has happened. Did she not take care of herself during pregnancy, did she smoke too much, or is what has happened the result of a punishment for sins? It is most important to be aware of the need for the parents to ask such questions, but at the same time never to have a moralizing attitude.

Through the years the parents need continuous guidance. There are always new problems arising which have to be discussed in detail, for instance concerning medical problems such as surgery, or resulting from educational or social difficulties. Very often it can be hard for the parents to look at the problems in a realistic way, and it can be impossible for them to accept the situation for a long time, particularly if the child is also mentally retarded. Overprotection can then be the result. Parents give all their care and attention to the child and do not think the child capable of managing for himself to the extent that he actually can. The mother—or both parents—can, through the years, be more dependent on the child than vice versa. Overdependence on professional support should also be avoided. The family should be in control and should seek advice to facilitate their predicament.

The children are, as a rule, living in their homes with the parents responsible for day-to-day care. Close co-operation has to be established from the very first day, and they have to know what our aims are and what sort of treatment and care is needed to reach these aims. Without the parents in the team, very little is possible. If confidence is shown in them from the beginning, they can give valuable information concerning the reaction of the child in different situations. How often parents are right in their observations!

For many years, cerebral palsy and many other neurological impairments in childhood were regarded mainly as a medical problem. If the handicap was due to a motor disability, the orthopaedic surgeon was the one in charge of the treatment. Gradually, the paediatrician has become more and more involved, especially the child neurologist and habilitation doctor. Developmental aspects in treatment have become more important. The needs of the growing child are better understood and so is the importance of an early diagnosis, early training and support to the parents.

Further management and care

In the overall management of the child with cerebral palsy the early years of life are of great importance. During these years it is necessary to consider feeding and communication, motor, intellectual, perceptual and emotional development, and to try to compensate for the handicap if necessary.

The motor handicap can in itself make it difficult for the child to feed and communicate, to move around, to crawl, walk, jump, to grasp and handle toys, to control speech, turn the head towards a sound and put things into the mouth; and therefore therapy is important for guidance and stimulation of motor skills.

Often the first difficulty experienced is with feeding. Attention needs to be given to the position in which the child is fed, the degree of sensitivity of the oral reflexes and the texture of the food. Even with skill and patience, feeding can be a source of frustration rather than pleasure for parents and child. It is postulated, but not proved, that facilitation of feeding mechanisms may permit improved speech articulation later. At least good feeding technique can make mealtimes less alarming, can lead to less drooling and can reduce the risk of aspiration. For older children with severe drooling problems, a lip sensor can be used as a teaching aid (Huskie *et al.*, 1979). Several surgical approaches to this problem are described (Chait & Kessler, 1979; Crysdale, 1980), but at present most would regard such procedures as a last resort.

The management of, and the help to, the handicapped child is closely integrated in therapy, playing and daily life activities. The child is first of all a member of a family and must be cared for in the family as much as possible, together with the parents, siblings, their peers, relatives and neighbours. Through the years the child should try to be involved in the same activities as other children, for example going to the local nursery school. But all the time the handicapped child must be prepared for a life in society, and society must be taught to accept the handicapped. In order to do this it is necessary to have an organization with professionals responsible for total care and management.

Firstly, the child must be motivated for the aims we are working for. It is important to find out how to encourage the child to be as independent as possible; and the members of the team must find the same motivation. The teaching situation is adjusted to age and development.

Secondly, we must consider the environment; advice must be relevant to where the child lives and plays and with whom he will interact. The attitudes of other children need attention, including their understanding of the handicap and the limits that result from it. Children can learn to play with a child in a wheelchair who cannot move his arms and hands well, who is difficult to communicate with because of hearing defects or lack of speech, and who is on a different 'eye level'. Information and guidance are of great importance.

Thirdly, what materials should be used? Toys the child is interested in may need to be adjusted to make it possible for the severely handicapped child to play with them. Equipment may be needed for communication, for proper seating (Rang *et al.*, 1981; Fulford *et al.*, 1982). Equipment should be designed to be useful and at the same time look attractive, both to the child and to those interacting with him. Motor and perceptual skills can be taught at the same time.

Fourthly, methods must be adjusted so that they fit the child, the parents and professionals. The method, of course, also has to be changed as the child grows, when he moves into other surroundings and when he meets other people.

When school starts, it is important to make an accurate evaluation of the abilities and difficulties of the child. With motor handicaps such as walking difficulties and impairment of hand function, often combined with perceptual disorders and communication problems such as a marked dysarthria, it is essential to try to foresee problems that may arise during the years to come. A physical disability is both a technical or practical problem and a social or educational one. The effect of a motor disability combined with one or two secondary disabilities adds up to a complex situation, often demanding highly specific individual solutions. This is particularly true when planning vocational training. Concentration disturbances, limited social skills, slow working pace, poor memory and unevenness in intelligence can make it difficult for many young people with cerebral palsy to live independently and obtain employment later on.

In addition to information and instructions given by different members of the assessment team, it is helpful for the parents to be given some literature about cerebral palsy. Very often parents' organizations or societies print small booklets giving brief facts on special topics, such as where to get social support, or where special courses for parents are given and how local habilitation services are organized. Some of these societies arrange meetings or workshops for parents and professionals. It is also an advantage for parents of handicapped children to share experiences with other parents and to realize that they are not the only ones to have problems. Sometimes this can be a way out of isolation, and a help in accepting the situation, and perhaps developing a more positive view of it.

Treatment

Our ambition is always to give adequate therapy which in the future will make it possible for the handicapped person to live an independent life and earn his own living. In the beginning, we do not know how much the child can attain. We know for certain that through the years the teaching programme has to be changed and adjusted over and over again, depending on the next problem to be solved.

Through the years, many 'systems of treatment' for cerebral palsy have appeared, some of them claiming to give very good results, even a complete 'cure' of the handicap. There has up to now been no confirmation, neither on theoretical grounds nor on the basis of scientific studies, that one system of treatment is superior to another. They all have their merits and demerits.

The first to work out a special training programme for children with cerebral palsy was W.M. Phelps (an orthopaedic surgeon in the United States). His programme included active and passive movements, training of balance and general fitness. Deformities were controlled with splints and he also constructed special equipment for 'activities of daily living'. Many of his ideas are still used, especially his training programme before and after surgery.

It was not until the beginning of the 1950s that therapists became interested in motor development and understood how to take this into consideration in the training programme. The best known system and techniques were worked out by Karel and Bertha Bobath (1980). They base their treatment on the observation that there is an overaction of tonic reflex activity, especially during the first years of life, and also later on in the child with dystonic cerebral palsy. Their treatment has as its aim an inhibition of abnormal tone and reflex patterns, and then the facilitating of the more mature postural reflexes. This can best be done in activities of daily living, feeding, playing and moving around. It is very important to give the parents information and give them proper instruction in the 'handling' of their child. Also, the child must be active himself and be able to obtain the sensation of normal tone and movements. Sensory stimuli are used for 'feedback' and to guide the more normal motor activities.

The Bobath method is most often used during the early years of life but can also help the older child, especially in the training of hemiplegic children.

Proprioceptive neuromuscular facilitation (PNF) has also proved to be useful. Diagonal and rotational motor patterns are facilitated through sensory stimuli, such as touch and pressure, muscle contraction against resistance or stretch, traction and compression. Modified, the PNF technique can sometimes be of use in the treatment of cerebral palsy, especially in the ataxic form.

In previous years, an orthopaedic surgeon was often responsible for the overall care of children with cerebral palsy. Today, he is an important member of the team. In spite of adequate physiotherapy, an imbalance of brain control of muscle function often develops, leading to contractures and deformities which have to be corrected in selected children by surgery. This is especially the case in the spastic syndromes. Intensive physiotherapy before and after an operation is essential to give a good result. For some 20% of all spastic children, surgery will become necessary mostly for correction of an equinus foot, adductor spasm, or contractures of the knee or hip. This should be carried out as late in growth as possible. Surgery on the upper limbs is less frequently needed. Splints and braces are nowadays mostly used after operation to prevent relapses and never to correct a contracture, although serial plastering has a place for tight tendo Achillis.

From what has already been said, it is clear that 'treatment' is best integrated with ordinary activities. In younger children, motor skills are trained when the child is playing with toys, building with blocks, playing with sand and water, painting, and so on. All this is a complement to regular physiotherapy. It is important to make use of the normal steps in child development and the child's interest in his own body, in dressing and undressing, and in exploring his surroundings. In doing all this the child has to be guided in ways of getting around difficulties which otherwise would be frustrating. At the same time, he must not be helped with everything he does. He must be shown ways of succeeding in what he wants to do. This can often mean the use of some kind of technical aid which needs teaching to handle (Figs 4.1–4.3). In all this the physiotherapist very often is acting more as a 'consultant' than as the one who is giving therapy.

When the child grows older, more teaching is given by the occupational therapist. She is responsible for teaching activities of daily living (ADL), for adaptation of the child's surroundings—e.g. at home and in the school—and for technical aids. She also takes an active part in vocational planning and training. In this work she will make contact with engineers, teachers and social workers, and she may be the link with the rest of the habilitation team.

Perceptual disorders

It is well known that childen with cerebral palsy have perceptual disorders more frequently than the non-handicapped and that these problems have repercussions for education. The difficulties can be due to brain damage

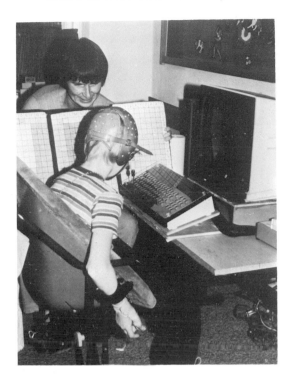

Fig. 4.1. Use of computerized synthetic speech.

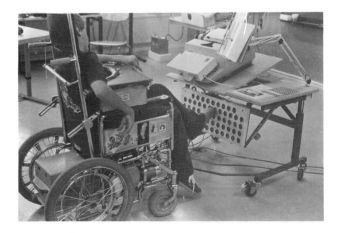

Fig. 4.2. Typing using foot operated keys.

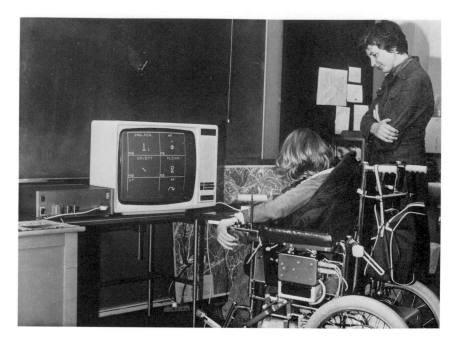

Fig. 4.3. Learning to communicate using Blissymbolics which have been projected on to the television screen with the words above (Swedish).

or to visual, hearing and sensory impairments, or to lack of practice because of the handicap. The cerebral palsied child very often does not obtain the same information or experience from his surroundings as other children. The repetition of motor skills seen in healthy children can be impossible for the handicapped child. He will not learn about distance and depth, or about the strength and force he must use to lift an object or to push a chair across the room. He will not learn to estimate the position and movement of his own body in the room. Even if he learns to crawl and walk, he often does this later than other children. It takes more effort to repeat a movement, and it takes a longer time than normal to obtain the same amount of information as ordinary children.

This lack of information about the world around can, in combination with motor difficulties, cause disorders in all fields of perception. There will be problems with eye–hand co-ordination, and in discerning a figure against the background because he cannot explore the environment, and this will also affect spatial relationships.

It is important to make an early diagnosis of perceptual disorders, and this can be made in different ways. A preliminary assessment of any problems may be obtained by observation. How does the child dress and play? How does the child move and at what rate? What is his ability to concentrate? Special testing procedures can be used, for example Marianne Frostig's test or Jean Ayres Southern California Sensory Integration test.

As a compensation for the lack of early information from the environment, the child with cerebral palsy needs, during the pre-school years, a more systematic and comprehensive teaching programme than the ordinary nursery school usually provides. The staff, who have not had experience with disabled children, must have their attention drawn to the child's special needs and difficulties. They must be given proper information and also continuous support from the team of professionals. The children with more complicated problems often need education in a special school, hopefully for possible integration later on in the normal school. Special education within local schools is another possible approach (Anderson, 1973; Hegarty *et al.*, 1981, 1982).

School age

It is important for the cerebral palsied child to live as much as possible at home and join in ordinary activities. This is also so during the school years. However, very often special arrangements have to be made to ensure this. Potential problems must be diagnosed and planned for long before the start of schooling, and the teacher must be well informed in advance. Although basic teacher training can include a certain amount of instruction concerning disabilities, the knowledge thus acquired is superficial, and it is not surprising that a teacher may feel at a loss when a handicapped child appears in the class. In order to give direct support to the school teacher, it is desirable that a trained teacher is a member of the habilitation team and can act as a consultant. The teacher must have a broad experience of problems connected with both technical aids and teaching methods.

To make it possible for the more severely handicapped child to attend an ordinary class it may be necessary to adjust the school building and the surroundings so that he can move about in a wheelchair. Sometimes the child also needs an assistant to help him in the classroom. It can also be necessary to alter the school working methods or provide special technical aids or adapt material of different kinds, depending on the problems the disorder causes.

Over the years, methods of facilitating schooling have developed and there is today considerable knowledge on how to adapt working materials (for instance the typewriter and computer), how to simplify them for pupils with perceptual disorders and how to select suitable teaching aids. We know the importance of attitudes towards the handicapped child, from the teacher, the other pupils and the parents in helping the handicapped child integrate with the rest of the class.

We also know that for a small group of severely handicapped children with cerebral palsy the medical and/or the educational problems are so considerable that special arrangements have to be taken, for shorter or longer periods, in a special class or school. 'Integration' must always be a dynamic process monitored through the years by the habilitation team.

Vocational planning

It is of course a truism to say that the possibility for the adult with cerebral palsy to obtain employment depends on his education. But it is important to consider this, especially today when handicapped children are more and more integrated into ordinary schools. The population with cerebral palsy is not a big one, especially those who are severely handicapped. Expertise within normal educational and vocational programmes cannot be expected. They must be helped and guided by the professionals in the rehabilitation team. All the time there must be co-operation between medical, educational and social services. Specialized further education is sometimes a desirable option.

Julius Cohen (1976) says:

> For any disabled individual, the total life programme must be geared to bring the person to an optimal level of performance as an adult. This level will be dependent upon the extent of the disability, the handicap which results from the individual's and society's perception of that disability and their reaction to it, and the extent to which the person and society are able and willing to utilize and capitalise on the individual's abilities.

The ideal society does not yet exist, however, and it is still difficult for the severely disabled person to find employment for which he is educated and trained. Factors to be considered include available accommodation, transport and access to services. Lack of these can cause major problems so that the individual will not get the job for which he has been trained.

To try to solve the problems there must be very close co-operation between the rehabilitation team and educational and social sectors. Many of the activities in ADL training and social training are guided from both sides. Vocational guidance starts early and it is important to try to find jobs in which the young boy or girl can first obtain experience and practice and then employment, perhaps after further education. The social situation must be discussed, as well as the potential for independence, possibly with help. Can they get this in the same town in which they are employed? If this is not planned for in a realistic way and at an early stage, much of the work done will come to nothing.

Social and psychosexual needs of handicapped people need to be planned for by education and provision of such facilities as youth clubs, holiday schemes and short-term care arrangements. These are not easily accepted by parents but are essential considerations both for the handicapped person and the family (Anderson & Clarke, 1982).

Chapter 4

APPENDIX

by Ena Davies

Intervention to help the handicapped child with feeding

Feeding problems are often an indication of future handicap. Early intervention is indicated for the baby who may be at risk of speech and language disorders; there is no purpose in delaying therapy until speech is noticeably absent. Much valuable time is lost in waiting. The early mother–child bonding that is strengthened in the closeness of feeding is disrupted by problems created by neurological disorders. The anxiety that the baby does not receive adequate nourishment for survival overrides what should be a pleasurable activity.

The floppy baby who cannot sustain muscle tone for sucking and swallowing may need to be fed by naso-gastric tube—a protracted procedure for mother and infant. There has not been any investigation into the long-term effects of tube feeding on phonological development, although there seems to be an increased risk of middle-ear infection and subsequent deafness. Conversely, the hypertonic baby will extend in spasm, choking as the head is thrown back out of alignment, making each feeding session a misery.

Management of feeding problems is multidisciplinary. The physiotherapist will advise on handling, the speech, occupational therapist or nurse will help facilitate chewing, sucking and swallowing, and the nurse or dietitian may be asked to plan an appropriate diet. The expertise needs to be drawn together by one person to provide an integrated programme that the mother or care-giver can follow, not as separate, and perhaps conflicting, idiosyncratic ideas.

Handling

Confidence in handling the baby is the first prerequisite for the mother learning to cope with the problem of handicap. Finnie's book, *Handling the Young Cerebral Palsied Child at Home* (1974), is an excellent manual for professionals and parents. So, too, is Levitt's eclectic approach to management, *Treatment of Cerebral Palsy and Motor Delay* (1977). Both provide graphic examples of positioning, seating, and development of head, hand and eye control, which are relevant to the acquisition of all other skills.

Feeding

Positioning is of primary importance, not only to facilitate control over chewing, sucking and swallowing (Mueller, 1972; Cordle, 1974; Morris, 1977a, b; Warner, 1981), but also to strengthen the mother–child bonding which occurs naturally in this situation. This bonding may be inhibited by the mother's anxiety (Clezy, 1978). It appears that mothers verbalize very little whilst the baby is actively engaged in feeding, commenting only on the lulls in feeding activity with 'Have you had enough?' or 'What's the matter?' (Snow, 1977). However, Snow (1977) also reports an increase in verbalization when mother and baby are able to maintain eye contact. This is an important factor to bear in mind when considering the most beneficial position for feeding the handicapped child, for whom every opportunity should be exploited.

The aim is to support the child in as near normal a position as possible. By cradling the baby's head in the crook of the mother's arm, the 'all-or-nothing' response of total extension may be controlled. Alternatively, the baby may be fed seated astride the mother's lap, supported by a pillow placed against a wall or table behind him. Whilst freeing the mother's hands to assist the baby's lip closure and swallowing, this has the added advantage of encouraging eye contact.

For the baby who is a poor feeder, unable to maintain the muscle tone to sustain sucking, the opening in the teat may be enlarged, to reduce the level of fatigue.

Introduction of semi-solids and solids into the diet may be delayed because of the mother's concern that the baby may choke. Whilst the baby continues to be fed a liquid diet, the immature patterns will persist. The consistency of the feed can be thickened (gradually) to accustom the baby to the new texture, and spoon feeding may be introduced gradually. The spoon should be placed alternately into one side of the mouth, then to the other, almost into the cheek pouch. Food placed directly on to the tongue will only be sucked up into the roof of the mouth into a soggy mass. Firm pressure is needed to depress the tongue tip, to inhibit the anterior thrusting associated with sucking. Babies and children with neurological disorders often have a pathological 'bite reflex' stimulated by placing utensils (or fingers) in the mouth. This is often painful and difficult to release and may be associated with subluxation of the jaw. It can be released by tilting the head back slightly to reduce the flexor spasm. Because of the extreme discomfort and inherent danger of the bite reflex, it is preferable to try to desensitize the mouth by touch with a finger prior to feeding and to use unbreakable polythene spoons and beakers as a safety measure (suggested suppliers in the United Kingdom:

Mothercare and The Spastics Society).

Lip closure and swallowing may be facilitated by depressing the baby's upper lip and elevating the lower lip by using the index and second finger of the mother's hand. Mature swallowing can be passively assisted by firm pressure upward and backward at the base of the tongue.

In collaboration with the physiotherapist and occupational therapist, a programme of independent feeding can be initiated as soon as the child can cope adequately with the food in his mouth.

Drinking as a progression from sucking can be introduced at about 6 months. Pliable plastic beakers with double handles are recommended for this purpose. The rim of the beaker should be placed well back into the child's mouth, over the tongue tip to depress the anterior thrusting. As the liquid contacts the back of the tongue, automatic swallowing will occur. The handicapped child will be unable to inhibit swallowing to take in air, so the onus of responsibility rests with the person who is giving the drink to monitor the rate of intake. Self-monitoring will take place when the child is able to drink unaided.

Straws are advocated for older infants for drinking, because they encourage lip seal, retraction of the tongue and palatal closure—all beneficial for subsequent articulatory skills. Polythene straws are more appropriate as they do not disintegrate under pressure. The gauge and length of the straw may be altered according to the child's ability to sustain oral pressure to draw liquid into the mouth. Initially, this action may need to be supported by helping the child to maintain lip seal. Colouring the liquid with blackcurrant or orange, according to taste, is a useful incentive, as the child can see the level of the liquid rising in the straw. It is often easier and more discreet for the handicapped youngster to carry a polythene straw than to run the risk of social embarrassment with inappropriate cups or glasses.

Dribbling is a common and distressing symptom of neurological disorders. If feeding programmes are initiated early, then the problem can be minimized. For those children who are unable to co-ordinate the movements for swallowing, various forms of intervention have been tried with varying degrees of success, viz.

1   behaviour modification—accompanied by reward or audible reminder (Jones & Ketteridge, 1981);
2   drug therapy (e.g. Probanthin);
3   training aids
    (a)   palatal prosthesis (Ellis & Flack, 1979; Hardcastle, 1974),
    (b)   lip aids—the Exeter lip sensor (Huskie *et al.*, 1981);
4   surgical resection of the salivary ducts.

References and further reading

Anderson, E.M. (1973) *The Disabled Schoolchild. A Study of Integration in Primary Schools*. Methuen, London.

Anderson, E.M. & Clarke, L. (1982) *Disability in Adolescence*. Methuen, London.

Bleck, E.E. (1979) *Orthopaedic Management of Cerebral Palsy*. (Saunders Monographs in Clinical Orthopaedics No. 2) W.B. Saunders, Philadelphia.

Bobath, K. (1980) A neurophysiological basis for the treatment of cerebral palsy. *Clinics in Developmental Medicine*, **75**, S.I.M.P., Heinemann, London.

Chait, L.A. & Kessler, E. (1979) An anti-drooling operation in cerebral palsy. *South African Medical Journal*, **56**, 676–678.

Christensen, E. & Melchior, J. (1967) Cerebral palsy—a clinical and neuropathological study. *Clinics in Developmental Medicine*, **25**, S.I.M.P., Heinemann, London.

Clezy, G. (1978) Modification of the mother–child interchange. British Journal of Disorders of Communication.

Cohen, J.S. (1976) Vocational guidance and employment. In *Cerebral Palsy* (ed. W.M. Cruickshank). Syracuse University Press, Syracuse.

Cordle, M. (1974) *Feeding can be Fun*. The Spastics Society, London.

Crysdale, W.S. The drooling patient: evaluation and current surgical options. *Laryngoscope*, **90**, 775–783.

Ellis, R.E. & Flack, F.C. (1979) *Palato-Glossal Malfunction*. (Monograph) College of Speech Therapists, London.

Finnie, N. (1974) *Handling the Young Cerebral Palsied Child at Home*, 2nd edn. Heinemann, London.

Freeman, R.D. (1970) Psychiatric problems in adolescents with cerebral palsy. *Developmental Medicine and Child Neurology*, **12**, 64–70.

Fulford, G.E., Cairns, T.P. & Sloane, Y. (1982) Sitting problems of children with cerebral palsy. *Developmental Medicine and Child Neurology*, **24**, 48–53.

Gillberg, Ch. Neuropsychiatric aspects of perceptual, motor and attentional deficits in seven year old Swedish children. *Abstracts of Uppsala Dissertations from the Faculty of Medicine*.

Hagberg, B., Hagberg, G. & Olow, I. (1977) The panorama of cerebral palsy in Swedish children born 1954–1974. *Neuropadiatrie*, **8**, Suppl., 516–521.

Hagberg, B., Hagberg, G. & Olow, I. (1982) Gains and hazards of intensive neonatal care: an analysis from Swedish cerebral palsy epidemiology. *Developmental Medicine and Child Neurology*, **24**, 13–19.

Hagerty, S., Pocklington, K. & Lucas, D. (1982) *Educating Pupils with Special Needs in the Ordinary School*. NFER–Nelson Publishing, Windsor.

Hardcastle, W.J. (1974) Instrumental investigations of lingual activity during speech. *Phonetica*, **29**, 129–157.

Harris, M.M. & Dignam, P.F. (1980) A non-surgical method of reducing drooling in cerebral palsied children. *Developmental Medicine and Child Neurology*, **22**, 293–299.

Holt, K.S. (1977) *Developmental Paediatrics*. (Postgraduate Paediatrics Series) Butterworths, London.

Huskie, C.F., Ellis, R.E., Flack, F.C., Selley, W.G. & Curle, H.J. (1981) Clinical application of the Exeter Lip Sensor. *Bulletin of the College Speech Therapists*, **329**, 10–12.

Ingram, T.T.S. (1964) *Paediatric Aspects of Cerebral Palsy*. Livingstone, Edinburgh.

Ingram, T.T.S. (1982) *Integration in Action. Case Studies in the Integration of Pupils with Special Needs*. NFER–Nelson Publishing Windsor.

Jones, M. & Ketteridge, K. (1981) The design of behaviour modification aids for severely disturbed children. *Distech 81*, The Spastics Society, London.

Kalverboer, A.F. (1975) *A Neurobehavioural Study in Pre-School Children.* Heinemann, London.

Krusen, F., Kottke, F. & Ellwood, P. (1965) *Handbook of Physical Medicine and Rehabilitation.* W.B. Saunders, Philadelphia.

Lagergren, J. (1981) Children with motor handicaps. Epidemiological, medical and socio-paediatric aspects of motor handicapped children in a Swedish county. *Acta Paediatrica Scandinavica*, Suppl. 289.

Levitt, S. (1977) *Treatment of Cerebral Palsy and Motor Delay.* Blackwell Scientific, Oxford.

Levitt, S., ed. (1984) *Paediatric Development Therapy.* Blackwell Scientific, Oxford.

Levitt, S. & Miller, C. (1973) The inter-relationship of speech therapy and physiotherapy in children with neurodevelopmental disorders. *Developmental Medicine and Child Neurology*, **15**, 188–193.

Mathews, D., Kruse, R. & Shaw, V. (1962) *The Science of Physical Education for Handicapped Children.* Harper & Brothers Publ, New York.

Morris, S.E. (1977a) Body language at mealtimes. In *Mealtimes for Severely and Profoundly Handicapped Persons: New Concepts and Attitudes* (ed. Perske). University Park Press, Baltimore.

Morris, S.E. (1977b) *Program Guidelines for Children with Feeding Problems.* Childcraft Education Corp., New Jersey.

Mueller, H.A. (1972) Facilitating feeding and pre-speech. In *Physical Therapy Services in the Developmental Disabilities* (eds P.H. Pearson and C.E. Williams). Charles C. Thomas, Springfield.

Nelson, K.B. & Ellenberg, J.H. (1982) Children who outgrew cerebral palsy. *Paediatrics*, **69**, 529–536.

Newman, J. (1976) *Swimming for Children with Physical and Sensory Impairments. Methods and Techniques for Therapy and Recreation.* Charles C. Thomas, Springfield.

Nielsen, H.H. (1966) *A Psychological Study of Cerebral Palsied Children.* Munksgaard, Copenhagen.

Rang, M., Douglas, G., Bennett, G.C. Koreska, J. (1981) Seating for children with cerebral palsy. *Journal of Pediatric Orthopedics*, **1**, 279–287.

Rapp, D.L. (1979) Meldreth dribble-control project. *Child: Care, Health and Development*, **5**, 143–149.

Scherzer, A.L. & Ischarnuter, I. (1982) *Early Diagnosis and Therapy in Cerebral Palsy: a Primer on Infant Developmental Problems.* Marcel Decker, New York.

Scrutton, D., ed. (1984) Management of the motor disorders of children with cerebral palsy. *Clinics in Developmental Medicine*, **90**, S.I.M.P., Heinemann, London.

Silverman, F. (1980) *Communication for the Speechless.* Prentice Hall, New Jersey.

Smith, V. & Keen, J., eds (1979) *Visual Handicap in Children.* Heinemann, London.

Snow, C.E. (1977) The development of conversation between mothers and babies. *Journal of Child Language*, **4**, 1–22.

Thompson, G.H., Rubin, I.L. & Bilenker, R.M. (1983) *Comprehensive Management of Cerebral Palsy.* Grune and Stratton, New York.

Thomson, R.J. & Quinn, A.N. (1979) *Developmental Disabilities. Etiologies, Manifestations, Diagnoses and Treatments.* Oxford University Press, Oxford.

Vanderheiden, G.C. (1978) *Non Vocal Communication. Resource Book.* University Park Press, Baltimore.

Warner, J. (1981) *Helping the Handicapped Child with Early Feeding*. Photographic Teaching Materials. Winslow, Buckingham.

Wing, E. & Roussounis, H. (1983) A changing pattern of cerebral palsy and its implications for the early detection of motor disorders in childhood. *Child: Care, Health and Development*, **9**, 227–232.

Chapter 5
The Management of Children with Spina Bifida and Associated Hydrocephalus

Robert Minns

Neonatal assessment

Usually, the infant with spina bifida is transferred within hours of birth to a regional centre where comprehensive assessment can be carried out as soon as possible.

The parents should be allowed to see and nurse the child immediately after delivery, and they should be told sympathetically by a paediatrician that the child has a spina bifida and that further details of the severity of this will be communicated to them after a full assessment has been done. The lesion should be covered with sterile gauze moistened in normal saline, and held in place lightly by means of an elastic bandage (Netelast). The baby is then placed in a portable incubator in the prone position and sent, along with details of the birth history, with the father, to the paediatric ward which will have been notified of the impending admission. In rare circumstances when neither parent can accompany the baby, the surgical possibilities are discussed and signed parental consent is obtained for procedures which they understand and accept. A comprehensive assessment is necessary, because sometimes the worst-looking lesions may have minimal neurological involvement and therefore a better prognosis than smaller lesions.

History

(Birth history and family history.) Firstly, details are obtained about maternal health, contraception, and previous pregnancies. The history of the recent pregnancy is searched for any illness, drugs, irradiation, cigarettes and alcohol, or rashes. The gestation is noted, and place of delivery, duration of the labour, and whether or not the membranes were ruptured, as well as the presentation and mode of delivery. Birth weight, the child's condition at birth and whether resuscitation was required are recorded. An expanded family tree should be attempted at this point. This may be added to at a later date when the parents have consulted older members of the family. The ethnic background, social conditions and place of residence should all be noted.

82

Delivery of one-fifth of spina bifida infants is accompanied by malpresentation. Approximately 10% require forceps to aid delivery, and a further 10% require caesarian section (Stark & Drummond, 1970). A difficult delivery may result in additional injury as a result of disproportion between the baby's large head from hydrocephalus and the maternal pelvis. Extreme increases in intracranial pressure may then occur during delivery.

Pathological effects of a traumatic birth may cause further intracranial or extracranial injury such as fractures or brachial plexus palsies. Injury may also be sustained to the myelomeningocoele sac and either rupture a cystic lesion with the additional likelihood of infection, or compress the plaque. Colonization of the lesion with staphylococci or coliforms is likely during delivery if the sac is ruptured, with consequent ascending meningitis and ventriculitis.

Examination

The examination should be conducted when the infant is warm (over 35°C). The child may have become cold during transfer and consequently have sluggish movements. Gamgee or silver foil in a heated incubator will prevent or remedy the situation quickly. The infant should not be fed until the assessment is concluded. During the examination there is again a risk of chilling. Although one wants a complete assessment, it has to be done whilst avoiding direct pressure on the back lesion either from the cot or the examiner's hand. The examination should therefore be conducted with the child lying on its side or with the infant's back supported away from the lesion.

The general condition is noted, as well as the colour, respirations, cry, temperature and level of activity. The respiratory and cardiovascular systems, abdomen, the number of vessels in the cord, the genitalia, and facies are examined, and any other genetic stigmata, or associated malformations are looked for.

Lesions

Firstly, the anatomical level is noted, and the size of the lesion is measured. Its condition is recorded: whether it is an 'open' or 'closed' lesion, whether it is leaking cerebrospinal fluid (CSF) or not, and the size of the neural plate. The open myelomeningocoele (myelocoele, rachischisis) has exposed cord, and the neurological lesion is a cord lesion. The spinal cord is elevated onto the roof of the sac as a flat neural plate and the central

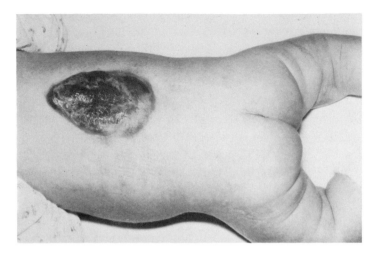

Fig. 5.1. Open myelomeningocoele.

canal is seen opening onto it at the upper end of the lesion, and may or may not be dripping CSF. The splayed-out central canal may be seen lengthways, or alternatively if there has been a longitudinal hemisection of the cord at a higher level, one-half of the central canal will be seen flattened on either side of the lesion (Fig. 5.1). The roots of the cauda equina are often seen at the lower end of the lesion through the membrane which is fused pia and arachnoid and surrounds the plate. The membrane may be thick or thin. The adjoining skin may be haemangiomatous and discoloured and joins the dura. Most of the open myelomeningocoeles are large, as much as 10 cm in diameter, while the closed myelomeningocoeles tend to be somewhat smaller and avoid the thoracolumbar junction where 60% of the open ones are found. Large cervical lesions which are open myelomeningocoeles are probably incompatible with life for more than a short period because there is early paralysis of respiratory musculature.

A closed myelomeningocoele is covered by a combination of skin and membrane, and the neural tube is closed. When they occur in the thoracic region, they are described as syringomyelocoeles if there is cystic dilatation of the central canal. The posterior cord which protrudes through the bony defect is covered by the meningeal sac and gives rise to a pedunculated lesion.

The upper end of both the open and closed lesion tends to coincide with the vertebral lesion on X-ray, but the vertebral lesion is often more extensive distally than the sac.

Meningocoeles have the spinal cord in a normal position and there is no disruption of the neural elements (Fig. 5.2). The sac contains only CSF and is mostly covered by thick membrane, or altered skin. Occasionally it is covered by normal skin. There may be pigmentation or haemangiomatous skin in the area. Like the closed lesions, meningocoeles tend to avoid the thoracolumbar junction. To be sure that it is a meningocoele there should not be any neurological deficit found in the lower limbs and at surgery no neural elements are identified. Meningocoeles are associated with hydrocephalus, but less so than myelomeningocoeles.

Rarely, there are multiple spina bifida lesions. Not infrequently a high level lesion is associated with a spina bifida oculta. Exceptionally, an anterior encephalocoele may co-exist with two spinal lesions. In about half the infants with myelomeningocele there is evidence of duplication of the cord (diplomyelia) and this may give the appearance of two separate lesions. They occur caudally in particular, and are enclosed within a single dural tube. Other pathological variants which are known to occur with myelomeningocoele include hydromyelia (dilatation of the central canal), syringomyelia, or diastematomyelia (where the two halves of the cord are separated by a fibrous band or cartilage or bony spur arising from a vertebral body). Hemimyelomeningocoeles have only half of the cord involved at the plaque level, and lipomas of the filum, dura, or leptomeninges are not uncommon (Emery & Lendon, 1973). Open myelomeningocoele lesions are usually flat at birth and gradually become elevated because of accumulation of the CSF within the lesion.

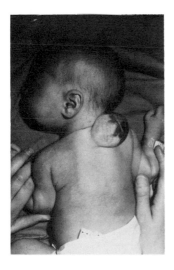

Fig. 5.2. Dorsal meningocoele.

Cranial nerves and upper limbs

The cranial nerves are examined in the usual way, particularly looking at eye movements, facial movements, tongue, palatal and other brain stem functions. The upper limbs' muscle power (and movements), tone (and posture), reflexes and sensation should all be normal unless the myelomeningocoele is in the cervical region, in which case asymmetries and dwarfing will be evident.

Cranium

The head circumference is measured, remembering that the occipito-frontal circumference (OFC) may be normal despite considerable ventricular dilatation. Usually a head circumference above the 90th centile is consistent with a cortical mantle of less than 25 mm (Lorber, 1971). Signs of intracranial pressure are looked for, including sutural separation, and in particular the lambdoidal sutures are palpated as they separate early with raised intracranial pressure. The state of the anterior and posterior fontanelle, their size, tension, and pulsatility, are noted (remembering that one can have a hydrocephalic microcephalic infant).

Lower limbs: motor testing

If the child is active, then a lot of information can be obtained by merely watching the child's spontaneous movements which occur against gravity or in a horizontal plane. One also needs to isolate the individual muscle groups in the lower limbs and trunk by stimulating the child on the face, or chest, and then observing individual movements. By adding resistance, one obtains a clinical estimation of muscle power according to the MRC gradings (MRC 0 is no muscle power, MRC 1 is evidence of muscle contraction with no joint movement, MRC 2 is active movement with gravity eliminated, MRC 3 is active movement against gravity, MRC 4 is active movement against gravity and added resistance, and MRC 5 is normal muscle power). It is important to remember not to stimulate the lower limbs in assessing voluntary muscle power, as subsequent movements may simply reflect 'isolated cord' activity. The baby will need to be positioned in different ways to observe these different muscle groups. Fingertip pressure is the only additional resistance that is generally needed, and Stark & Drummond (1972) have shown that this correlates well with EMG assessments. Such an assessment of the muscle power in the lower limbs may require some time, patience and experience of this sort of examination in the new-born. It also requires a thorough knowledge of the myotome levels (Table 5.1). It should also be appreciated that in the early neonatal period the levels of paralysis may change quickly, and what is present immediately after birth may be different by one or two neural segments, after 24 hours. Certainly, the pre-natal effects of traction on a cord which is anchored by the spina bifida lesion, or by the shearing forces during delivery, may influence the neurological level. Also, post-natally, if the lesion is allowed to become desiccated or infected, there will be further loss of neurological function.

The neurological motor level referred to is the last normally functioning neurosegmental level. This may be difficult to define if there is a sloping lesion, that is, a progressive fall off in muscle power from MRC 5 to MRC 1 over several consecutive segments of the cord. The motor levels and function of the lower limbs are usually different from adult paraplegics who usually have a transected cord. The patterns of paralysis have been outlined by Stark as of two basic types.

Type I lesions. There is total loss of cord function below a certain level, that is, there is lower motor neurone paralysis, absent sensation and loss of reflexes. These constitute about 30% of all myelomeningocoeles. Such a pattern may be consequent on a total rachischisis lesion with obliteration of all active elements in the cord below a certain level, or it may be consequent on ischaemic infarction of the lower part of the cord below the lesion, secondary to pressure effects.

There are three varieties of the **type II lesion**. In type IIA lesions a section of the cord is obliterated by the myelomeningocoele, so that the affected roots corresponding to this section of the cord will be associated with lower motor neurone signs. Segments below this will show reflex activity and, because of preservation of the spinal reticular formation, will show features of the isolated cord. Isolated cord features include:

1 spontaneous spinal myoclonus (spinal epilepsy)
2 dermatome to myotome responses
3 crossed adductor responses
4 brisk flexor withdrawal with oscillation
5 spastic individual muscles
6 loss of reciprocal inhibition
7 reflexes present in the toes, hamstrings, and tibialus anterior
8 no extensor activity
9 flexor pattern of tone if there is a long segment
10 ankle reflex preserved
11 spastic pelvic floor and bladder neck

Table 5.1.

Muscle power	MRC			
	R	L	R	L
T8−10 upper abdo				
11−12 lower abdo				
12 Psoas				
3/4 Adductors				
3/4 Quadriceps				
4 Tib. ant.				
L−S 5/1 Hamstr. med.				
5/1 Abductors				
5/1 Long Ext.				
5/1 Peronei				
S 1/2 Calf				
1/2 Hamstr. lat.				
1/2 Glut. max.				
1/2 F.H.L.				
1/2 F.D.L.				
2/3 Intrinsics				
Reflexes				
Abdo.				
Cremasteric				
K.J.				
A.J.				
L.H.				
Anal				
Crossed ext.				
Flexion				
Motor level				
Vol.				
Isol. cord				
Sensory level				
Central				
Isol. cord				

12   deformity due to unopposed muscles and spastic muscles

13   wide afferent field and crossed flexor responses

The neurosegmental level and the corresponding deformity with either a type I or type II lesion is seen in Table 5.2.

Type IIB lesions are virtually transections of the cord and in these there is a very long 'isolated cord' segment with much evidence of reflex activity on stimulation. Type IIC lesions are those where some of the long corticospinal tracts pass through the spina bifida lesion undisturbed, and some are involved in the dysplastic process. Assessment of the lower

Table 5.2. The neurosegmental level and corresponding deformity in type I or type II lesions

Neurological level	Deformity	Orthotic requirement
T8–T12	Bulging (paradoxical with respiration) abdomen. (Type I lower limbs straight, undeformed.) Hip flexed/abducted—externally rotated. scoliosis, kyphosis, lordosis.	Wheelchair mostly. Thoracic extension on above knee calipers. Tripod crutches, 'walker' (up to 3 yrs) standing frame (up to 12 months).
T12–L1	Kyphosis, flexion of hip.	Wheelchair mostly. Above knee calipers and pelvic band.
L1–2	Hips flexed, adducted, dislocated.	Wheelchair predominantly (to L3). Above knee calipers and pelvic band.
(L3) L4	Flexed hips (dislocated), extended knees (recurvatum), bilateral talipes—calcaneo-varus or equino varus.	Below knee calipers ± aid.
L5	Toes extended. Calcaneus, calcaneo-valgus, flexion knee.	Below knee calipers (to S1) ± aid.
S2	Rocker-bottom foot (valgus) with vertical talus.	No appliance.
S3	'Flat bottomed' patulous anus, cavus feet, claw toes.	No appliance.

limbs is the only way to determine which are involved and which are not. A further possible sub-group includes those with an incomplete conus lesion.

About 5% of lesions are hemimyelomeningocoeles, where one leg is involved and the other is normal. This is convenient from the point of view of the bladder, because, with the bilateral innervation of the bladder, half of the cord can be involved yet normal function may persist. However, there is often a spinal deformity (kyphoscoliosis) associated with these lesions.

Mechanism of deformity. Deformity occurs in two ways. Firstly, muscle imbalance may occur across joints. There may be normal functioning of motor activity in one group of muscles but the antagonists are flaccid. There may be spastic muscles as agonists and normal functioning or flaccid antagonists, for example, at the hip joint if innervation is normal, or if there is total paresis of flexors and extensors there will be no deformity or dislocation.

If imbalance occurs between the upper and lower innervation of the muscles about the hip joint—for example, flexors and adductors (L1 to 3) acting normally, and gluteal extensors and abductors (L5 to S2) paralysed—there will be a resultant dislocation. Therefore L4 lesions show invariably dislocated hips at birth, and L2 or L5 lesions dislocate later from increasing contractures. Similarly, at the knee joint, deformity may occur because of imbalance between extension L3/4 (quadriceps) and flexion L5/S1. If there are strong extensors, but flaccid paralysis of the flexors there will be a tendency for recurvatum and 'knee-back' to occur with dislocation of the knee. Likewise, at the ankle joint, active L4 muscles and paralysis of L5 muscles will cause a talipes deformity. The presence of talipes with a type I lesion is understandable, but not infrequently talipes occurs with a high level paraplegia and the mechanics of this may be either because (i) at some time in intra-uterine life the neurological motor level may have been L4, and then with the relative movement of the cord proximally with respect to the vertebrae, particularly in the last trimester, there may have been severing of the nerve roots so that at birth a high level paraplegia is evident with talipes positioning; or (ii) there may have always been a high-level paraplegia from early intra-uterine life, with the talipes position being a result of intra-uterine positional deformity. Figures 5.3 and 5.4, for example, show hips flexed, knees extended, and feet approximating the side of the face, in a child with T10 paraplegia and breech delivery with, finally, a positional talipes equino-varus.

The second mechanism of deformity is one of position. This positional deformity may occur antenatally as described above, or may occur postnatally (e.g. equinus) as a result of the infant lying supine with weakness in the dorsiflexors of the ankle joint enhancing this deformity. Similarly, with weight bearing on paralysed feet, there is a tendency to produce valgus at the subtalar joint, that is, 'position' overrides the neurological picture.

The paralysed lower limbs with absent psoas will tend to fall into a pithed frog position with secondary positional external rotation deformity, making the fitting of AK callipers difficult later.

Deformity, therefore, may result from imbalance of muscle actions with or without secondary positional deformity superimposed. Not only that, but the antenatal positional deformity may be totally different from

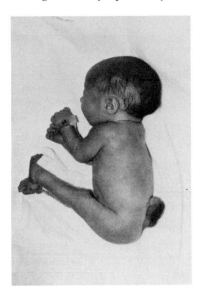

Fig. 5.3. Secondary (intra uterine) positional deformity in child with high level paraplegia.

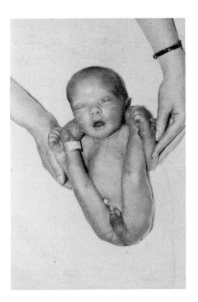

Fig. 5.4. Same child as in Fig. 5.3. Breech intrauterine position simulated.

the positional deformity that occurs postnatally in the same patient.
After one has determined the voluntary motor level and, if present, the
isolated cord level, fixed deformities are noted and measured in the usual
way (that is, by joint angles or linear measurements of limitation) and are
photographed for recording purposes. This motor level and the assessment of motor function is charted for both the right and the left lower
limbs.

Lower limbs: sensory testing

Sensory testing is next done (some people prefer to do this first) and
again it is best done when the child is awake. As with motor levels, the
lowest normal sensory segment is determined, and testing is done in the
conventional way by means of a sterile needle and a knowledge of the
dermatomes of the lower limbs. With practice, this can be done quite
accurately by proceeding down the front of the abdomen and lower limbs,
over the dorsum of the feet to the plantar surfaces, and then with the
child in the prone position, proceeding up the posterior aspect of the
lower limbs to the buttocks and anal area. The child is watched for
evidence of sensation: crying, grimacing, etc. The sensory dermatomes
are charted, in the same way as motor function, and may show evidence of
isolated cord activity. The sensory level is in most infants similar to the
motor level by one or two segments.

Investigations
These include bacteriological swabs on the lesion, the umbilicus, nose and
throat; and X-rays of the skull, spine and hips. X-ray of the skull may
show lacunar anomaly, which is very common and is associated with a
thin skull. These are apparent circular areas, in which the calcification is
defective. It does not result from raised intracranial pressure *in utero*, nor
is it a result of compression by the gyri and sulci on the inner table. It
disappears at about 6 weeks or so and is usually associated with myelomeningocoeles. X-ray of the hips may confirm any dislocation. X-ray
of the spine is undertaken after special radio-opaque skin pencils have
marked out the lesion, or sterile wires (pipe cleaners) are placed about
the lesion. This gives an indication of the extent of the lesion in relation
to the extent of the vertebral defect, and the degree of separation of the
spinous processes in the antero-posterior X-ray. The absence of anterior
notching of the vertebral bodies is seen in the lateral film which indicates
the site of the lesion. In addition to this, the spine X-ray may show
diastomatomyelic bony spurs, often with narrow disc spaces, malformed

vertebrae including hemi-vertebrae, wedged vertebrae, fused and malformed laminae, widening of the spinal canal, and abnormal curvatures
such as kyphosis, scoliosis or lordosis.

About half the infants with myelomeningocoele will have either
kyphoscoliosis or lordosis. Those with kyphosis tend to have extensive
rachischisis lesions, underlying major vertebral abnormalities, and do not
survive. A bowstring deformity develops as a result of lost erector spinae
function where there are active diaphragm and psoas muscles (Drennan,
1970). When scoliosis is present at birth it is consequent on anomalous
vertebral features such as hemi-vertebrae, which may fuse with adjacent
transverse processes of the ribs. Higher level scoliotics tend to also have
some kyphosis, and lower level scoliotics have some additional lordosis,
although it is seldom present at birth. The result of spinal curves is a tilt
of the pelvis, deformity of the chest and shortening of trunk.

Clinical photographs are taken of the back lesion, and of the lower
limbs, for filing in the child's case notes. An ultrasound of the head is
done using 'real time' ultrasound as most spina bifida children will have
some degree of ventricular dilatation present at birth. The ultrasound can
be introduced through the anterior fontanelle or through the posterior
fontanelle.

At present, we scan the whole spine and any 'closed' lesion with
ultrasound. CT scanning of the spine is also sometimes undertaken.
Where a closed myelomeningocoele, or meningocoele is present, ultrasound may prove useful in identifying the contents of the sac prior to
surgery.

Most of the defects in children with spina bifida are a consequence of
the back lesion itself, but there are occasionally associated abnormalities.
Mongoloid features often necessitate chromosomal analysis but usually
prove normal unless there is the rarely encountered 18 trisomy syndrome
(Passage *et al.*, 1966). A mongoloid slant to the eyes and other facial
features become more normal over the succeeding weeks. There are
sometimes other related odd facial appearances, single palmar creases,
imperforate anus, congenital heart defects, such as patent ductus arterio-
sis, or transposition with VSD, Klippel-Feil anomalies or genito-urinary
abnormalities such as hypospadias, or undescended testes. Horseshoe
kidneys and pelvic or cystic kidneys also occur.

Management decision

A selective policy operates in Edinburgh, and while the decision to treat
actively is an individual one for each patient, certain features are gener-

ally accepted as being associated with a bad prognosis in terms of intellectual and physical handicap. These features are:
1   a motor level at L2 or above;
2   spinal abnormalities such as curvatures, and absent, wedged, fused
or hemi-vertebrae;
3   gross hydrocephalus at birth.
If there are associated problems such as prematurity or severe respiratory
problems which preclude general anaesthesia, cyanotic congenital heart
disease, severe birth asphyxia, or intestinal atresia, such deficits are a
further contra-indication to intervention. On the other hand, parental
wishes may override the above.

Though the above criteria are not rigid, it is usually accepted in our
practice that any of the three major adverse factors mitigate against active
intervention. It is accepted that this is based as far as possible on existing
follow-up studies which have pointed to such features as being bad prognostic indicators. The recommendation to 'select out' is a medical one
and analagous to most other situations in medicine where indications for
or against operation are based rationally on statistical probability from
follow-up series.

After this full assessment a management decision is made. There
follows a most important communication in the interview with the child's
parents and, if possible, grandparents.

Firstly, the nature of the condition is explained. Secondly, an outline
of how this has arisen is given, in particular stressing that nothing the
parents could have done or failed to do would have influenced the child's
condition. Next, the consequences of the spina bifida lesion are spelt out
as they have been found in the child. At the same time, it is explained that
there is a single fundamental defect which is responsible for the multisystem disorder and there are not numerous congenital abnormalities.
One explains the prognosis relative to the child's examination, and
follows up with an explanation that all such children can be actively
treated. The medical opinion may be that in this particular child one
would be prolonging extreme suffering and treatment should not be
further pursued. It is also stressed to the parent that closure is not a
curative operation anyway and that, while failure to close the back may
result in ascending meningitis, one cannot guarantee optimum results in
any child 'selected in'.

It is essential to involve the parents in the decision-making process,
without asking them to make a decision for or against operation themselves. It is probably better put to them that they either agree or disagree

with the medical recommendation. If the recommendation is for 'selection out' then it is stressed that the child is allowed to die in peace naturally without pain or discomfort, and that there is no question of euthanasia, either actively or passively.

Management of infants not for active treatment

These infants are nursed in the paediatric ward, with full nursing care in the form of dressing changes to the spina bifida lesion, nursed in an isolette or incubator, and kept warm. The baby is dressed as a normal neonate and routine observations are kept. The child is fed on demand with a full strength formula, and the parents and close relatives visit as desired. The ward sister and the nursing staff are encouraged to maintain a close contact with the family. If there is obvious distress from pain associated with the back lesion (the exposed neural tissue if often exquisitely tender and in addition cerebral irritability may be present), analgesia or sedation is used when necessary in strict pharmacological doses. Support for the parents is organized by the medical social worker to the unit, and the family doctor is informed. Depending on the parents' wishes, the hospital chaplain or their own priest or minister will be contacted and advised. Should hydrocephalus develop rapidly with obvious head enlargement, distention of the fontanelle or scalp veins, ventricular puncture may be necessary to relieve the raised intracranial pressure.

With such a policy some infants will undoubtedly survive and their spina bifida lesion will epithelialize. It is important, therefore, to ensure that the child does not survive with more handicap than he would have had, had he been treated from birth. When, according to the clinical signs and symptoms of raised pressure and the ultrasound assessment, CSF shunting is needed, a CSF shunt is inserted and treatment should continue in full thereafter. There is no place for second class treatment once the original decision not to treat actively has been reversed. It is our experience that by this time (about 6 weeks) the parents as well have recognized the 'fighting spirit' of their infant and are happy for this change of policy. Such a policy will often be fraught with additional complications, such as infection of the back lesion itself which may supervene in the interim. *Staph. pyogenes* may form loculated pus at the membrane–skin junction and this will not only prejudice the remaining viable cord segments, but any shunt which is inserted to control hydrocephalus.

Operative closure of the spina bifida lesion

It is our practice to close the spina bifida lesions within the first 24 hours
of life if possible. If the lesion is a 'closed' one, while there is no urgency,
there is no advantage in delaying closure more than a few days. Heimburger (1972) has showed that closure after 48 hours was associated with
a greater mortality and morbidity, but in a recent report (Charney *et al.*,
1983) it is suggested that neurological function is not prejudiced by delayed or late closure up to 10 months later. They also maintain that more
accurate assessment of the lower limbs, as described above, can be
performed. In the new-born period it is possible for an examiner with
experience in assessing dermatome and myotome function in the lower
limbs to make an accurate assessment of new-borns. It is also of practical
neurosurgical importance that lesions left for several weeks are considerably harder to close accurately because the tissue planes sclerose and are
harder to identify.

The technique has been described by Smith (1965) and Zachary &
Sharrard (1967). First of all, an elliptical incision is made around the sac,
the skin is mobilized into the flanks by blunt dissection and the neural
plate separated from the surrounding skin and membranes. The spinal
canal is explored for lesions which can compress the cord, and the membrane is excised completely, leaving no part of the covering membranes
which might later develop dermoids. The open dura is identified and
mobilized, and neural tissue is replaced in the spinal canal. The dura is
usually closed. If the defect is large, it is left open, no muscle flaps are
fashioned and the skin is secured. Obtaining skin closure without undue
tension for large lesions may involve the plastic surgeon. The buttock skin
is not used because of its anaesthetic nature and closure may be done by
means of relaxing incisions or rotating skin flaps, or by fracturing the
laminae to bring the skin over without subsequent necrosis. Drainage of
the wound is not necessary and no antibiotic cover is usually given.

Post-operatively, the child is nursed in an incubator, prone or side-
lying. It is better that the lesion is protected by a dressing. This dressing
usually takes the form of a non-adherent (e.g. Melolin) layer, covered by
hypa-fix, a porous adhesive dressing that has some mobility. At about 2
to 3 days post-operatively, the wound is inspected, and then inspected
every other day until the sutures are removed. The same dressing is kept
in place and sutures removed between 7 and 10 days post-operatively,
depending on whether there is any tension in the suture line.

Urinary retention may be a problem. If it is, an indwelling catheter
will be necessary. On occasion, infants are born with grossly hydrone-

phrotic kidneys from the effects of their neuropathic bladder *in utero*. An indwelling catheter has resolved this renal distention within 2–3 weeks. On other occasions, the retrograde pressure effects from the neuropathic bladder on the compound papillae of the newborn result in renal tubular damage with the passage of large volumes of dilute urine.

Complications of the back closure can be expected where the operative closure itself was difficult and required grafting, or where there was severe tearing of the sac pre-operatively. Wound breakdown, because of tension within the sutures or necrosis at the edges, may necessitate grafting. If, prior to the operation, significant hydrocephalus with raised pressure is communicated freely to the back lesion, undue tension will be transmitted to the wound; certainly if there is a post-operative leak of CSF, this will delay healing considerably, and an early shunt or ventriculostomy reservoir will be required to reduce the CSF pressure.

Infection of the wound with *Staph. aureus*, or coliforms, will necessitate treatment with gentamycin and cloxacillin, at 5 mg/kg/day and 50 mg/kg/day respectively, unless otherwise dictated by bacteriological sensitivities. Careful monitoring of the CSF by means of cisternal or ventricular puncture may be necessary in any symptomatic child.

Hydrocephalus

More than 95% of spina bifida children will have hydrocephalus to some degree, and about 30% of these will undergo an early spontaneous arrest of their ventricular dilatation and not have a further problem. The cause for the hydrocephalus is the Type II Arnold–Chiari malformation. The pathological features of this have been well described by Variend & Emery (1973, 1974). They consist of herniation of the brain stem and vermis through the foramen magnum so that the fourth ventricle opens into the cervical spinal cord. The cerebellum itself is small and deformed, and there is pressure on the mid-brain, causing it to distort with buckling or kinking of the aqueduct. While in-depth descriptions of the course of the vessels, cranial nerves, etc. have been described in this condition, in summary the pathological findings are indistinguishable from an intra-uterine encephalopathy where brain swelling has resulted in a downward movement of the hind-brain through the foramen magnum. Therefore, one can expect, and does see, isolated Arnold–Chiari malformations at post-mortem without associated spina bifida lesions. Instead of the distorting pressure coming from above, in spina bifida lesions, the effect is possibly from a downward traction of the brain stem because of the fixed cord in conjunction with the myelomeningocoele (Penfield & Coburn, 1938). An alternative postulate by Barry *et al.* (1957) ascribes the coning from an overgrowth of neural tissue (encephalocranial disproportion).

The Arnold—Chiari malformation may result in hydrocephalus by obstructing CSF flow, or by interfering with venous drainage in the posterior fossa. It may also compress the upper cervical spinal cord, with progressive quadriparesis. Neurosurgical operations are sometimes successful in reversing this deterioration by releasing posterior dural bands and dividing multiple adhesions over the dorsal surface of the cervical cord. If obstruction to the CSF flow occurs at the foramen magnum, there is communicating hydrocephalus between the spinal and ventricular CSF, but no absorption at the arachnoid villi because of the absence of CSF flow over the brain surface. Communicating hydrocephalus occurs in one-third of infants with myelomeningocoeles (Milhorat, 1972).

If obstruction occurs at the aqueduct of Sylvius, then 'internal hydrocephalus' results in the lateral and third ventricles. If the obstruction occurs at the outlet of the fourth ventricle from closely adherent tonsils, then a symmetrical four ventricle hydrocephalus will result.

As the posterior fossa is rich in venous sinuses and large veins, Andeweg (1976) postulates that the Arnold—Chiari malformation may encroach on the diameter of these large venous chambers, disproportionately increasing the pressure on the arterial side of the circuit and enhancing arterial blood flow at all points, including the choroidal arterioles with enhanced CSF production.

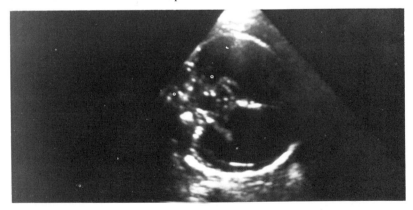

Fig. 5.5. Ultrasound in late pregnancy showing dilated ventricles with a thin rim of residual brain tissue, and pulsating choroid plexus in real time.

Although hydrocephalus is usually present at birth, there may not be a significant increase in the OFC. Hydrocephalus at birth in myelomeningocoele has varied from 50% to 90% in published series because of the previous difficulty in diagnosing hydrocephalus without invasive techniques. However, with ultrasound scanning, well over 95% will be shown to have some degree of hydrocephalus.

After the lesion closure on the back there is usually a rapid progression in the head circumference and in ventricular dilatation. This takes the form of a step-wise increase in the OFC, representing phases of compensation and decompensation, as the increased CSF volume and pressure interact with alternative CSF pathways of absorption. The usual sequence of events in the development of this hydrocephalus associated with myelomeningocoele, or any other hydrocephalus, is initially small or normal-sized ventricles with high pressure, then, following Laplaces' formula, as the radius of any sphere increases the pressure will relatively decrease within the sphere. Therefore, the second phase is one of ventricular enlargement with still high pressure, and then one of grossly enlarged ventricles with the pressure now dropping. In between these last two stages there are probably phases of intermittent pressure.

Two-thirds of CSF is produced by the choroid plexus; the other third is a result of 'brain lymph' and descends from the extra-cellular spaces of the brain through the ependymal pores into the ventricle. Thus, under situations of raised ventricular pressure, it is postulated that CSF can be made to reverse this direction in the hope of finding alternative CSF absorptive sites. Another effect of the raised ventricular pressure is to recanalize narrowed parts of the Aqueduct of Sylvius, or those areas where membranous obstructions to flow exist. The hydrocephalus increases rapidly after the closure of the back lesion for a number of possible reasons. First of all, any possible leak from an open lesion is now precluded, and similarly, for those communicating types, there is now no chance of increasing the distensibility of this CSF containing sac at the back. In addition, because of the closure, rapid increases in raised pressure can no longer be damped by the myelomeningocoele sac and these high pressure pulses will be communicated to the ventricular walls and cause them to distend. Williams (1971) has postulated that there is an upward movement of CSF past the Arnold–Chiari malformation on straining, followed by a fall in pressure in the lumbar region on relaxation, creating a differential pressure which enhances further hind-brain impaction.

Hydrocephalus may therefore be considered as 'active hydrocephalus' or 'arrested hydrocephalus'. The active hydrocephalus, as mentioned before, goes through various phases of very high pressure in small or normal ventricles, high pressure in large ventricles or relatively lower pressure in huge ventricles with the intermediate phase of intermittent pressure. Hydrocephalus is not synonomous with raised intracranial pressure. CSF shunts are for treating pressure (pressure devices or pressure shunts) and not for treating hydrocephalus *per se*. The effects of active hydrocephalus are the effects of expansion of the CSF compartment (as distinct from the brain or blood compartment) and this pressure results in a dilatation of the ventricular system and a breakdown in the septum pellucidum. While the brain is virtually incompressable (because it is largely water), it does have visco-elastic properties, and in response to pressure it shows deformation and displacement (herniations) and pressure decay (atrophy). The herniations and displacements take the form of foramen magnum impaction, tentorial herniation and cingulate gyrus herniation. While many of the classical signs of each of these are an indication of impending death in the adult world, young children frequently present with such signs, indicating the greater capacity for distortion of the infant's brain compared to the adult. Apnoea, hypotonia and stridor are not infrequent with active ventricular pressure in childhood, but are signs classically attributed to foramen magnum impaction. Similarly, with tentorial herniation, a paralysis of upward gaze is a very frequent phenomenon and indicates movement of the brain against the tentorial edge. Third nerve lesions, pupillary abnormalities, nystagmus and hippus are other frequently encountered signs of pressure in children.

Pressure atrophy results in thinning of the palium (cortical mantle) which is normally more than 35 mm at the vertex at birth. Next, a disruption of the ependymal lining of the ventricles occurs with a rediffusion of CSF into the white matter of the brain, interstitial oedema, and this is responsible for the periventricular hypodensity seen on CT scans in children with active hydrocephalus. This eventually leads to demyelination and axonal destruction within the white matter of the hemispheres, with sparing of the grey matter (Weller *et al.*, 1969; Rubin *et al.*, 1972).

The signs of acutely raised intracranial pressure in children depend on which intracranial compartment is being expanded and on the age of the child (because of the buffering ability) and the rapidity with which it develops. The signs and symptoms of active hydrocephalus (CSF compartment) are initially different from those of increasing pressure within the brain compartment (fits, coma, decerebration and loss of homeostasis). Initially, when the pressure increases within the ventricular compartment, buffering comes into play if time is available, and this takes the form of displacement of the CSF into the distensible spinal subarachnoid space (which is not therefore available to those with myelomeningocoele); as a result of this increased pressure, there is increased absorption across the arachnoid villi. The second buffer is that of reducing cerebral blood volume by collapsing cerebral veins with increasing venous resistance or by lowering cerebral perfusion pressure. The third buffer is that of increasing the OFC, available to children under the age of 18 months. So the signs of neonatal active hydrocephalus are buffering signs, and when this is exhausted, the herniations occur with their additional signs.

The signs of active hydrocephalus in infancy are an increasing OFC, bulging non-pulsatile anterior fontanelle and splayed sutures both clinically and radiologically. McEwan's sign of the 'crackpot' skull, scalp and retinal venous distention, intracranial bruit (Korotoff sounds), hypertension and brachycardia may be found. The child's scalp will be tight and the skin shiny. 'Sunsetting' is due to pressure on the tectum of the mid-brain, from tentorial herniation at the supra-pineal recess of the third ventricle (Shallat *et al.*, 1973). False localizing signs may also appear and these can take the form of anosmia and hemianopia, cranial nerve V to VII dysfunction, but mostly VIth cranial nerve lesions with convergent strabismus. Long-standing pressure will give rise to depression of the orbital roofs. Papilloedema is infrequently encountered in the early years, due to raised pressure, although chronic atrophic papilloedema is frequently a consequence of these children's pressure problems. The signs of herniation include extensor hypertonus, head retraction, obligatory tonic neck reflexes, opisthotonus progressing to decerebration and total homeostatic collapse.

The principle underlying the management of acute hydrocephalus is to allow dilatation of the ventricles to occur, hoping for spontaneous arrest, but not to allow the ventricular dilatation to proceed to a point where the cortical mantle is so thin that intellectual retardation will be the inevitable result. During the course of this ventricular dilatation, daily or second-daily ultrasound scanning of the head is undertaken, obtaining both coronal and saggital views on a sector scan, and an estimate of the radiological 'ventricular index'. By means of centimetre markers on the scan, sequential scans will allow intervention at an optimal time. Alternatively, a bifrontal ratio or ratios of corneal transventricular diameters divided by transcalvarial diameter at the level of the head of the caudate nucleus and also at the level of the mid-glomus of the choroid plexus in the ventricular atria, are normally 0.32 and 0.51 in newborns. A further ratio in the parasagittal plane—the occipital cortical mantle divided by the frontal cortical mantle should be 0.78 in non-hydrocephalic newborns. These methods are a means of following the progress of hydrocephalus (Poland *et al.*, 1985). It remains a useful observational exercise to have daily head circumference measurements recorded and these are plotted weekly on a percentile chart. It is the usual practice to obtain a CT scan or MRI scan of the head sometime during this period, to obtain a better view of the posterior fossa, particularly if the fourth ventricle is not visible on ultrasonography. It will also provide more accurate evidence of the dimensions of the posterior fossa, the attenuated density pattern (i.e. periventricular haloes which reflect raised pressure, although this is rare in infants), and the tightness or otherwise of the cortical subarachnoid space. While the ultrasound will show the ventriculomegaly, it may be less useful in recognizing parenchymal oedema, although it may show reduction in pulsation of the cerebral arteries consequent on the raised pressure.

A skull X-ray shows growth of the cranial vault and the size of the posterior fossa with possibly some evidence of a Dandy−Walker cyst (Raimondi *et al.*, 1969). It also shows sutural separation.

A CSF shunt can be avoided in about one-third of children. Shunting will be required early in those who at first assessment have a cortical mantle of less than 15 mm or a recorded ventricular pressure in excess of 20 mm of mercury using fontanometers or intraventricular or surface catheter methods (Minns, 1984). The remainder, those with a mantle between 16 and 25 mm, will need continued careful observation with ultrasounds and some two-thirds of those will eventually require a shunt. For those with a cortical mantle of more than 26 mm, two-thirds will eventually escape a shunt. It is suggested that complications from the CSF shunting occur less frequently when the shunt is inserted late in the neonatal period (Lorber, 1969). For some years, the service in Edinburgh for children with spina bifida was co-ordinated by a full-time research paediatrician. The experience gained has been incorporated into the work of the paediatric neurology department, with developments in the understanding of complications and of their management. The latter is now co-ordinated by the paediatric neurology department which offers facilities to investigate the former.

Discharge and out-patient follow-up

Prior to discharge, orthopaedic consultation should be sought, so that the orthopaedic surgeon with special responsibility for the spina bifida children will have an opportunity to carry out an orthopaedic assessment in the new-born period, record the child's joint angles, deformities, muscle power, and view the X-rays of the hips. It is our practice to splint prophylactically the hips which are subluxed or at risk (e.g. L4 lesions) by means of a modified Pavlic harness, which has the advantage of being a dynamic harness and allows maximum movement of the lower limbs while keeping the hips abducted (Fig. 5.6). The only orthopaedic surgery that may be necessary in the neonatal period is for the calcaneo-valgus foot deformity, where there are dorsiflexors working unopposed. Treatment is to tenotomize the dorsiflexors in the new-born period. This can be done in the ward's treatment room and frequently needs to be repeated once or twice.

Some families will be unable to cope immediately with the anxieties of looking after their own child with a severe handicap, and for this reason their discharge from the paediatric ward may need to be staggered. Initially, the parents take the child home for a day or two, and gradually increase this with their confidence in handling the child.

Immediately prior to the child's discharge, the medical or senior nursing staff on the unit will sit down with these parents and advise them of the dos and don'ts of which they should be aware. The valve is shown to them, and they learn to recognize its normal feel and how to palpate it if

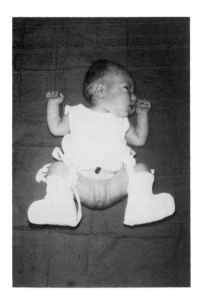

Fig. 5.6. Modified Pavlic harness.

the child becomes symptomatic. They are advised how to express the bladder, how often, and how much pressure to exert, and the symptoms to be expected should a urine infection occur are discussed. Other points raised include the avoidance of excessive weight gain; the predisposition to, and management of constipation; care of nappy area; avoidance of tightly fitting clothing, footwear, and heavy bedding; the necessity to check for pressure sores and where these are most likely to occur. They are advised that vigilance is needed to prevent cold injury in anaesthetic limbs during the winter, and that excess sunlight on scars should be avoided in the summer. Any painless swelling of the limbs should alert the parents to a possible fracture (and they should notify it immediately), and in particular, they are advised against the use of hot water bottles in the child's bed. Immunization is discussed. Pertussis and measles vaccines should not be recommended, and parents are supplied with a booklet which they can read at their leisure on spina bifida generally.

Some mothers may prefer to 'live in' for a few days prior to the child's discharge to acquire more confidence in handling their new spina bifida child. Emotional support is most important and this has been detailed by MacKeith (1973). The parents are advised of an early home visit by the medical social worker to the unit and the family doctor is notified. The parents realize at this first discharge (which is usually at 3−4 weeks of age) that they have ready access to the facilities of the paediatric unit at any time.

It is impressed on the parents that most children with spina bifida will require regular, lifelong out-patient follow-up. The first out-patient appointment is within a month of discharge.

Out-patient follow-up of the spina bifida child is by the same paediatric unit. Initially, care is supervised mostly by the hospital unit. Gradually, other aspects of the child's care and health surveillance are undertaken by the general practitioner and the community paediatric services. It is important, however, to maintain a paediatric base and centralize the care for these children from both an in-patient and out-patient point of view. The follow-up clinics are 'combined clinics' and in Edinburgh this clinic consists of a neuro-paediatrician, a senior clinical medical officer responsible for the physical handicap school that most of the children will attend, an orthopaedic surgeon, a peripatetic stoma-therapist/catheter nurse, physiotherapist, occupational therapist, and social worker. The facilities of real-time ultrasound, neurophysiology services, laboratory services, non-invasive out-patient ICP recording in selected children (Cosman *et al.*, 1979) and the fitting of urinary aids and appliances are all to hand. From this clinic, a letter is dispatched to the family doctor about the child's multisystem involvement, the timing of various surgical and investigative procedures, and any liaison that is required between the hospital and the community therapists, psychologists or other personnel.

At the first combined clinic appointment, genetic counselling of the parents will generally be undertaken by a paediatrician, so that if the couple have had a previous spina bifida child, the risk of a further affected child is advised to be about 1 in 20. Following two affected children, the risk becomes 1 in 6. Prevention using periconceptional vitamins in subsequent pregnancies is discussed, though the present evidence is still uncertain.

The management and treatment of the complications of spina bifida are discussed in Book 2. These include the neuropathic bladder and bowel, spinal deformities, sensory loss and orthopaedic management.

Education and progress after school

Many children attend normal nursery and normal schools, and their place of education frequently depends on local facilities. In the educational assessment of these children it is important to realize that tests such as the Stanford–Binet are verbally biased and these children may appear more intelligent than they sometimes are. A WPPSI and Bender test may be more appropriate.

The characteristics of learning disorders in spina bifida children include hyperverbal performance, poor comprehension, inappropriate use of language, difficulty with visuo-spatial perception (particularly figure ground), poor body image, visual motor inco-ordination (dysgraphia), dyspraxia, and maturational deficits (delayed dominance). For the present adult spina bifida population who attended school up to 1963 in the UK, about half attended normal local authority or private schools, for both primary and secondary education. Approximately equal numbers attended schools for those with physical handicap or multiple handicap.

In terms of secondary school qualification in this cohort, one patient obtained one A level, and two two A levels, seven did a certificate of 6th year studies in Scotland, and 19 obtained higher certificates. O levels at a C+ grading were obtained by 43 individuals, and the mean number of O level passes obtained by these 43 was 3.6. In terms of the total number of adults and teenagers with spina bifida this represented a mean number of O levels at any grade of 1.8 per person. The presence of O levels correlated negatively with the degree of handicap.

Full- or part-time secondary education was undertaken by some 40% of the spina bifida adults, and qualifications obtained by 27%. Again, the number of qualifications correlated negatively with the degree of handicap ($P < 0.05$). In addition, training courses feature largely in the self-education of spina bifida adults and they are thought to be useful and to lead to better employment prospects.

Over 70% of all teenagers and adults live at home with parents or a guardian, and less than 20% are independently accommodated. Twice as many would prefer an independent existence. In terms of activities of daily living, which is a net result of their several handicaps, 56% were completely independent, 39% partially dependent, and 5% totally dependent on support from other adults. More than 80% claim to spend less than an hour a day on their personal care, although it is likely that this may prove to be an underestimate if they should be actually timed.

Occupational therapy clearly has an important part to play in their personal and social independence skills. At the combined spina bifida clinics, a cyclostyled questionnaire is completed for each patient, questioning whether they have any difficulties with bathing, using the toilet, face washing, cleaning their teeth, feeding, preparing a snack, dressing, managing their urinary appliances, buttons and tight fastenings, callipers, and bed; and it also asks about the access to and suitability of their house and transport. The occupational therapist will visit the home to recommend necessary modifications, such as a downstairs toilet, wide passageways, ramps, bath hoists or plunge baths, telephone, washing machine, dishwasher, etc. Functional independence is assessed as (i) fully independent; (ii) dependent in one or two areas; (iii) dependent in three or more areas. One might think that leisure activities in spina bifida adults, because of their physical handicap, would be largely mental or artistic, or musical. However, this is not so. The majority have combined physical and musical pastimes, including non-specific activities with a social flavour, e.g. church activities, driving, bird watching. Twenty-eight per cent of adults with spina bifida have a predominantly sporting or physical interest as their main leisure activity. Interestingly, over 80% enjoy leisure activity not specifically for the disabled, although many also join clubs for disabled drivers, wheelchair dancing, wheelchair fishing, wheelchair basketball, and archery and table tennis. Clearly, the intellectual dimension makes for differences between this group of adults and those with traumatic paraplegias. However, one feels that, for the future, emphasis should be applied equally to their physical training and independence, as well as to their formal education.

One difficult problem at the present time is the continuity of care once the child leaves paediatric supervision and school. Most spina bifida adults do not prefer medical supervision by a 'traumatic paraplegia' service, but again much depends on available local facilities. Each child at present is treated individually and if he has a multisystem disorder which requires several disciplines for follow-up, such as orthopaedic plus neurological plus urological, then this adolescent is referred to an Adult Spinal Paralysis Service. If, however, only one system needs review, e.g. bladder function, then he will be referred for follow-up to an adult urologist. Where only a watching brief is required and no intervention anticipated, the general practitioner is asked to maintain an annual surveillance.

References

Anderveg, J. (1976) *The cause of hydrocephalus.* Bronder–Offset BV, Rotterdam.

Barry, A., Patten, B.M. & Stewart, B.H. (1957) Possible factors in development of the Arnold–Chiari malformation. *Journal of Neurosurgery*, **14**, 285–301.

Charney, E.B., Sutton, L.N., Bruce, D.A. & Schut, L.B. (1983) Myelomeningocele newborn management: time for parental decision. *Zeitschrift für Kinderchirurgie*, **38**, Suppl. 2, 90–93.

Cosman, E.R., Zervas, N.T., Chapman, P.H., Cosman, B.J. & Arnold, M.A. (1979) A telemetric pressure sensor for ventricular shunt systems. *Surgical Neurology*, **11**, 287–294.

Drennan, J.C. (1970) The role of muscles in the development of human lumbar kyphosis. *Developmental Medicine and Child Neurology*, Suppl. 22, 33–38.

Emery, J.L. & Lendon, R.G. (1973) The local cord lesion in neurospinal dysraphism (meningomyelocele). *Journal of Pathology*, **110**, 83–96.

Heimburger, R.F. (1972) Early repair of myelomeningocele. *Journal of Neurosurgery*, **37**, 594–600.

Lorber, J. (1969) Ventriculo-cardiac shunts in the first week of life. *Developmental Medicine and Child Neurology*, Suppl. 20, 13–22.

Lorber, J. (1971) Medical and surgical aspects in the treatment of congenital hydrocephalus. *Neuropadiatrie*, **3**, 239–246.

Mackeith, R.C. (1973) The feelings and behaviour of parents of handicapped children. *Developmental Medicine and Child Neurology*, **15**, 524–527.

Milhorat, T.H. (1972) *Hydrocephalus and the cerebrospinal fluid.* Williams and Wilkins, Baltimore.

Minns R.A. (1984) Intracranial pressure monitoring. *Archives of Disease in Childhood*, **59**(5), 486–488.

Passage, E., True, C.W., Sueoka, W.T., Baumgartner, N.R. & Keer, K.R. (1966) Malformations of the central nervous system in trisomy-18 syndrome. *Journal of Pediatrics*, **69**, 771–778.

Penfield, W. & Coburn, D.F. (1938) Arnold–Chiari malformation and its treatment. *Archives of Neurology and Psychiatry*, **40**, 328–336.

Raimondi, A.J., Samuelson, G.H., Yarzagaray, L. & Norton, T. (1969) Atresia of the foramina Luschkae and Magendie: the Dandy-Walker-cyst. *Journal of Neurosurgery*, **31**, 202–216.

Rubin, R.C., Hochwald, G., Liwnicz, B., Tiell, M., Mizutani, H. & Shulman K. (1972) The effect of severe hydrocephalus on size and number of brain cells. *Developmental Medicine and Child Neurology*, Suppl. 27, 117–120.

Shallat, R.F., Pawl, R.P. & Jerva, M.J. (1973) Significance of upward gaze palsy (Parinaud's syndrome) in hydrocephalus due to shunt malfunction. *Journal of Neurosurgery*, **38**, 717–721.

Smith, E.D. (1965) *Spina Bifida and Total Care of the Spinal Myelomeningocele*. Charles C. Thomas, Springfield, Illinois.

Stark, G.D. & Drummond, M. (1970) Spina bifida as an obstetric problem. *Developmental Medicine and Child Neurology*, Suppl. 22, 157–160.

Stark, G.D. & Drummond, M. (1972) Neonatal electromyography and nerve conduction studies in myelomeningocele. *Neuropadiatrie*, **3**, 409–420.

Variend, S. & Emery, J.L. (1973) The weight of the cerebellum in children with myelomeningocele. *Developmental Medicine and Child Neurology*, Suppl. 29, 77–83.

Variend, S. & Emery, J.L. (1974) The pathology of the central lobes of the cerebellum in children with myelomeningocele. *Developmental Medicine and Child Neurology*, Suppl. 32, 99–106.

Williams, B. (1971) Further thoughts on the valvular action of the Arnold–Chiari malformation. *Developmental Medicine and Child Neurology*, Suppl. 25, 105–112.

Zachary, R.B. & Sharrard, W.J.W. (1967) Spinal dysraphism. *Postgraduate Medical Journal*, **43**, Suppl. 1, 731–754.

Chapter 6
Orthopaedic Management of Children with Neurological Disorders

Charles Galasko

The orthopaedic management of children with neurological disorders is aimed at obtaining the optimum quality of life within their disability by preventing deformity or treating it when it has occurred. The prevention and management of scoliosis may be associated with an increased life expectancy but orthopaedic treatment will not do anything for the underlying neurological disorder.

Prevention and treatment

Ideally, children should be treated via a multidisciplinary approach. The members of the team will depend on the disease. For example, in spina bifida, a team could consist of paediatric surgeon, urologist, orthopaedic surgeon, physiotherapist, occupational therapist, orthotist and social worker; whereas in cerebral palsy, essential members of the team must include the paediatric neurologist or paediatrician, speech therapist, teacher, orthopaedic surgeon, orthotist, occupational therapist, physiotherapist and social worker and, depending on the associated abnormalities, the child may require help with hearing, vision or perceptual difficulties. The therapist must be specifically trained. A child with severe cerebral palsy should not be treated in a routine physiotherapy department but requires physiotherapists who have special postgraduate training in the management of cerebral palsy.

The value of the multidisciplinary approach is that it leads to an earlier and more accurate diagnosis, a more accurate assessment of the prognosis and the earlier recognition and treatment of deformity.

Assessment

Before embarking upon treatment, these children require a detailed assessment. This includes an assessment of their overall functional capability (Table 6.1), a detailed assessment of their muscle power, the range of movement of each joint and measurement of any joint contrac-

Table 6.1. Functional assessment

1.	Walks; climbs stairs without assistance
2.	Walks; climbs stairs with aid of rail
3.	Walks; climbs stairs slowly with aid of rail
4.	Walks; unable to climb stairs
5.	Walks; unable to get out of chair without arms
6.	Walks with assistance or callipers
7.	In wheelchair; can roll chair
8.	In wheelchair; unable to perform chair activities
9.	In wheelchair; sits with support; minimal activities
10.	In bed; unable to perform activities of daily living

tures. All deformities must be noted and the ability of the child to co-operate determined. This will depend on the intelligence of the child, his or her physical development, the psychological approach of the child and the family, and the age of the child. This assessment is usually carried out by the physiotherapist. As part of our initial assessment we obtain an erect antero-posterior X-ray of the spine, an X-ray of the pelvis, and lung function tests.

The deformities vary in the different diseases, and they will be discussed separately.

Development of deformity

Deformity results from an interaction between several forces: neurological, postural and gravitational (Fulford & Brown, 1976; Fulford *et al.*, 1982). Neurological mechanisms include unequal forces of movement and tone, as in cerebral palsy, or through weakness as in neuromuscular conditions. Postural mechanisms may be intrinsic, e.g. hemivertebrae in spinal dysraphism, or extrinsic, e.g. wheelchair footrest at the wrong height. Gravitational forces lead the inactive body to become moulded into the most commonly adopted posture. The extreme example of this is the wind-swept posture of children with severe cerebral palsy or spinal muscular atrophy (Table 6.2).

If there is muscle imbalance (Fig. 6.1) (e.g. in poliomyelitis or Duchenne dystrophy), correction of the imbalance will correct the deformity. Techniques include tendon division (tenotomy), elongation, transfer and/or neurectomy. The results of these procedures for children with cerebral palsy is less easy to predict, as the problems tend to be from unequal forces of movement and tone. Though surgery on tendons and

Table 6.2.

	No. of patients	Scoliosis	CDH	Foot deformity	Knee contracture	Hip contracture	Misc.
Duchenne dystrophy	47	9	0	27	14	10	2
Misc. dystrophies	45	9	5	20	5	7	1
Neuropathies	22	4	2	15	2	2	2
Spinal muscle atrophy	45	23	2	16	10	8	4
Congenital myopathies	17	6	2	6	3	2	0
Total	176	51	11	84	34	29	9

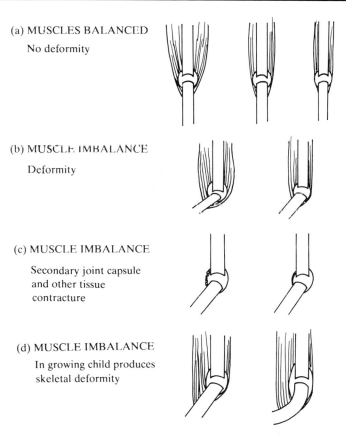

(a) MUSCLES BALANCED

No deformity

(b) MUSCLE IMBALANCE

Deformity

(c) MUSCLE IMBALANCE

Secondary joint capsule and other tissue contracture

(d) MUSCLE IMBALANCE

In growing child produces skeletal deformity

Fig. 6.1. (a) Providing the agonists and antagonists acting on a joint are balanced, deformity tends not to occur, irrespective of whether the muscles are hypertrophied, normal or weak.

(b) If there is imbalance between the muscles, the joint is pulled in the direction of the more powerful muscle. This occurs irrespective of whether one muscle is spastic and the other is normal, one is normal and the antagonist is weak or whether both muscles are weak but one is more powerful.

(c) The redundant capsule and ligaments fibrose on the contracted side of the joint producing secondary joint contractures. At this stage rebalancing the muscles will not correct the deformity; a soft tissue release is also required.

(d) In the growing child, if the muscles attach distal to a growth plate, the bone will tend to be deformed in the direction of the more powerful muscles.

nerves can be very successful, the effect may only be temporary. Surgery may change the balance of movement and tone in such a way as to release previously weak muscle groups which may become overactive. Also, division of tendons and/or peripheral nerves in the groin may lead to a loss of stability at the hip. Ideally, surgical intervention should be carefully planned in discussion with the patient and family, physicians and physiotherapist. On the one hand, the most enduring results are obtained from surgery near the end of growth. On the other hand, persisting deformity may lead to secondary changes, e.g. subluxation or dislocation of the hip. There is a need for prospective trials on the best method of preventing hip subluxation and dislocation. Equinovarus deformity may respond to serial plastering and intermittent wearing of splints during times of activity (Jones, 1982), so long as this is combined with experienced physiotherapy treatment.

If deformity has been present for some time, fibrosis and shortening of the joint capsule and ligaments on the contracted side of the joint occur. Balancing of muscles alone will not improve the deformity. The contracted tissue must also be surgically divided. At all times the functional purpose of intervention must be considered as opposed to cosmetic results.

If the muscle insertion is distal to a growth plate in a child, the bone will be bent in the direction of the more powerful forces. Balancing muscles and releasing contractures will not suffice. An osteotomy or arthrodesis will be needed to correct the deformity.

Cerebral palsy

General considerations
Cerebral palsy is a disorder of posture, movement and tone due to a non-progressive lesion of the immature brain. It is associated with a high incidence of speech defects, deafness, blindness, perceptual difficulty, mental retardation and epilepsy, but there is no primary visceral involvement. Orthopaedic management plays an important role in the total management of the child. It must not be carried out in isolation but should be regarded as part of the continuing treatment programme. In general terms, the more severely affected the child the higher the incidence of musculo-skeletal deformities and the greater their severity. Most of the deformities should be managed conservatively by physiotherapy or splintage. Surgery is only indicated where correction of the deformity can

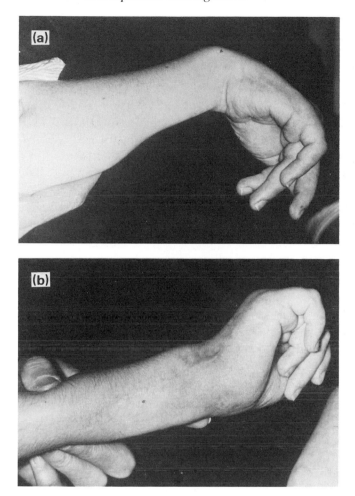

Fig. 6.2. Cerebral palsy. (a) Flexion deformity of the wrist: the patient has very poor finger flexion. (b) Following a flexor to extensor transfer, the wrist is slightly extended and finger flexion has markedly improved.

be expected to be associated with improved function, or to prevent progressive dysfunction. Hundreds of operations have been described, many of which are no longer in use, and only a few will be discussed.

Flexion deformity of the wrist

A flexor to extensor transfer may improve the position of the wrist and give better hand function. It is impossible to flex the fingers normally when the wrist is maximally flexed. When the wrist is in the neutral or slightly dorsiflexed position, finger flexion is improved and a more powerful grip results (Fig. 6.2).

Thumb in palm deformity

A flexed adducted thumb interferes with hand function (Fig. 6.3). Release of this deformity can be associated with improved function of the hand. However, this needs to be done during the first few years of life. Once a child has reached the age of 4–5 years and has not used a hand, he/she is unlikely to use that hand even if the positional abnormality responsible for the failure to use the limb is corrected. It seems as if the cerebral connections must be established within the first 2–3 years of life.

Scoliosis

This occurs commonly. In general terms, the more severely affected the child and the greater the degree of mental retardation, the worse the

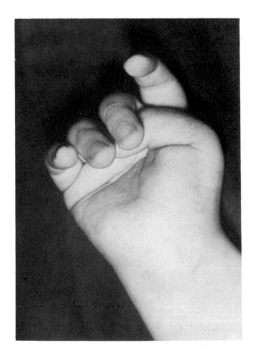

Fig. 6.3. Child with cerebral palsy. Thumb in palm abnormality, interfering with the use of the hand.

curve. In the severely affected, mentally retarded, immobile child, surgery is contraindicated (Fig. 6.4). Treatment is limited to providing the child with the optimum chair; a moulded insert often is extremely helpful. In the less severely affected patients a spinal support may be used.

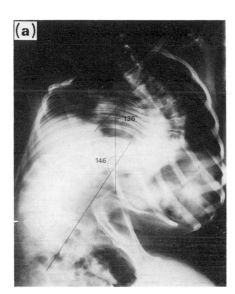 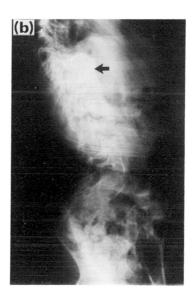

Fig. 6.4. Severely mentally retarded child with cerebral palsy. (a) Antero-posterior X-ray shows a gross scoliosis, with a double curve and marked pelvic obliquity. (b) Lateral X-ray of the spine. The severity of the deformity is such that a cranial view of one of the vertebrae can be seen on the lateral X-ray (*arrowed*).

Progressive scoliosis in the less severely affected child should be treated by surgical correction.

Dislocation of the hip
This is easier to prevent than to treat and is due to imbalance of movement and tone, the spastic flexors and adductors overpowering the extensors and abductors. Secondary bony deformity with acetabular dysplasia, coxa valga and increasing femoral anteversion usually develops. It may also be secondary to pelvic obliquity due to scoliosis (Fig. 6.5), an adduction contracture of the same side or abduction contracture of the

contralateral hip. Serial X-rays of the pelvis will show progressive sub-luxation of the hips, usually associated with a valgus femoral neck before the hip dislocates. Prevention is by night splinting during growth or early muscle balance procedures, particularly an adductor release, if necessary supplemented by release of the ilio-psoas and rectus femoris, upper femoral varus derotation osteotomy and a pelvic osteotomy when required.

A dislocated hip (Fig. 6.6) is treated by reduction, correction of pelvic obliquity, pelvic osteotomy to correct acetabular dysplasia, varus derotation femoral osteotomy, and tendon releases to balance the muscles. Whereas dislocated hips in spina bifida are often asymptomatic, in cerebral palsy they may be associated with pain. Such major reconstructive surgery is only warranted in patients who are able to walk, or in whom the dislocation makes sitting uncomfortable. There is no indication for surgery in patients confined to a wheelchair or bed whose dislocated hip is asymptomatic.

Once growth has ceased, if a dislocated hip produces discomfort in a severely affected patient who is confined to a wheelchair or bed, it may be treated by excision of the proximal femur, but this is not always successful. If there is an associated scoliosis, the scoliosis and pelvic obliquity must be corrected before dealing with the dislocated hip, otherwise recurrence is common.

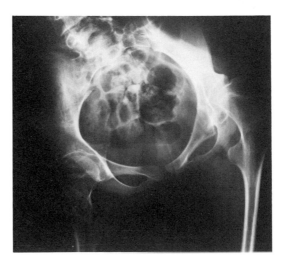

Fig. 6.5. Cerebral palsy. There is marked pelvic obliquity secondary to scoliosis. The left hip is subluxed. The patient requires correction of the pelvic obliquity as well as reconstruction of the hip joint.

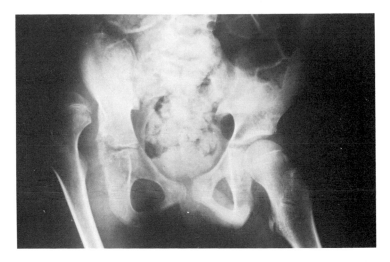

Fig. 6.6. Dislocated hip joint in a severely mentally retarded child with athetoid cerebral palsy. The child was unable to stand or walk and appeared to be comfortable, both in the sitting and lying position. Movement of the child was not associated with pain or tenderness at the hip joint. There was no indication for surgery in this child.

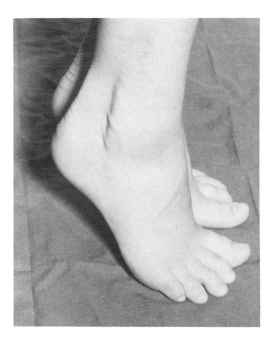

Fig. 6.7. Cerebral palsy associated with bilateral severe equinus deformity of the ankles. Elongation of the tendo Achillis was required.

Contractures

Contractures of the knee and ankles occur commonly in cerebral palsy (Fig. 6.7). Where indicated, regular stretching exercises or serial plastering should be carried out in an attempt to prevent these deformities. Surgery is only indicated if the deformity interferes with gait, and physiotherapy, orthoses and muscle relaxants have failed to control the deformity. Before surgery is carried out, careful assessment is required to ensure that the patient will be able to co-operate with physiotherapy following surgical correction.

The common surgical procedures are release or transfer of the hip adductors; release, elongation or transfer of the hamstring tendons; elongation of the tendo Achillis and transfer of the tibialis posterior tendon, although other procedures may be indicated.

Down's syndrome

Dislocation of the hip can occur. Capsular laxity is prominent and usually there is no recognizable muscle imbalance. Bony changes are minimal unless the dislocation is long standing and there is no pelvic obliquity. The treatment is to repair the capsular laxity and to create a compensatory bony deformity with acetabular coverage and a varus femoral neck. These children stand an increased risk of dislocation of their cervical spines, probably resulting from capsular and ligamentous laxity.

Spina bifida

Spina bifida occulta

Spina bifida occulta is rarely associated with orthopaedic deformities, but if they occur they are usually due to traction on a nerve root. Frequently, this is accompanied by an external manifestation, such as a hairy patch, dimple or lipoma overlying the lumbo-sacral junction. Such nerve root tethering may present with inequality of foot development (Fig. 6.8).

Meningocoele

This requires closure at birth. Neurological complications are uncommon.

Myelomeningocoele

General considerations

Most of the orthopaedic complications develop in children with myelo-

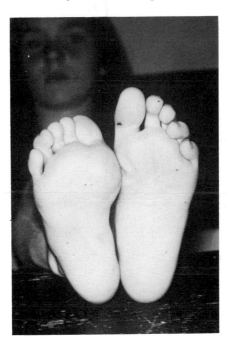

Fig. 6.8. Unequal foot growth due to traction on nerve root.

meningocoele. The neurological level often can be diagnosed at birth, by careful observation of which muscle groups are functioning and by assessment of the deformities that are present (Table 6.3).

The higher the lesion, the worse the prognosis and the greater the eventual disability. Whereas the dystrophies, atrophies and myopathies are purely motor disturbances, spina bifida also is associated with severe sensory and visceral disturbances. As a result of loss of sphincter control, the patients develop urinary retention with overflow incontinence, hydro-ureter, hydronephrosis and pylonephritis. Urinary drainage, often in the form of a urinary diversion, may be required.

Approximately 50% of the more severely affected patients develop hydrocephalus once the defect has been closed, and require the insertion of a valve to drain the excess CSF.

These children also have anaesthetic feet. Training of the parents initially, and the patient subsequently, in the care of the feet is an essential part of their management.

Mobilization

Most patients have normal or powerful musculature in their shoulder

Table 6.3.

Level of lesion	Deformity	Due to unopposed action of
L1	Kyphosis	Abdominal muscles + gravity
	Flexion of hip	Psoas
L2	Flexion + adduction of hip—dislocated	Psoas + adductors
L3	Flexion + adduction of hip	Psoas + adductors
	Genu recurvatum	Quadriceps
L4	Flexion + adduction of hip	Psoas, adductors + rectus femoris
	Genu recurvatum	Quadriceps
	Calcaneo-varus	Tibialis Anterior
L5	Flexion of hip	Psoas + rectus femoris
	Calcaneus	Tibialis anterior + peronei
S1	Clawing of toes	Long toe flexors

girdle, upper limbs and upper trunk. Those severely affected by myelo-meningocoeles have virtually no power in their lower limbs. They can walk either with a swivel walker or callipers. The advantage of the swivel walker (or clicker) is that the upper limbs are free. The disadvantages are that although children find it easy to control, teenagers and adults often find great difficulty in using the device; secondly, unless there are railings to allow the patient to lever themselves up a step, the patient can only walk on an absolutely level surface. The alternative is the provision of callipers. Because the hip musculature is usually grossly deficient, the patients require long leg callipers, with a trunk support and pelvic hinge. Younger children are provided with a rollator, older patients with a pair of crutches. The disadvantage is that the upper limbs are not free but are required for the external support. The main advantage is that the patients may be able to manage stairs. The reciprocating gait orthosis may prove to be extremely useful in these patients.

Spinal deformities

These occur commonly in the severely affected child. Kyphosis (Fig. 6.9) is a major problem and, because of pressure, may make it impossible to use a calliper, swivel walker or a standing frame, and may make sitting

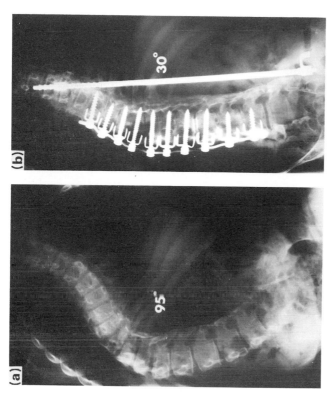

Fig. 6.10. Spina bifida (courtesy of Mr McMaster, Edinburgh). (a) Age 11 years: the curve measured 95°. (b) One year 3 months post-operation: following anterior correction with Dwyer instrumentation and a subsequent posterior correction with Harrington instrumentation, the curve has been corrected to 30°.

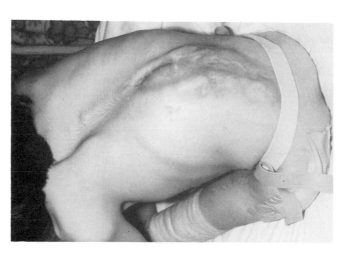

Fig. 6.9. Spina bifida. Note the kyphosis. The overlying skin is thin. This combination is likely to lead to skin breakdown if the orthosis rubs against the kyphus.

uncomfortable. When this does occur, surgical excision of the kyphus is required.

Scoliosis is another frequent complication. The curves are often very severe, and a combined anterior correction and fusion using Dwyer instrumentation and a posterior fusion with Harrington or Luque instrumentation is indicated (Fig. 6.10). Unlike patients with Duchenne dystrophy, the vast majority of patients with severe spina bifida have adequate pulmonary function to withstand this major surgery.

Lower limb deformities

Dislocation of the hip commonly develops in patients with a high lumbar lesion. This is due to the unopposed action of the ilio-psoas, rectus femoris and adductor group of muscles. Secondary acetabular dysplasia usually develops. Open reduction of the dislocation, pelvic osteotomy, transfer of the ilio-psoas tendon and release of the other tight tendons, including a contralateral abductor release if necessary, are required.

Recurvatum deformity of the knees may occur as a result of the unopposed action of the quadriceps muscle in patients with a mid-lumbar lesion, and in lower lumbar lesions calcaneus deformities occur due to the unopposed action of tibialis anterior. The latter may be associated with an inversion deformity unless the invertor effect is balanced by the peronei. Clawing of the toes may be the only skeletal deformity with sacral lesions, due to the unopposed action of the long flexor tendons, but these children will have loss of bladder and rectal control.

Plaster casts, which are frequently applied following reconstructive surgery, must be very well padded to avoid the development of pressure sores in patients with anaesthetic limbs. There is a high incidence of stress fractures when the plaster casts are removed and mobilization is commenced.

Spinal muscular atrophy

Orthopaedic management is usually required in the intermediate variety, but only rarely indicated in the mild variety (Kugelberg–Welander syndrome) where the children are already ambulant and should be encouraged to remain so, or in the severe form (Werdnig–Hoffman disease) when the patient usually dies within the first year of life.

Mobilization

Most of the children with intermediate spinal muscular atrophy are unable to walk when first seen. Usually, it is not possible to provide callipers until the child is 3–4 years of age, and during this period, active physiotherapy is encouraged, provided that the child will co-operate and has sufficient power in the upper limbs to control a rollator. Callipers can be fitted when the child is 3–4 years of age (Fig. 6.11). Older patients may be mobilized without the use of a rollator or crutches. Unlike Duchenne dystrophy, patients with spinal muscular atrophy can be mobilized even though they have been chairbound for months and even years.

Scoliosis
Like Duchenne dystrophy, the most important deformity in these children is their scoliosis. A curve is already present in nearly half the patients when first seen at our clinic. It is our policy to obtain an erect (sitting) antero-posterior X-ray of their spine at 6-monthly intervals.

Curves of less than 20° are watched. Progressive curves or curves greater than 20° are treated by bracing until the child is old enough for surgical correction and spinal fusion (Fig. 6.12). The type of bracing

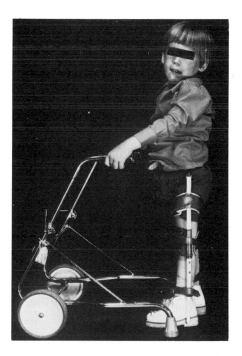

Fig. 6.11. Spinal muscle atrophy. This patient, who was confined to a wheelchair, has been mobilized with the use of callipers and a rollator.

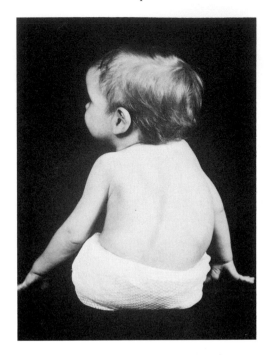

Fig. 6.12. Spinal muscle atrophy. At the age of 19 months, this patient had a scoliosis measuring 63°.

depends on the age of the child. In the first 2–3 years of life a plaster-zote jacket may suffice. In older children moulded orthoses are usually enough, and curves greater than 70° may need periods of immobilization in a plaster jacket. If bracing does not hold the curve, earlier surgery may be required.

Hips
Unlike Duchenne dystrophy, dislocation of the hips does occur in spinal muscular atrophy, although much less frequently than in spina bifida or cerebral palsy. The dislocation is secondary to muscle imbalance and is preceded by progressive subluxation. Serial X-rays will indicate which hips are at risk. Dislocation can usually be prevented by balancing the musculature (which often requires release of the hip flexors and adductors) and a varus upper femoral osteotomy. Dislocated hips require open reduction and muscle balancing procedures. Flexion contractures of the hip (Fig. 6.13) can interfere with mobilization and may require surgical

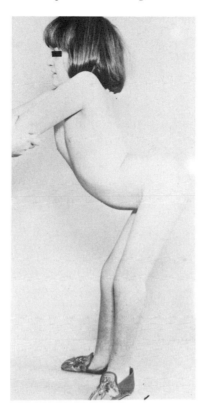

Fig. 6.13. Spinal muscle atrophy. Note the gross fixed flexion deformities of the hips which made walking impossible.

correction. Regular prone lying should be encouraged in an attempt to prevent these deformities.

Knees and feet

The principles of management are similar to Duchenne dystrophy (see below). Regular stretching exercises are encouraged. If the tendo Achillis is becoming tight, night splints are provided. Once the deformities occur they should be treated by surgical release.

Friedreich's ataxia and ataxia telangiectasia

This is commonly associated with scoliosis and pes cavus. The scoliosis frequently requires surgical correction to allow comfortable sitting (Fig.

6.14), whereas the cavus may only require treatment if the patient is ambulatory. Ataxia telangiectasia is also frequently associated with scoliosis, which may require surgical correction for comfortable sitting.

Neuropathy

This group includes a variety of conditions. In hypertrophic neuropathy (peroneal muscular atrophy, Charcot–Marie–Tooth syndrome, HMSN type 1), pes cavus is often noted in early childhood before the onset of symptoms. Later, there is involvement of the hand with difficulty in fine manipulation. In the neuronal type of peroneal muscular atrophy (HMSN type 2), there is marked atrophy of muscle and there may be an associated pes cavus. The commonest early symptom is difficulty with walking, but the onset may not be until middle age and the patient may have excelled at sports in his youth. In hypertrophic neuropathy of infancy (Dejerine–Sottos, HMSN type 3), the onset usually is very early in life, with delay in early motor milestones, and walking may only be achieved by the 3rd or 4th year.

Overall, the commonest orthopaedic problem is foot deformity. This may be in the form of pes cavus (Fig. 6.15), but equinus and equino-varus deformities also occur. The latter are treated by soft tissue releases, whereas a significant cavus deformity requires wedge tarsectomy. Scoliosis may also occur in polyneuropathy and the management is similar to that for spinal muscle atrophy.

Sensory neuropathies may present with trophic ulceration (Fig. 6.16).

Duchenne dystrophy

This condition is associated with progressive and rapid increase in weakness, the majority of boys losing the ability to walk independently between the age of 7 and 9 years. Most die in their late teens. Discussion with the parents of boys attending our muscle clinic indicates that there are four main areas of concern where orthopaedic management may help.

Early diagnosis

Many of the parents felt that the diagnosis was missed for months or years. In several instances, they were initially reassured that their son would grow out of his stumbling gait and frequent falls. The diagnosis is

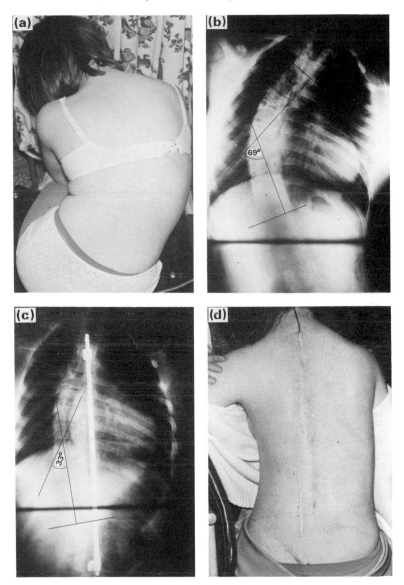

Fig. 6.14. (a) Patient with Friedreich's ataxia. The scoliosis has extended to the pelvis resulting in obliquity. Her complaint was of pain under the right buttock, so that she was unable to sit comfortably for any length of time. (b) The curve measured 69°. (c) Following posterior correction with Harrington instrumentation and bone graft, the curve was reduced to 33°. (d) She developed a pseudarthrosis and required a second exploration with further grafting 6 months later. Following the consolidation of the bone graft, her spine looked clinically straight, her pelvis was horizontal, she was able to sit comfortably for hours and was able to return to her studies.

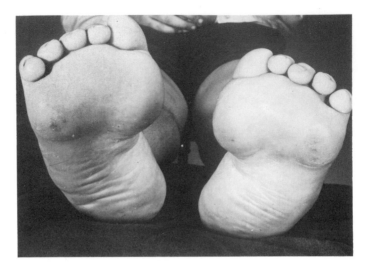

Fig. 6.15. Patient with peroneal muscle atrophy. The patient has developed pes cavus. Note the high arch, the prominent metatarsal heads in the forefoot with the overlying callosities and clawing of the toes. He complained of pain under the forefeet which settled following triple arthrodeses with correction of the deformities.

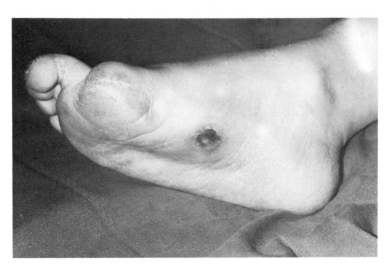

Fig. 6.16. Sensory neuropathy. Note the trophic ulcer on the medial side of the foot. The big toe had been amputated for a previous trophic ulcer that would not heal.

unlikely to be missed if the possibility of muscular dystrophy is considered when a boy is late in walking, is clumsy, or when walking deteriorates. Demonstration of proximal weakness by Gower's sign is especially useful.

Mobilization

Many parents stated that the morale of their son deteriorated significantly when he lost the ability to walk independently. Provision of callipers can maintain weight bearing for an additional 2−4 years (Fig. 6.17). However, the callipers must be fitted before the boy goes off his feet. It is not possible to mobilize a child with Duchenne dystrophy once he is chairbound. Callipers should be prescribed when the child is starting to have difficulty climbing stairs or getting out of a chair (Table 6.1). Once the callipers have been provided, the child uses them for 15−30 minutes each evening and as he starts to go off his feet he gradually becomes more dependent on them.

Frequently, the children cease to be able to walk independently after

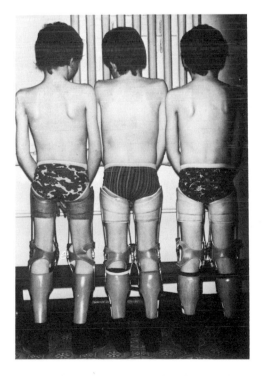

Fig. 6.17. Three brothers with Duchenne dystrophy who have been kept mobile with the use of cosmetic callipers.

they have been confined to bed for an intercurrent illness, following an operation or as a result of injury. In general terms, these children should never be confined to bed. Fractures should be treated by plaster of Paris casts and immediate mobilization. If a child is operated on in the morning he should be stood up with help from the physiotherapist that afternoon. If surgery is carried out in the afternoon, he should be up the following morning.

Not every child nor every family will accept callipers. They slow down the patient and some centres prefer to prescribe a powered chair to allow the boy to keep up with his peers. Learning to use callipers requires a lot of effort, and unless the family will co-operate the child will never succeed.

Scoliosis

This is the most important and most serious deformity that can occur in a child with neuromuscular disease. It is not just a cosmetic deformity but is associated with significant disability. In neuromuscular disease, the scoliosis eventually involves the pelvis and results in an increasing pelvic

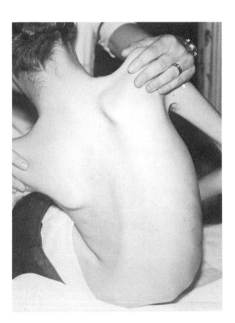

Fig. 6.18. Duchenne dystrophy. This patient has developed gross scoliosis with secondary pelvic obliquity so that when he sits his weight is taken on the lumbar spine. He is unable to sit without support and sitting is extremely uncomfortable.

obliquity. The patient can no longer sit squarely and weight is increasingly taken on one buttock and, as the deformity increases, on the lumbar spine (Fig. 6.18). Sitting becomes uncomfortable and the patient is confined to bed, not because of the underlying neuromuscular disease, but as a result of the progressive scoliosis.

Neuromuscular scoliosis tends to progress more rapidly than idiopathic scoliosis and continues to deteriorate after growth has ceased, perhaps due to the effect of gravity on the weakened trunk musculature. If bracing is used, it must be continued for the remainder of the patient's life.

Table 6.4. Scoliosis in Duchenne dystrophy: curve when patient first presented at muscle clinic.

Age (years)	Curve (degrees)
3	0
$3\frac{1}{2}$	0
4	0—10*
$4\frac{1}{2}$	0
5	0 10*
$5\frac{1}{2}$	0
6	0—15*
$6\frac{1}{2}$	0
7	0
$7\frac{1}{2}$	0
8	10
$8\frac{1}{2}$	7
9	12
$9\frac{1}{2}$	10
10	18
$10\frac{1}{2}$	16
11	10
$11\frac{1}{2}$	10
12	11
$12\frac{1}{2}$	18
13	13
$13\frac{1}{2}$	44
14	85
$14\frac{1}{2}$	79
15	65
$15\frac{1}{2}$	70
16	80
$16\frac{1}{2}$	85
17	100

*One patient.

Secondly, scoliosis is associated with diminished lung function. As the curve deteriorates there is progressive pulmonary insufficiency. Treatment of the scoliosis does not improve lung function but prevents further deterioration due to the progressive deformity.

Prevention

The scoliosis increases with increasing age (Table 6.4). Under the age of 8 years scoliosis is uncommon. This is thought to be due to the lordotic posture adopted by patients who are still mobile (Fig. 6.19). Once the child is confined to a wheelchair, the curve deteriorates rapidly. Provision of callipers not only maintains mobility but also seems to maintain the lordotic posture and shows down the development of scoliosis (Table 6.5). Standing for 2−3 hours per day in the callipers, standing frame or tilt table, even when the patient is no longer mobile, may protect the spine.

Many centres have tried to modify the wheelchair to maintain a lordotic posture (Fig. 6.20). If the back of the chair is made to recline at about 20−25° and is made from soft material that wraps around the trunk,

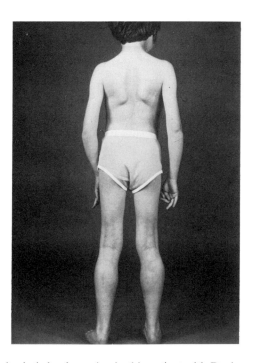

Fig. 6.19. Note the lordotic lumbar spine in this patient with Duchenne dystrophy.

Table 6.5. Scoliosis in Duchenne dystrophy: at $13\frac{1}{2}$ years plus

State of mobility	Curve (degrees)
Confined to wheelchair; no spinal support	68
Confined to chair; modified chair and/or corset	51
Mobile with callipers	7

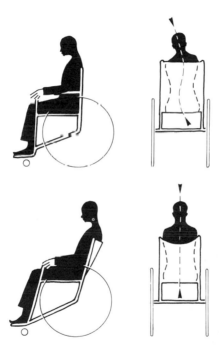

Fig. 6.20. The majority of wheelchairs are made with a straight back. Children with neuromuscular disease tend to lean to the side. This list is aggravated by the effect of gravity on the weak trunk musculature, producing a scoliosis. There is some relationship between the side of the scoliosis and the handedness of the child. If the chair is modified so that the back is reclining and is made of soft material, the patient can lean back against the chair, the fabric wrapping around the trunk and holding it straight. This tends to prevent the development of scoliosis, but the patient is further from his table and work benches, and the environment must be altered so that he can make optimum use of the chair.

when the child leans back against the chair, it will support the spine and hold it straight. However, this design of chair has definite disadvantages. Because the patient is reclining he is further away from his work surfaces both at school and at home. These surfaces need to be raised to his level, but most of the schools for the physically handicapped will not co-operate so that the patient has to lean forwards adopting a kyphotic posture and putting his spine at risk. Secondly, when leaning backwards, the patient is further away from the wheels and finds it more difficult to control the chair manually. The wheels cannot be moved backwards as this will upset the balance of the chair, but this can be obviated by providing a power-driven chair.

In many instances, the arms of the chair are removed to allow the child easier access to the wheels. This results in further lack of support to the trunk, and the child leans to one side, starting the scoliotic process (Fig. 6.21). It is essential that arm rests are fitted to the chair at all times to provide maximum support.

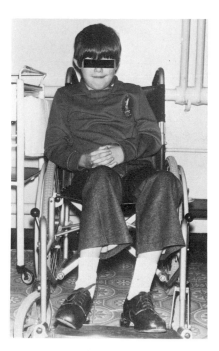

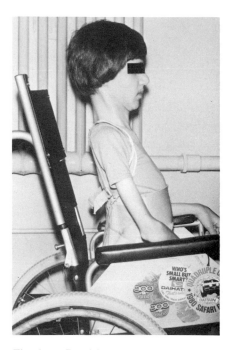

Fig. 6.21. The list to the side is worsened when the arms of the chair are removed, the patient leaning on the wheel of the chair.

Fig. 6.22. Provision of a surgical corset or other forms of spinal support may help maintain the lumbar lordosis.

A variety of corsets and jackets have also been tried (Fig. 6.22). They may slow down the scoliotic process, but do not halt it. There are inherent difficulties with these orthoses. Because the children are sedentary they are more difficult to fit and tend to ride up. If they are too well-fitting, they may interfere with respiration which often is diaphragmatic. Other devices include traction on a neck halter and a suspension jacket that is fixed to the side of the chair.

Treatment

Once the curve has developed, the use of a modified chair, corsets, jackets or braces may slow the progression of the curve if it is less than $30-40°$, but the curve tends to deteriorate rapidly once it is greater than $60-70°$. Moulded chair insets (Fig. 6.23) have been tried, but many children find them uncomfortable.

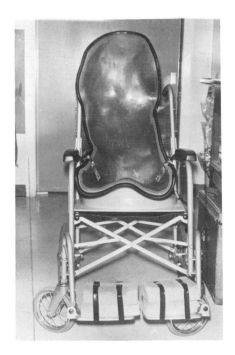

Fig.6.23. Moulded wheelchair. These tend to be more successful in cerebral palsy than in the dystrophies, most of the dystrophy children finding them uncomfortable.

In most neurological disorders, the optimum choice of treatment for a progressive or major curve is surgery. However, in Duchenne dystrophy, by the time the curve warrants surgical correction the patient is no longer fit for surgery because of progressive deterioration in lung function (Fig. 6.24). Therefore, the question of prophylactic surgery has been raised. Is it ethical to stabilize the spine of a child with Duchenne dystrophy, when he is first confined to a chair and when his lung function is adequate for major spinal surgery, but before he has developed a deformity that requires operation, when it is known that such surgery may be associated with a definite albeit small mortality? This question has not yet been settled but in the author's opinion it is an important question in the management of these children, since the development of scoliosis is the most significant factor in their quality of life. A minority of parents stated that they were not keen on 'prophylactic' surgery, yet they were unable to look after their son once he had developed a gross scoliosis. He could not be sat up without support or discomfort. The recent development of the Luque system (Fig. 6.25) (Luque, 1982; Taddinco, 1982) has made 'prophylactic' surgery a much better proposition, and in the author's opinion is now the optimum method of preventing scoliosis in these children. The operation should be carried out shortly after they lose independent mobility, when the curve is 20−30° or less, and when their lung function is adequate for what is a very extensive procedure.

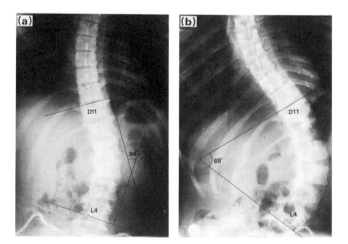

Fig. 6.24. Duchenne dystrophy. (a) When first seen, the scoliosis measured 34°. (b) Nine months later, the curve had deteriorated to 68°. Surgical correction was not possible due to his grossly restricted pulmonary function.

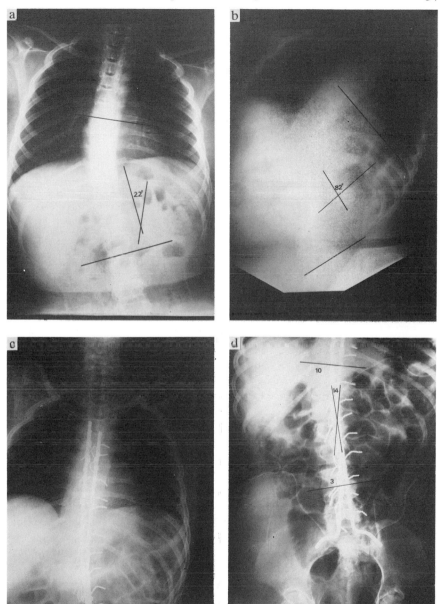

The treatment of the gross curve (Fig. 6.18) is unsatisfactory. Attempts have been made to pad the chair or provide moulded inserts, but these usually fail and the boys may be virtually confined to bed as a result of their progressive deformity.

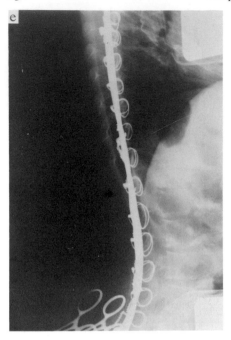

Fig. 6.25. Rapid progression of scoliosis in a boy with Duchenne muscular dystrophy. (a) Curve of 22°. (b) The curve has deteriorated to 82°. (c) and (d) Fortunately he was still fit for surgery. The spine has been stabilized using Luque rods. The curve has been corrected to 14° and the rods have been fixed to the spine, using sublaminal wires from D4 to the pelvis. The stabilization should extend from the upper dorsal spine to either the pelvis or the sacrum. (e) A lumbar lordosis must be moulded into the rods to prevent a 'flat-back', which will interfere with comfortable sitting.

Contractures

Mobile patients

The development of contractures in a mobile patient makes walking even more difficult in a child with inherent muscle weakness (Fig. 6.26) and may make the fitting of callipers impossible.

Contractures should be avoided or minimized by physiotherapy, in the form of daily prone lying and stretching exercises to the knees and ankles. The parents should be taught these exercises so that they can be carried out daily. If the tendo Achillis or hamstrings become tight, night splints should be provided.

Once the contractures have developed, surgical correction should be considered. The commonest is the development of an equinus or equino-varus deformity, which usually can be corrected by simple elongation of the tendo Achillis. The development of flexion contractures of the hips or knees will require release or elongation of the relevant tendons. Where possible, the contractures should be corrected under a single anaesthetic.

All contractures must be corrected before a child is fitted with callipers. If the patient is losing the ability to walk, long leg plaster casts are applied and the patients mobilized in the casts until the callipers are ready.

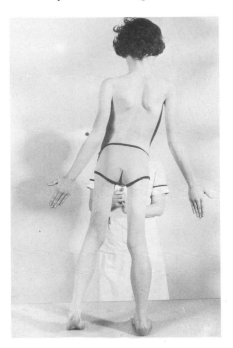

Fig. 6.26. Unilateral equinus in a patient with Duchenne dystrophy. The equinus has affected his balance and gait. Following lengthening of the tendo Achillis, he showed a marked improvement in gait.

Chairbound patients

Most of the contractures develop after the patient has gone off his feet. Flexion contractures of the hips and knees always occur and seem to be of little significance. Flexion of the hip is not associated with dislocation in Duchenne dystrophy and contractures of the hip or knee do not produce symptoms unless attempts are made to correct them forcibly.

On the other hand, deformities of the feet are significant. Progressive equino-varus is associated with pain, which occasionally may be due to a stress fracture of an osteoporotic bone, pressure sores over bony prominences and inability to fit footwear (Fig. 6.27). Attempts have been made to prevent the development of equinus or equino-varus by providing adequate support using foot plates which hold the foot in a slightly dorsiflexed position (Fig. 6.28). Night splints to hold the foot in the neutral or slightly dorsiflexed position and lightweight moulded day splints which fit into the shoes and hold the feet in this position are also useful.

Modification of the foot plates (Fig. 6.28) may make the chair slightly more inconvenient to use and some families do not like them. If this is

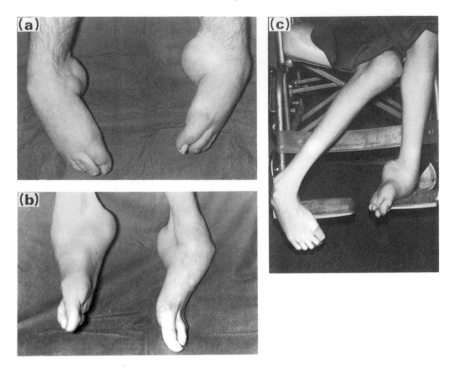

Fig. 6.27. Foot deformity in wheelchair-bound patients with Duchenne dystrophy.
(a) This patient complained of pain as a result of stress fractures affecting both talus
bones. (b) This patient developed localized tenderness over the prominent
talonavicular area with incipient ulceration. (c) The parents were unable to fit
footwear on this patient.

the case, moulded day and night splints should be used. Unfortunately,
some of the boys remove the foot plates completely, so that they can use
their feet to propel the chair. This leads to rapid progression of the deformity and should be avoided by providing powered chairs.

If the deformity is producing symptoms, surgical correction is indicated. Patients whose lung function is inadequate for major spinal
surgery usually have sufficient pulmonary function for foot correction. By
this stage, elongation of the tendo Achillis may not be sufficient and
elongation or transfer of the tibialis posterior tendon with tenotomy of
the tendons of flexor hallucis longus and flexor digitorum longus and a posterior capsulotomy of the ankle joint may be required. Post-operatively,
the limb is immobilized in a below-knee plaster cast until the wounds
have healed, following which splints are worn to prevent a recurrence of
the deformity.

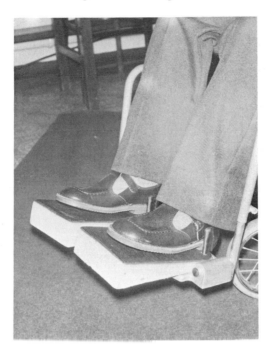

Fig. 6.28. Wedges fitted to the footplate to hold the feet in the neutral or slightly dorsiflexed position.

Other dystrophies, myopathies and atrophies

This section covers a large number of conditions that require orthopaedic management but occur less often than Duchenne dystrophy or spinal muscle atrophy. The orthopaedic problems differ in the different conditions. For example, congenital dystrophy is associated with a very high incidence of scoliosis (Fig. 6.29), hip dislocation and contractures (Fig. 6.30) which may already be present at birth, whereas in scapulo-humeral and facio-scapulo-humeral dystrophy the main problem is abduction of the shoulders (Fig. 6.31). Many of these patients learn trick manoeuvres, but abduction of the shoulders can be helped by stabilizing their scapulae to the chest wall. This minimizes the winging of the scapulae and allows the residual musculature optimum mechanical advantage. Most of the patients with a congenital myopathy are mobile, their commonest deformities being scoliosis (Fig. 6.32) and foot deformities. The principles of treatment are similar to those for spinal muscle atrophy. However, there may be an associated myocardial myopathy.

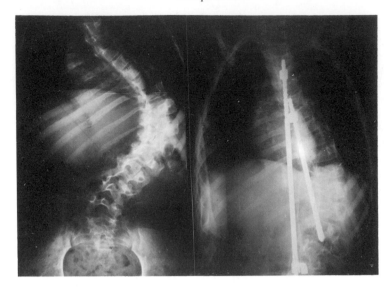

Fig. 6.29. Congenital muscle dystrophy. The curve extended from D7 to L3 and measured 105°. Following posterior fusion with the insertion of two Harrington rods, the curve has been corrected to 55°.

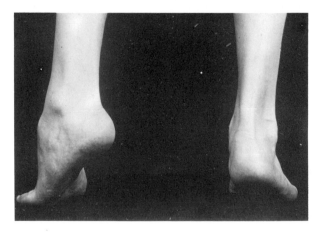

Fig. 6.30. Congenital muscle dystrophy. There is a gross equinus deformity on the left associated with slight varus. On the right there is an equinus deformity. These deformities require surgical correction.

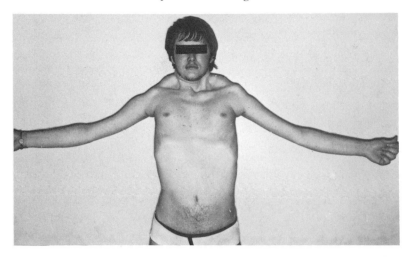

Fig. 6.31. Facio-scapulo-humeral dystrophy. The patient is unable to abduct his shoulders to more than 70°. Note the hypertrophied trapezius muscles. Following the stabilization of his scapula, by fixing it to the chest wall, he was able to abduct beyond 90°.

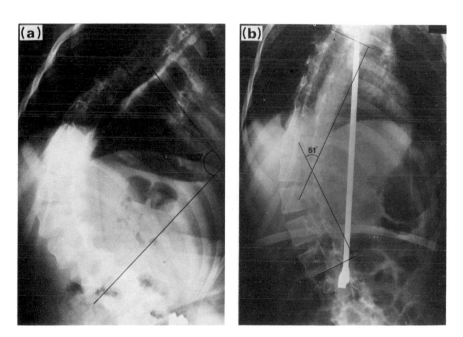

Fig. 6.32. (a) Congenital myopathy. The scoliotic curve extends from D6 to L3 and measured 100°. (b) Following posterior correction with Harrington instrumentation and bone graft, the curve measured 51°.

General discussion

Deformities occur commonly in neurological disorders. They are usually secondary to disorders of posture, movement and tone, and gravitational factors or muscle imbalance, but the incidence and type of deformity vary in the different conditions.

The most significant deformity is scoliosis. Progressive neurological scoliosis produces increasing respiratory insufficiency and involves the pelvis producing pelvic obliquity and difficulty with sitting. Attempts have been made to control the scoliosis by wheelchair design and the use of spinal supports. Unfortunately, in Duchenne dystrophy, once the curve has deteriorated to the degree that surgical correction is required, the patient's pulmonary function will not allow major surgery. This occurs much less frequently in the other neuromuscular conditions. Because the curve continues to deteriorate after growth, the earlier that surgical correction is carried out the better, providing that the vertebrae are sufficiently developed.

Subluxation/dislocation of the hip is the next most significant disorder. It occurs most frequently in cerebral palsy and myelodysplasia, but does occur in other conditions. If it is associated with pelvic obliquity and/or scoliosis, the latter must be corrected first. The treatment differs in flaccid and spastic paralysis. In spastic paralysis the muscles must be balanced by division or transfer of the adductors and release of the ilio-psoas, whereas in flaccid paralysis an ilio-psoas transfer is usually required. In both, secondary bony deformity of the pelvis and/or femur require correction by pelvic and/or upper femoral osteotomy.

Where possible, dislocation should be avoided by night splinting, by the use of a pommel in the chair to prevent adduction of the hip and by surgically correcting progressive subluxation.

Kyphosis is likely to warrant surgical correction only in myelodysplasia, although minor degrees occur in many of the other neurological conditions.

Contractures can occur at any joint. Contractures of the upper limb rarely require surgical correction except in cerebral palsy.

Contractures develop most often in the feet and ankles. The commonest are equinus and equino-varus deformities but any type of deformity can occur. In Duchenne dystrophy, the deformity is usually an equinus or equino-varus; in spinal muscle atrophy, equino-varus or calcaneo-valgus deformities occur. In the other myopathies, the deformity is usually equinus or equino-varus, whereas in peroneal muscular atrophy

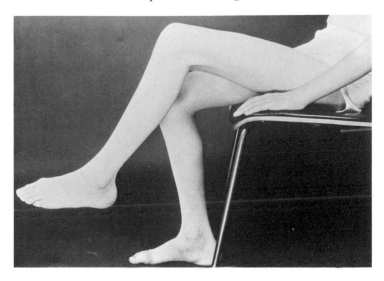

Fig. 6.33. Eighty degrees fixed flexion deformity of the left knee joint. Note the contracted hamstrings. Surgical release of the contracted structures, with gradual extension of the knee in serial plasters, was required to prevent traction on the tibial and common peroneal nerves.

It frequently is a pes cavus. In cerebral palsy, equinus is the commonest deformity but varus and valgus deformities occur. In many conditions, these deformities can be prevented or minimized by physiotherapy and night splints. The latter should be avoided in spina bifida because of the risk of trophic ulceration in the anaesthetic foot.

Contractures of the hip and knees occur less frequently. They always develop in children confined to a wheelchair but under these circumstances rarely produce problems. Regular stretching exercises and prone lying may help prevent their occurrence. If they occur, do not respond to physiotherapy and interfere with gait, surgical correction is indicated (Fig. 6.33).

Finally, it must be emphasized that the orthopaedic management is part of the continuing treatment of these children. This is particularly the case in myelodysplasia and cerebral palsy, but is also true in the other neurological conditions. Isolated orthopaedic surgery is of little value. It must be associated with a careful assessment, pre-operative physiotherapy programme, and detailed post-operative rehabilitation. It forms part of the overall management of the child.

Orthopaedic surgery can do nothing to cure the underlying neurological condition. It is aimed at preventing deformity or correcting it when it does occur. Major reconstruction surgery in these patients should not be undertaken purely for cosmetic reasons. It should be done to aid mobility, alleviate discomfort and improve the quality of life of these children.

Our technique of spinal stabilization has altered during the past 2—3 years. We now rarely use Harrington instrumentation in neuromuscular scoliosis, but usually use a modified Luque technique (Fig. 6.25), supplemented by anterior correction and stabilization when indicated. The advantage of the multiple level sublaminal wire fixation is that it obviates the need for a post-operative plaster of Paris jacket.

Acknowledgements

I am grateful to the Department of Medical Illustration, Royal Manchester Children's Hospital, for the illustrations, and to Mr M. McMaster, Edinburgh, for Fig. 6.10.

References and further reading

Bleck, E.E. (1979) *Orthopaedic Management of Cerebral Palsy.* W.B. Saunders, Philadelphia.

Breed, A.L. & Ibler, I. (1982) The motorized wheelchair: new freedom, new responsibility and new problems. *Developmental Medicine and Child Neurology*, **24**, 366—371.

Bobath, B. (1967) The very early treatment of cerebral palsy. *Developmental Medicine and Child Neurology*, **9**, 373—390.

Dickson, R.A. (1983) Scoliosis in the community. *British Medical Journal*, **286**, 615—618.

Drennan, J.C. (1983) *Orthopaedic Management of Neuromuscular Disorders.* Lippincott, New York.

Fulford, G.E. & Brown J.K. (1976) Position as a cause of deformity in children with cerebral palsy. *Developmental Medicine and Child Neurology*, **18**, 305—314.

Fulford, G.E., Cairns, T.P. & Sloan, Y. (1982) Sitting problems of children with cerebral palsy. *Developmental Medicine and Child Neurology*, **24**, 48—53.

Jones, M. (1982) *Serial Splinting in Hemiplegic Cerebral Palsy.* Association of Paediatric Chartered Physiotherapists, London.

Luque, E.R. (1982) The anatomic basis and development of segmental spinal instrumentation. *Spine*, **7**, 256—259.

Nichel, V.L. (1982) *Orthopaedic Rehabilitation.* Churchill Livingstone, Edinburgh.

Pollock, G.A. & Stark, G. (1969) Long-term results in the management of 67 children with cerebral palsy. *Developmental Medicine and Child Neurology*, **1**, 279—287.

Rang, M., Douglas, G., Bennet, G.C. & Koreska, J. (1981) Seating for children with cerebral palsy. *Journal of Pediatric Orthopedics*, **1**, 279—287

Samilson, R.L. (1975) Orthopaedic aspects of cerebral palsy. *Clinics in Developmental Medicine*, **52/53**. S.I.M.P., Heinemann, London.

Sandifer, P.H. (1967) *Neurology in Orthopaedics.* Butterworths, London.

Schultz-Hurlburt, B. & Tervo, R.C. (1982) Wheelchair users at a children's rehabilitation center: attributes and management. *Developmental Medicine and Child Neurology*, **24**, 54–60.

Staheli, L.T. (1983) Orthopaedics in adolescence. *Developmental Medicine and Child Neurology*, **25**, 806–818.

Taddinco, R.F. (1982) Segmental spinal instrumentation in the management of neuromuscular spinal deformity. *Spine*, **7**, 305–311.

Williams, P.F. (1982) *Orthopaedic Management in Childhood*. Blackwell Scientific, Oxford.

Chapter 7
Rehabilitation Engineering

Nigel Ring

A definition

Rehabilitation engineering may be defined as 'the application of engineering technology to the habilitation or rehabilitation of the handicapped person'. Thus, rehabilitation engineering includes such diverse activities as the management of incontinence, mobility, communication, assistance with employment, and the prevention of pressure sores.

The role of the rehabilitation engineer

The key to any successful programme of rehabilitation is team-work. Thus, the role of the rehabilitation engineer is to work within a team alongside doctors, therapists, nurses, psychologists and social workers. His contribution will, inevitably, vary from case to case. However, his particular expertise may be relevant at various stages. In assessment, he may help quantify the current status of the patient; in training, he may provide or modify equipment that allows particular functions to be developed; in treatment, he may provide equipment to supplement or complement natural body functions or to allow an increased level of independence to be achieved.

His involvement in the team is vital, since it is only when he has a personal appreciation of the problem faced by the patient, whether physical, mental or social, that he is able to contribute effectively to improving the situation. If he is held 'in the wings', only being involved when the others have decided upon the course of rehabilitation to be adopted, his usefulness is restricted by the interpretation of the problem as seen through the eyes of those who have only limited technological knowledge. If, however, he is recognized as a full member of the clinical team, the programme of rehabilitation can be prescribed, if appropriate, to include the application of, say, microelectronics or modern materials. Naturally, not all patients should be exposed to the latest technological advances, but each should have the opportunity, if appropriate.

The other benefit of his close involvement in the team is to ensure that his 'feet are kept on the ground'. An engineering approach often centres on the fulfilment of a functional requirement, the satisfaction of a performance specification. However, important as this is in rehabilitation, such an approach does not represent the whole picture. The method of interfacing equipment to the child, the ability to present equipment in a way that is aesthetically pleasing, and the necessity of obtaining the user's confidence are all aspects that must be considered by the engineer at the outset. Ultimate success depends upon the person's willingness to use the equipment. If the item of equipment lives in the 'cupboard under the stairs' it can hardly be called 'successful', however elegant the engineer might consider his design to be.

The criteria for success

There are five factors: function, reliability, weight, cost and cosmesis.

Function

Through discussion between clinical personnel, the patient and his escorts, such as parents, some functional specification must be agreed. It is almost inevitable that compromises will have to be imposed and the engineer should alert his colleagues to these at an early stage. For instance, a wheelchair that has to be stowed in the boot of a car must not be so heavy or unwieldly that an escort cannot lift it. Once the final design has been agreed and the equipment built, it is the engineer's responsibility to ensure that it meets the functional specification and that the patient can interact with it in an appropriate way.

Reliability

We have all experienced the frustration of a car that will not start in cold weather. For a handicapped person who relies on a piece of apparatus, the frustration of unreliability is even greater. Unfortunately, equipment that is produced in small quantities (as is inevitable in rehabilitation) can rarely undergo exhaustive reliability and acceptance tests, due to economic restraints. Thus, unreliability must always be a possibility. To counter this, the engineer must ensure satisfactory service back-up at a level that is appropriate to the patient's dependency on the equipment.

Weight

By definition, apparatus used in the rehabilitation field has a close involvement with human beings. Frequently, the item of equipment is worn
on the body or has to be carried by the user or a third party. Under such
circumstances, weight is a vital consideration, and the possible cost
penalty of incorporating appropriate light weight materials may be a small
consideration in comparison with the energy saving for the user.

Cost

Cost is a topic that the engineer, probably more than any of his clinical
colleagues, is best equipped to monitor. Frequently in health care, especially in a nationalized health system, economic considerations do not
receive a great deal of attention in the prescription process: particularly,
the high cost of labour may be overlooked. Through his training, the
engineer should have a good appreciation of cost factors, and may frequently be able to demonstrate how an apparently expensive item of
equipment may be justified economically if set against, say, the saving of
a therapist's time. Further reference will be made to this in the consideration of bio-feedback training. Also, an apparently cheap piece of apparatus, judged by its simplicity, may be uneconomic to produce if a therapist
has to spend many hours making it. An example of this may be seen in
many therapy departments, where simple aids and orthoses are made by
the therapists themselves to save purchasing off-the-shelf items.

Cosmesis

Reference has already been made to appearance and its role in contri-
buting to acceptance of the device by the patient. Cosmesis or appearance
may be considered under two headings: static and dynamic. An artificial
arm wearer may, for instance, use his prosthesis purely as a sleeve filler,
in which case he is most concerned about the static appearance and
texture of the artificial hand and fingers. If, however, he requires a
functional arm, operation may require gross shoulder movements (to
operate the control cables) which, being unnatural, make him conspicuous
in public. Under such circumstances, the functional effectiveness of the
hand takes priority over the social response that the user receives.

Provision of service

Health care is full of examples of equipment that have been the brain-children of individuals but have never been widely applied. One only has to consider the number of surgical tools or items of orthotic equipment that carry individuals' names and are used only locally, and compare these with essentially similar items used elsewhere under other names, to realize the truth of this statement. One of the most important roles of the rehabilitation engineer is to evaluate the approach, if novel, that he and his colleagues have adopted and to ensure its widespread application, if appropriate. This may involve the creation of a clinical service, the negotiation with manufacturers for production, or the arrangement of marketing and publicity procedures, to name a few alternatives. However, it is the engineer's responsibility to ensure that appropriate steps are taken to maximize the effectiveness of his approach. Failure to do so represents both an inefficient use of professional time and a moral irresponsibility to the disabled population.

In dealing with the topics listed below, the discussion will focus on principles rather than detail. The topics to be considered are: (i) mobility (ii) seating, (iii) communication, (iv) bio-feedback training, (v) orthotics and (vi) aids to daily living.

Mobility

The importance of independent mobility can hardly be overstressed. It is vital to ensure that any child has the ability to move himself between two locations of his own choice at the time he chooses if his ability to investigate and mature are not to be severely restricted. However, frequently this independence is not given sufficient priority compared with other aspects of his rehabilitation programme, it being easier to put him in a wheelchair and push him around according to functional need or an adult's convenience. The resulting lack of independence does not limit only his mobility. It also severely restricts his ability to learn about the relative positions of objects, the shape of space (i.e. by guiding himself through a doorway) and so on, which also has an effect on his hand-eye co-ordination. Further, his lack of ability to investigate may limit the development of communication, since it prevents the constant stimulus of new discoveries which lead to questioning and description. Thus, attempts should be made to provide some means of independent mobility at all ages and stages of development under as wide a range of situations as possible.

Throughout this section, attention will be paid only to wheeled mobility. Mobility provided by artificial legs has very limited application for the group of children being considered and the contribution of orthoses is considered later.

Categories of wheeled vehicles

The variety of wheeled vehicles is extremely wide. To the range of traditional wheelchairs (both self-propelled and electrically powered) must be added tricycles, saddle-walkers, various toys, prone trolleys and walking aids.

One decision to be faced at an early stage is the dilemma between self-propulsion and the use of external power. This decision should not be based purely on either the child's physical disability or economics. Provision of external power at an early age may allow ranges of travel and independence to be achieved that permit his personality to develop; if delayed, he may never retrieve the ground that is lost. The insistence upon self-propulsion to help build up arm and trunk muscles for, say, a spina bifida child must be balanced against the losses that may occur as a result of the very slow propulsion this opinion would cause. The ideal may be formal exercises, together with some combination of vehicle encompassing external power, self-propulsion and attendant operation. However, the range of vehicles to achieve this is likely to be both inconvenient and uneconomical.

In prescribing a particular mode of transport to satisfy the needs of a child the clinician should be aware of the child's physical ability, the likely progression of his condition and mobility needs, and of any external constraints, such as the home or school environment. Consider, as an example, the spina bifida child. His first vehicle should be available as soon as he has sitting balance and could be one of the small go-carts, such as the Chailey Go-cart (Fig. 7.1). He can then progress through the range of conventional wheelchairs until he reaches adulthood. Each must, of course, be matched to his particular needs, taking account not only of his physical dimensions but also of any protection that may be required to accommodate a spinal deformity, of any padding to protect his anaesthetic skin, and of any incontinence device he may be wearing.

In the event of the spina bifida child requiring to be prone (e.g. because of a decubitus ulcer or of spinal surgery) he should not be confined to bed. Provision of a self-propelled prone-trolley (Fig. 7.2) can maintain his independence and motivation, at least in an institutional environment where this larger vehicle can be accommodated.

The approach for a cerebral palsy child may be totally different. Depending on which end of the spastic-athetoid scale he lies, in terms of

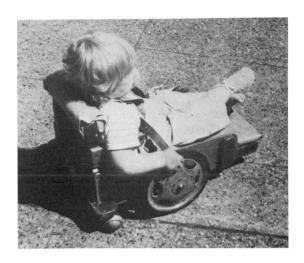

Fig. 7.1. The Chailey Go-cart provides self-propelled mobility for the young child.

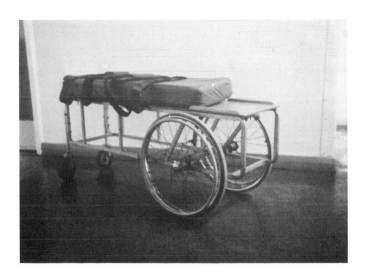

Fig. 7.2. A prone-trolley which is self-propelled retains independent mobility, e.g. post-operatively.

his limb and postural control, he may require minimal modification to a conventional tricycle or the construction of a sophisticated 'special'. The 'minimal modification' could be the addition of foot plates, perhaps with a side-steel to reduce plantar flexion (Fig. 7.3). The 'special' may be a prone-tricycle (Fig. 7.4) such as that developed at the Ontario Crippled Children's Center, in which the child rides prone with his hands centralized on the steering tiller and his feet harnessed to direct drive pedals.

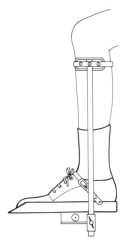

Fig. 7.3. A replacement tricycle pedal, with side steel, to control plantar flexion.

Psychologically, upright mobility may be advantageous and, for the athetoid child, the Chailey Walker (Fig. 7.5) is an example of a walking aid that gives partial support by load-bearing on the pectoralis muscles while allowing the poorly co-ordinated leg movement to provide propulsion.

Finally, brief mention was made above to the use of toys. Wherever possible, toys should be used since they provide a level of normality for the child which no wheelchair can ever achieve. The use of a tricycle has already been mentioned. However, it is sometimes possible to use ride-on toys or the like, especially for the young child.

Seating

At the beginning of the 1970s, comparatively little was known about the seating requirements of disabled people. Frequently, a severely disabled individual sat in a wheelchair supported by a variety of cushions, bandages, straps and so on. Within one decade, the importance of good

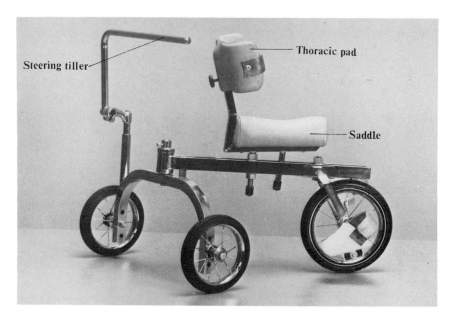

Fig. 7.4. Prone tricycle for athetoid children.

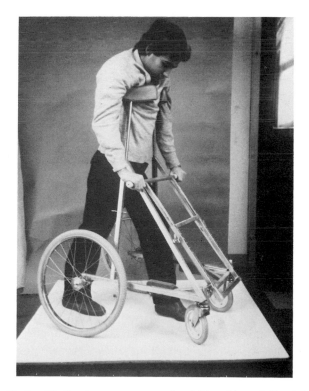

Fig. 7.5. The Chailey Walker increases postural stability without full weight relief.

seating not only became recognized but also resulted in a wide variety of products and techniques becoming available to satisfy individual needs. Why should this be?

The need for suitable seating may be encountered in a variety of situations. For instance, an ulcer may develop over the ischial tuberosity or sacrum as a result of prolonged sitting in one position. Pressure and underlying tissue shear must be relieved if healing is to be effected. Again, a speech-impaired individual may find it necessary to use a piece of equipment, such as a typewriter, in order to communicate. However, this can be achieved satisfactorily only if he is in a good position to use the keys and observe the typed output. Lack of suitable seating may seriously affect an individual's ability to lead his life to its maximum potential.

The purpose of special seating

There are four factors which may contribute to the need for special seating: (i) pressure relief, (ii) postural support, (iii) comfort and (iv) function. Clearly, there are many situations in which more than one of these factors may apply and the social requirements may also contribute to the total need.

In considering how to satisfy these functional needs, the clinical team must be clear that there is no unique solution that can be applied universally. The successful outcome depends largely upon the careful assessment and prescription of particular seating and this assessment takes time. The interaction between the child and an inanimate object always introduces potential danger points and this is critically true of a seat, especially when the person is paraplegic.

The reader is directed to the list of references for a more comprehensive discussion of the various aspects. Only general approaches and examples of different principles will be considered here.

Types of seating

In assessing a patient it is helpful to be aware of the possible seating systems which may be adopted. Figure 7.6 indicates the purposes for which different cushions and seating systems may be prescribed.

All systems contribute to improved comfort. The choice between a cushioning system and a supportive system is usually between the need for pressure control alone and the need for postural support with pressure control available. Also, since cushioning allows greater postural freedom

System	Application	Varieties/features
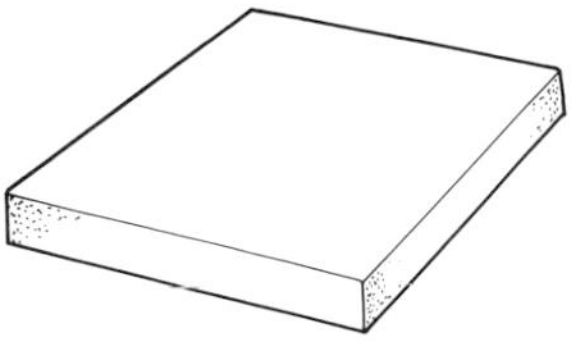	1. Comfort 2. Pressure distribution	1. Foam 2. Fluid filled (air, water etc.)
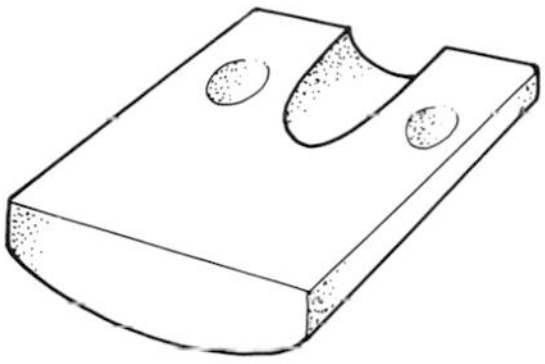	1. Comfort 2. Pressure relief 3. Pelvic support	1. Variable densities 2. Cut-away sections to relieve sacrum and ischial tuberosities. 3. Shaped to fit wheel-chair seat.
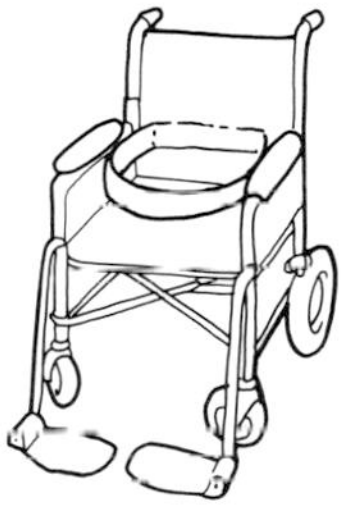	1. Comfort 2. Postural support 3. Functional positioning 4. Constraint of spasm	1. Bespoke 2. Lateral support pads. (alternative)
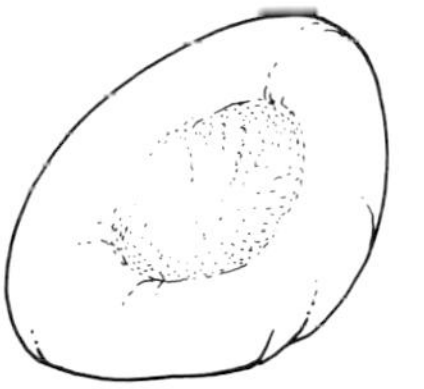	1. Comfort 2. Postural support	1. Single or multi compartment bags containing expanded polystyrene beads.
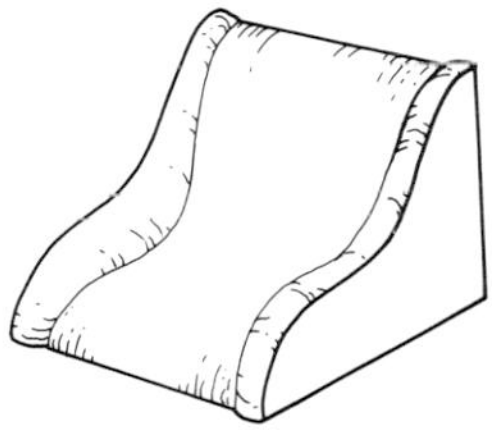	1. Comfort 2. Postural support 3. Pressure distribution or relief.	1. Bespoke. Often using timber and foam plastic.
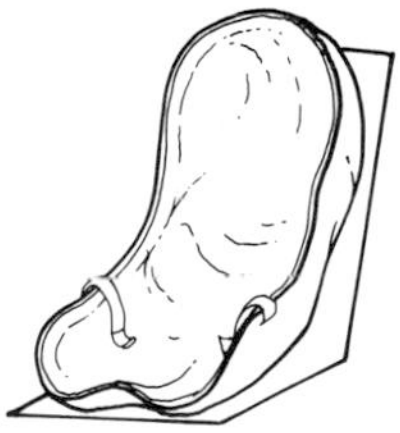	1. Comfort 2. Intimate postural support. 3. Specific pressure distribution-relief	1. Bespoke. Usually foam lined with semi-rigid plastic shell.

Fig. 7.6. Chart showing different seating requirements and solutions.

than other systems, it allows a correspondingly lower likelihood of the development of hip and knee flexion contractures.

The properties available from different cushions vary widely. Simple upholstery foam is suitable for general purpose comfort, provided the quality of the skin and underlying tissue is good. However, the cover may introduce a hammocking effect and cause localized pressure concentrations under the bony prominences.

More sophisticated cushions may be fluid-filled, to equalize pressure, or even have compartments that may be inflated to different air pressures, thus providing greater control of the pressures applied to different parts of the buttocks and thighs. One cushion, the Roho, achieves this with a matrix of inflatable pods which have a low transverse stiffness and thus reduce the shear forces on the underlying tissue (Fig. 7.7).

Where some postural support is a major requirement, the options range from a light harness to an intimate moulded seat, such as the Chailey Moulded Seat. Once again, careful assessment is essential in order to ensure that sufficient support is provided without imposing unnecessary restrictions of movement. The methods of manufacture of these seats are indicated in the references. The range of techniques available allows control of posture from minimal (for, say, the early stages of a degenerative neuromuscular condition) to highly supportive (such as may be needed to contain severe involuntary spasm).

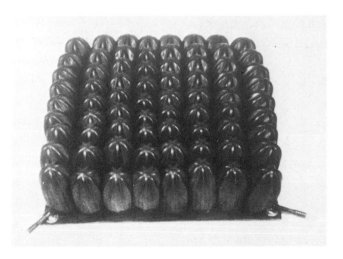

Fig. 7.7. The Roho cushion provides even pressure distribution and low shear forces across the supporting surface.

Assessment and prescription

The ultimate success of any system is determined at the assessment and prescription stages of treatment. Thus, it is important to allow sufficient time and have available appropriate facilities to give a thorough assessment. If either is not available the child should be referred to a specialist centre.

In 'extreme' cases, assessment should include an estimate of joint range and mobility, an inspection of skin quality in the vulnerable areas, examination of the spine, measurement of respiratory function, and so on. Detailed discussion must also take place about the manner of life that the child leads, such as the method of transport to school, use of wheelchair at home and school, and activities and hobbies which he may pursue. Some simple devices are available for use both during these assessments and at the fitting stage. In particular, simple inflatable pressure transducers are a 'must' for locating the high pressure areas and ensuring that pressure relief has been achieved by the seat.

If a postural support is prescribed, it may be necessary to take a cast of the child. This is best achieved using vacuum casting techniques widely used in the orthopaedic field. This achieves a negative impression of the child's shape while sitting fully clothed in the recommended posture and attitude.

Conclusion

The provision of suitable seating represents the foundation of much rehabilitation therapy and education. Accordingly, it is important that the provision of seating is given sufficient priority at an early stage in the rehabilitation process for children who are susceptible to pressure sores, or who have difficulties with postural control or associated manual functions.

Communication

The ability to speak is taken for granted by the vast majority of the population. For many, their only encounter with someone with speech impairment may come through contact with a 'stroke' patient. Nevertheless, tens of thousands of children have severely impaired speech to the extent of its being unsuitable as a means of communication. Undoubtedly the largest group are those with cerebral palsy.

The problem of communication and some of the alternative systems to speech that are available are discussed in Chapter 9. They include hand sign systems (Amer-Ind, British Sign Language, the Makaton Vocabulary and the Paget–Gorman Sign System) and symbol systems (Blissymbolics). The purpose of this section is to demonstrate how technology can be applied to assist communication, either in conjunction with some of the above alternatives, or through more socially acceptable means such as synthetic speech.

Speed
In order to identify the contribution that technology can make, it is important to compare the speeds of various forms of communication. Compared to speeds in excess of 150 words per minute for speech, the alternatives are very slow. Comparable figures, simplified for the sake of clarity, are: copy-typing 50–60 w.p.m.; typing (expressive mode) 10–18 w.p.m.; handwriting (expressive) 23 w.p.m. These figures are quoted from particular studies and the reader should refer to Foulds (1980) for details of the experimental conditions. All were conducted with able-bodied subjects. If we now consider a disabled person using one of the alternatives quoted above, speeds of perhaps 10 w.p.m. would be common. Such speeds would reflect both the limitation of the system and, to a greater extent, the severity of handicap of the individual. Nevertheless, even these speeds may seem rapid in comparison with some of the alternatives offered by technology.

Clearly, it is dangerous to generalize a very diverse population and range of options into a few short sentences, and then to draw conclusions. Nevertheless, technology is frequently a second-best option to some simpler form of communication, such as pencil and paper, and it should be clearly understood what contribution it will make before a particular item of equipment is prescribed. Despite that, however, there are many situations where a technological solution is the only viable one and accordingly is worthy of attention.

The I–S–D–O chain
Communication using technology may include up to four links in the chain between 'speaker' and 'hearer': (i) input, (ii) selector, (iii) display and (iv) output. Since each of these may contribute a short delay to the communication process, it is important that each component is carefully

considered in the context of a particular user's needs. Thus, the most vital step is, once again, the careful assessment of the user and this will be considered before the above categories are discussed in greater depth.

Assessment

Initially, the child must be assessed for his ability to understand language and to use it meaningfully. The process, which is typically carried out by a speech therapist, is described in Chapter 9. Once a system of communication has been prescribed, a further assessment must be carried out on the child to examine his physical ability. This is particularly important if the system prescribed may contain a technological component. This second assessment may include a physical examination similar to that used for seating, since postural control and position must be the first consideration in achieving a relationship between the child and his equipment. A record will also be made of his ability to control his head, hands, feet and eyes, since each of these has potential as a part of the body that may be used for interacting with the equipment.

In order to carry out the assessment, certain simple aids are useful. For instance, assessment of a child's ability to hold a gaze is best carried out using a piece of clear plastic on which a grid is drawn (Fig. 7.8). The assessor can then draw pictures or letters in the squares and, by viewing the child through the plastic, assess the child's ability to look at various squares, as directed.

For fine control, such as may be required to operate a key-board of switches, it is necessary to assess (i) range of motion of fingers, (ii) independence of finger control and (iii) strength. Various spring-loaded lever gauges are available for this purpose. For total arm movements, where a child may be able to make only gross movements, a series of grids may once again be used (Fig. 7.9). These grids, having different pitches, allow the accuracy and range of motion to be assessed and may well help the assessor to choose between direct access to, say, a letter-board, and indirect access through a series of carefully positioned switches or inputs.

Inputs

The first link in the I−S−D−O chain, the user input or interface, is in many ways the most important part of the prescription. Since this is the one point of contact between the child and the equipment, it is essential

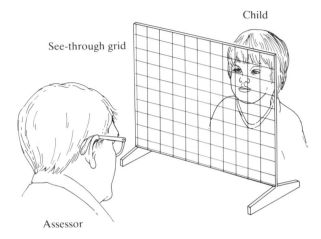

Fig. 7.8. Grid for assessing eye-gaze.

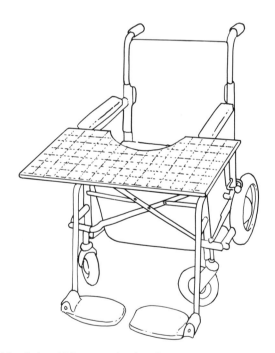

Fig. 7.9. Variable pitch grid for assessing hand control.

that it matches his abilities closely. From the assessment, knowledge will have been gained about his ability to control various body parts, the force he is able to apply, the speed at which he can move with accuracy, and so on. The input must be designed to optimize all these abilities and thus give the child the closest possible relationship with the equipment to the extent that he can, hopefully, view his communication system as an extension to his body and personality.

The interface may be either active or passive. One example of a passive interface is a head-pointer (Fig. 7.10) which allows head move-

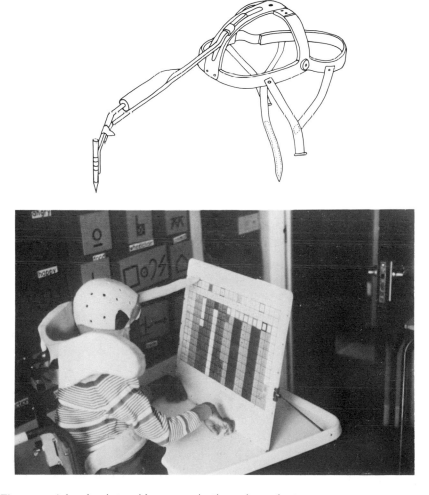

Fig. 7.10. A head-pointer aids communication using a chart.

ments to be used effectively to indicate a display or to operate a device. An active interface is, typically, one or more electric switches that operate an electrically powered piece of equipment. The choice of such an interface is frequently personal, since a child requiring technological assistance is unlikely to operate a standard input. The particular features to be considered when choosing an active interface are (i) the number of switches, (ii) the location of each switch and (iii) the force/excursion required for operation. The results of the assessment will help in making this choice. The range of switches that may be used is immense.

The role of the interface is not only as a means of transforming information from the user to the equipment. It is also a channel through which information may be fed back to the user about performance (Ring, 1977). Under such circumstances, the input provides a degree of 'feel', as for instance the steering wheel of a car provides information about the direction of the road wheels. Inclusion of this information enhances performance, since the user not only relies on his visual and auditory channels to monitor performance but also uses his tactile sense and proprioception.

Selector

The next link in the chain may be the selector. For instance, if a child can operate only one input switch and wishes to use a typewriter, it becomes necessary to use a scanning system in order to locate the particular letter (Fig. 7.11). When a switch is depressed an illuminated square scans through the alphabet until the desired letter is reached. Release then causes the typewriter to be activated. Thus, a time sequence has to be introduced to enable the child to anticipate the moment at which his letter will be available. This time is, of course, small compared to the total time required, and thus the selector makes the communication process extremely tedious, rates of only one word per minute being common.

Display

The selector may itself fulfil the role of the display, that part of the system which is observed by the third party. However, there are also occasions when the selector is personal to the child and the display is available for group use, enabling him to communicate in a group.

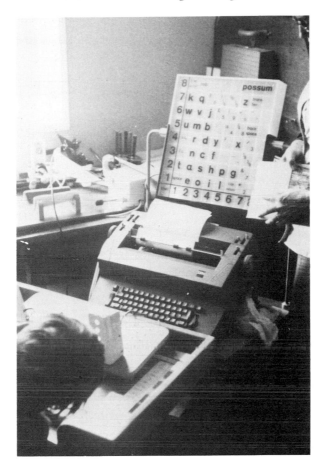

Fig. 7.11. A scanning board is used to produce a typewritten output from a small number of switches.

Output

The output is the final stage in the chain, whether typewritten script, final display or synthesized speech. It may be operated directly from the input (*viz.* a typewriter) or it may require the intermediate step of a selector and/or display, such as with the scanning selector already described.

Choice of equipment

The range of equipment available is already large and is rapidly increasing as microelectronics make an increasing impact. There is also a wide price range from a few pounds to several thousands of pounds. Thus, the recent development of Communication Centres is welcome and, where possible, assessment and prescription should be carried out in collaboration with such a centre.

The reader is referred to the Department of Health, London, or the International Project on Communication Aids for the Speech-Impaired, 25 Mortimer Street, London, for more detailed information. However, by way of example, a small range of approaches will be considered.

Alpha-numerics

One simple approach is through a display that shows the letters of the alphabet and selected words. This simple and cheap method of communication may be enhanced, at a price, by using a display board that contains electric switches. These are used to send a signal to a box of electronics and cause the selected letter or word to be displayed on a television screen or typewriter, such as with SPLINK (Fig. 7.12).

Pictographs

Selection of individual letters and words from a grid has severe limitations of speed and range of vocabulary, since each word requires on average five letters and the total number of words is limited by the size of the display board. One way of improving this situation is to use pictographs, such as Blissymbols. These are described in greater detail in Chapter 9. However, since each symbol conveys an idea or concept that is enhanced by or interpreted in the context of other symbols, the content of the communication is larger for each selection made than is the case with letters and words. Once again, direct selection by pointing to a grid is most rapid but, if this is impossible, the use of technology can allow the symbol to be selected by a coded input through a small number of switches, the output being, say, on a television screen or printer.

Synthetic speech

One of the many advantages of speech is the ability to communicate at a distance, or to a group. Thus, synthetic speech is an attractive option which should be considered. Currently, this is available only at an appreciable cost, but it is likely that prices will fall. Operation of a voice synthesizer may be either by direct selection (the words being printed on

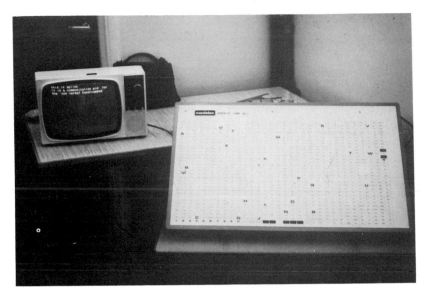

Fig 7.12. SPLINK (SPeech LINK) allows two or more people to communicate by using a touch sensitive board to put text on a TV screen.

the keys) or by a coded input. Also, complete sentences may be stored for recall and some intonation may be included.

Conclusion

Until recently, the severely speech-impaired were largely a 'forgotten' population. However, with the current technological revolution and the recent development of various alternative systems of communication, they can now face the future with greater confidence and optimism that their impairment will no longer isolate them totally from society.

Bio-feedback training

Much therapy for children with cerebral palsy and spina bifida is directed towards improving mobility and posture, each of which requires a continuous but unconscious monitoring of the positions of different parts of the body, such as head, trunk and limbs. However, the primary condition does, by its nature, imply some impairment of the normal proprioceptive mechanisms and/or their related neurological networks. Thus, through therapy, attempts are made to train the child to use control and monitoring procedures that differ from those normally associated with a given task or activity.

The person who has normal sensory mechanisms takes corrective action if the monitored information does not match his desired performance. For instance, when standing upright one does not overbalance because the balance mechanisms detect accelerations which indicate motion and initiate appropriate corrective action. However, when the sensory feedback mechanism is impaired, the appropriate correction does not take place. This is perhaps seen most dramatically in a child with athetoid cerebral palsy whose posture is rarely upright and whose limb movements are unco-ordinated. The purpose of bio-feedback training is to use an augmentative system to provide feedback that is readily recognizable and upon which the child can rely to help him make the necessary correction.

Augmented sensory feedback
Bio-feedback is frequently associated with the voluntary control of such functions as heart rate and galvanic response of the skin. However, the approach described here has little to do with such techniques and, following the work of Herman (1974), the term 'augmented sensory feedback' (ASF) is deemed more appropriate.

It has been shown in the fields of ergonomics and experimental psychology that man—machine operation is impaired if the delay between input and response exceeds 40 milliseconds. However, the operator is unaware of any delay at a conscious level until 70—100 milliseconds have elapsed. Thus, for the child who has poor head control, verbal correction to 'hold his head up' is inevitably received too late for him to reverse the signal that caused the incorrect response.

ASF provides additional information about the body's performance that can be readily interpreted by the child. For instance, if the head attitude is monitored continuously and the information presented virtually instantaneously in an easily recognized form, such as an audible tone whose frequency varies with angle of deviation, corrective action can be taken as soon as the tone indicates an unacceptable head angle.

Application
The apparatus to achieve ASF is generally simple, and can readily be accepted as an additional tool to support the physiotherapist's training programme. Typical applications include (i) head position training, as already quoted, (ii) balance, by monitoring the position of the centre of gravity of the body, (iii) identification and training of residual muscles

through electromyographic techniques and (iv) gait training, by monitoring the load applied to a limb and knee angle.

ASF may be used at various stages of rehabilitation. In assessment, it may help to indicate whether the ability to control particular muscles or make gross voluntary movements exists. In training, it may allow a child to learn what movements are required of him and whether any residual sensory feedback exists which can be used to monitor these movements. ASF may also be used as a 'prosthetic' feedback device which, like an artificial limb, provides on-going support to replace a deficit.

Second, the engineering aspects of the technique vary from extreme simplicity to sophisticated electronics. For example, if knee angle is of interest in teaching a spastic child to walk, a lightweight goniometer may be strapped to the knee as a transducer. The signal could be displayed in a variety of forms, but an auditory signal is frequently used since one's hearing readily detects change and is not normally used a great deal for other purposes during locomotion. The most efficient means of presenting the information to the child, e.g. through the visual, auditory or tactile senses, is a complex subject that has been widely researched in other applications. The ultimate choice, however, may well be decided by practical rather than theoretical considerations, such as the portability of the hardware.

Third, the technique should be seen as complementary rather than supplementary to traditional therapy. Used appropriately, it can significantly increase the rate of improvement in performance and the level of performance attained. Correctly chosen equipment can also be used to monitor progress automatically, thus freeing the therapist from being continuously with the patient.

Orthotics

Orthoses, those external supports which, when worn on the body, assist or resist residual body motions or replace impaired functions, are commonplace in any paediatric clinic at which neurologically impaired children are treated. They may be seen in various forms. For the spina bifida child, the orthosis may encompass all the major joints of both lower limbs, a bilateral hip−knee−ankle orthosis (HKAO) being the prescribed appliance. Children with spinal muscular atrophy may require spinal support, the thoraco-lumbar-sacral orthosis (TLSO). Children with cerebral palsy are frequently the recipients of ankle−foot orthoses (AFO).

Orthoses are available in many forms and, as with all aspects of prescription, careful assessment must be the starting point. It is essential

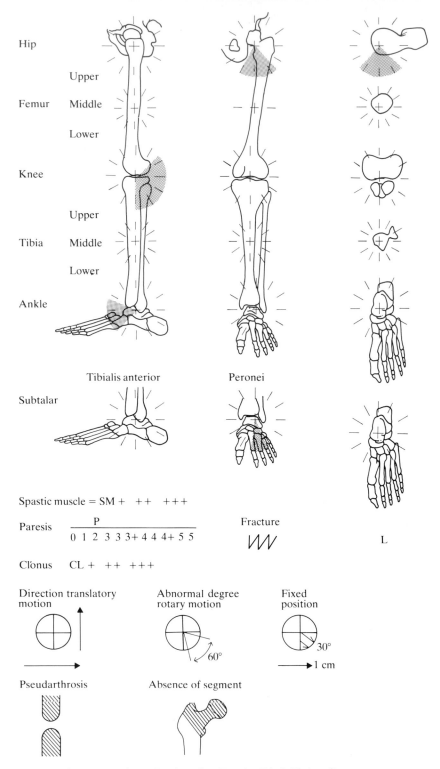

Fig. 7.13. Assessment form developed at Dundee Limb Fitting Centre.

that the individual child is carefully assessed and that his current status is accurately recorded. Each clinic has its own procedure and method of recording. Frequently, this involves the use of a diagram such as that used in Dundee, based on work carried out in the United States by the American Academy of Orthopedic Surgeons (Fig. 7.13). Such a chart quantifies variables, such as range of motion, in a way that allows good records to be maintained and ensures that no feature is forgotten in the assessment process.

In defining the current situation, the crucial factors to consider are (i) joint range, (ii) muscle strength and (iii) degree of spasticity. Additional information about the child's home and school environments and recreational interests also allow an accurate and appropriate prescription to be made.

Orthotic principles

An orthosis may fulfil one or more of the following functions: (i) total support to or restraint of one or more joints, (ii) assistive support to one or more joints, (iii) corrective support to one or more joints, (iv) total weight relief, (v) partial weight relief and (vi) mobility. The orthosis may also be 'rigid' or have some flexibility or free motion.

In order to achieve these functions, an appreciation of the force patterns which may be applied by an orthosis is important. Consider a spina bifida child with a high level lesion resulting in total paralysis of the lower limbs. It is desirable to support him in an upright attitude for two reasons. First, socially, so that he is able to look his peers 'in the eye'. Second, medically, an upright stance assists kidney drainage and the development of good quality bone. This is encouraged by the weight of his body being supported through his legs, the normal loading from muscle tone not being available.

In order to provide this support, a series of three-point loading patterns must be applied to each joint. For instance, the F forces in Fig. 7.14 support the knee, the P forces support the hip. The 'central' force in each case is applied over the joint being supported, the location of the other two forces being as remote as practical from the joint in order to increase the leverage and thus reduce the force at the point of contact with the body. Clearly, the ankle also needs supporting. However, its maximum extension does not correspond to the attitude required for an upright stance and thus the necessary restraint cannot be achieved with a simple three-point force system. It is necessary to have a more complex system that includes 'stops' at the appropriate angles.

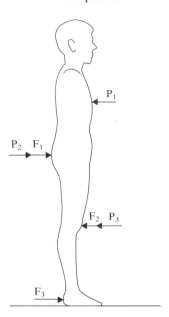

Fig. 7.14. The three-point force systems required to support the hip (P) and knee (F).

Additional forces may be required. For instance, torsional forces may be necessary to restrain or assist rotational motion around the long axis of a particular bone. Or, again, lateral forces may be required to support joints that are unstable in a direction perpendicular to the normal plane of motion.

Interfaces

Whenever force is to be applied to the body, great care should be taken with the design of interface at the point of application. For instance, the area of contact must be large enough to spread the load, thus reducing localized pressure. Since the methods depend upon the particular type of orthosis being used, the two common types will be considered briefly: (i) strut and (ii) shell.

The strut type of orthosis (Fig. 7.15) consists of an external structure or framework, attached to the limb or trunk by means of straps. These straps also provide the means of applying force to the body. This structure is substantially rigid, except at those points where joints are provided in line with the natural joints, allowing motion to take place under certain circumstances (e.g. when the joint is not locked) in one plane. The shell type of orthosis (Fig. 7.16), frequently formed from sheet plastic, partially

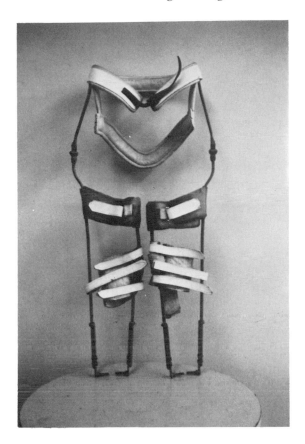

Fig. 7.15. A strut Hip Knee Ankle Foot Orthosis.

or totally envelopes the particular limb segment, providing an intimate fit. The stiffness of this construction depends upon the detailed configuration of the shell and can readily be tailored to be more or less flexible, according to the specific need. Thus, if appearance is of paramount importance, or if some flexibility is desirable, the shell type of orthosis is preferred.

Potentially, the shell type of orthosis is attractive since, by design, the configuration distributes the load over large areas. However, the comparative flexibility of these orthoses may make them unsuitable for application of high forces, such as the restraining forces required to contain strong spasm. If, under these circumstances, the strut type of orthosis is indicated, the straps through which the forces are applied must be well-padded with suitably enlarged areas over the contact surface. Strong

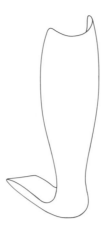

Fig. 7.16. A shell construction Ankle Foot Orthosis.

elastic may also be used to cushion the 'shock' for children with severe spasm.

Finally, in considering the force system and its method of input, it should be appreciated that some undesirable restraints may also, of necessity, be imposed. For instance, the distal attachment of the orthosis may be through spurs into the heel of the shoe. Thus, inversion and eversion of the ankle becomes blocked, even if that is not a prescribed restraint.

Dynamic orthoses
Brief mention was made above of the ability to build in flexibility or to use elastic. There are occasions, for instance with drop-foot, where some form of dynamic orthosis is desirable, incorporating a device to assist dorsiflexion. There are many ways of achieving this, from a simple toe spring to the use of functional electrical stimulation (FES), triggered by a heel-contact switch.

Walking machines
In recent years, particularly for spina bifida children, various alternatives (e.g. Taylor & Rocca, 1982) to conventional orthoses have been developed which, while providing structural support, encourage independent mobility without using crutches or a walking aid. The principle is that of a swinging gate. Under each foot there is a bearing with a vertical axis (Fig. 7.17). The plane containing these two axes is posterior to the centre of

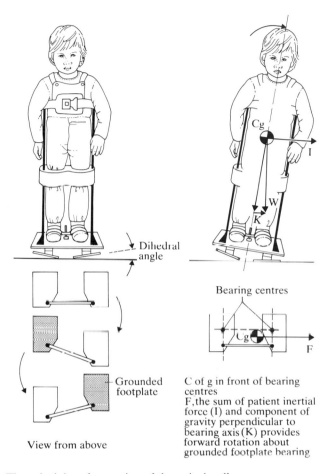

Dihedral angle

Grounded footplate

View from above

Bearing centres

C of g in front of bearing centres
F,the sum of patient inertial force (I) and component of gravity perpendicular to bearing axis (K) provides forward rotation about grounded footplate bearing

Fig. 7.17. The principles of operation of the swivel walker.

gravity of the body. The base plate under each foot is angled so that, by leaning sideways, the child achieves a position of stability with this plate on the ground. Since the axis of rotation through this foot is now tilted, the child's body swings in an arc until the contralateral foot strikes the ground. Leaning the other way allows a similar motion to take place in the opposite direction, forward progression being accomplished in a series of arcs. The advantages of such a device are independent mobility (on flat ground) and freedom for the hands to perform other functions, such as carrying.

Upper limb orthoses
Attention in this section has been focused primarily upon the lower limb.
Many of the principles also apply to upper limb orthoses. However, the
forces involved are considerably lower and the purpose of fitting an
orthosis is usually substantially different.

There are two main purposes for using an upper limb orthosis: therapy
and function. Therapeutically, it may be the means of exercising, say, a
hand or of releasing contractures in the fingers. Typically, these are
achieved by an intimate attachment of a cuff to the forearm. Then,
depending upon the application, a dorsal structure will be used to apply
loads to the fingers in order to encourage extension (Fig. 7.18), or a
palmar plate will be used to open this aspect of the hand (Fig. 7.19).

For the more proximal joints of the arm, the main purpose of an
orthosis when used for children with neurological conditions is to enable
the arm to function more effectively in placing the hand in a good
working position. Various approaches may be required. For those with
degenerative conditions, such as muscular dystrophy, improved function
may be achieved by using muscle power from elsewhere to supplement
the affected muscles. For instance, the shoulder muscles may be used to
provide assistance to biceps by means of a harness and cord that can
operate on an external structure around the arm.

One problem frequently encountered in neurological conditions is
involuntary movement. Such movements may take the form of a high

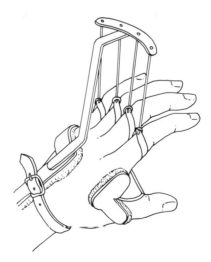

Fig. 7.18. Hand orthosis with metacarpophalangeal extension assist (after Anderson).

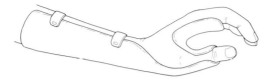

Fig. 7.19. Hand orthosis with palmar plate.

frequency low amplitude tremor, as with Friedreich's ataxia, or of a slower writing movement, as with athetoid cerebral palsy. Three approaches have been taken to treat these. The first attempts to restrain the undesirable motions of the limb by adding inertia, using weights as a bracelet, for example (Anderson, 1965). This reduces the frequency of tremor but also applies a load in the direction of gravity. Thus, it does not provide a uniform effect throughout the normal range of motion. An alternative approach is to use friction (Largent & Waylett, 1975). Here an orthosis is fitted which has adjustable friction at each of the joints corresponding to the anatomical joints. Potentially, this allows the restraining force to be applied equally in all directions. However, this approach is less than ideal since the level of restraining force has to be preset and the force required to initiate motion (the break-out force to overcome static friction) is greater than that required to maintain motion (the dynamic friction) (Fig. 7.20).

The third approach is to use viscous damping. This is attractive as a technique since the restraining force opposing motion is related to the speed of motion (Fig. 7.21). Thus, a high frequency tremor is restrained with a greater force than the underlying deliberate motion that the individual is trying to perform. This is analagous to filtering out the interference on the radio to allow the main signal to be heard. Although still in the research stage, the results of this approach look promising, the main limitation being the availability of suitable hardware.

Conclusion
The usefulness of orthoses to support or restrain body segments has been recognized for many centuries. Their ability to be tailored to particular needs has, even now, not yet been fully exploited. However, the population of potential beneficiaries represents one of the largest groups of rehabilitation patients and readers are urged to familiarize themselves with the topic if they are to be successful in their treatment of this group of children.

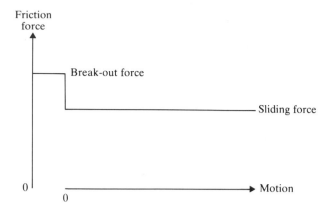

Fig. 7.20. Characteristic of friction force v. displacement.

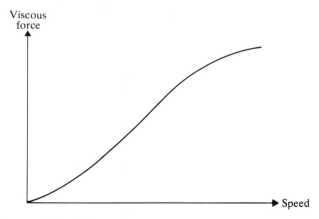

Fig. 7.21. Characteristic of viscous force v. speed.

Aids to daily living

The overall aim of any aid is to give a person a greater degree of independence, from independent mobility to independence in cleaning one's teeth.

The motivation to achieve independence varies both between two individuals in similar circumstances and also as a child grows up and becomes more self-conscious. So, while a young child is content to receive help in going to the lavatory, the young teenage girl demands independence in managing her monthly period.

The role of the rehabilitation engineer is seen in the adaptation of an existing article or the creation of something new. However, much has already been said about this role, so the observations that follow will be limited to those factors which affect the choice or design of an aid.

Assessment
As in the other areas discussed in this chapter, assessment must feature at an early stage in the prescriptive process. However, in the case of an aid, consideration should be given to various questions that cannot be answered solely by examining the child and defining his immediate needs. For instance, is the aid to be used in private or public? Is there any device on the market for the able-bodied which, with adaptation, would be suitable? What are the environmental limitations (e.g. door widths, stairs, etc.)? These and other questions must be answered if the aid is not going to be a 'white elephant'.

Prescription
After a careful assessment has been made, a particular aid or design for an aid can be suggested. At this stage, the interaction between the child, parents, therapist and engineer is vital since, unless the solution is very obvious, a little discussion and experimentation can save hours of frustration as well as excessive expense. For instance, if a child is unable to feed himself is it that the cutlery is wrong, or is it related to seat height or table height, or even that he does not want to? Naturally, if the last mentioned is the case, some 'selling' has to take place and the general appearance of the aid is particularly crucial.

Function and appearance may be conflicting criteria. For instance, for the arm amputee a split-hook may be most functional but an artificial hand more acceptable for cosmetic reasons. Thus, in each of the aspects of daily living outlined below, the reaction of the family, child's peer group and other people may well be the ultimate reason for acceptance or rejection.

Aspects of daily life
There are six aspects in which aids may be required: (i) personal care (hygiene and dressing), (ii) eating, (iii) control of the environment, (iv) education/employment, (v) mobility and (vi) recreation. In each of these aspects, priorities must be assigned to function and appearance (as already discussed), portability/manoeuverability and cost. From these con-

siderations, the choice of materials, the appropriate level of technology and the method of production will emerge.

Provision and evaluation

Once the aid has been designed and manufactured, two further steps must be carried out. First, the aid must be given to the patient with sufficient instruction concerning its use and maintenance to ensure that maximum benefit will result. Second, the aid must be evaluated against the original requirements to ensure that it satisfies the performance specified.

Conclusion

An aid, being a tool, must satisfy a need. Since it is prescribed to meet the needs of a particular child, the child's views must be sought as fully as possible at all stages. The success of an aid does not depend, in the final analysis, on its elegance in the eye of the clinician but upon its performance in the hands of the child. Failure to recognize this can result in the device being not an aid but a hindrance.

References and further reading

Seating

Key, A.G., Marley, M.T. & Wakefield, E. (1978/79) Pressure redistribution in wheelchair cushion for paraplegics: its application and evaluation. *Paraplegia*, **16**, 403–412.

Koreska, J. & Albisser, A.M. (1975) A new foam for the support of the physically handicapped. *Biomedical Engineering*, **10**(2), 56–58.

Nelham, R.L. (1981) Seating for the chairbound disabled person—a survey of seating equipment in the United Kingdom. *Journal of Biomedical Engineering*, **3**(4), 267–274.

Ring, N.D., ed. (1978) *Seating Systems for the Disabled*. Bio. Eng. Soc., London.

Ring, N.D., Nelham, R.L. & Pearson, F. (1978) Moulded supportive seating for the disabled. *Prosthetics and Orthotics International*, **2**, 30–34.

Souther, S.G., Carr, S.D. & Vintner, L.M. (1974) Wheelchair cushion to reduce pressure under bony prominences. *Archives of Physical Medicine and Rehabilitation*, **55**, 460–464.

Communication

Foulds, R.A. (1980) Communication rates for non-speech expression as a function of manual tasks and linguistic constraints. In *Proceedings of International Conference on Rehabilitation Engineering, Toronto*. National Research Council of Canada, Ottawa.

Ring, N.D. (1977) Specification of interfaces. In *Proceedings of Workshop on Communication*. National Research Council of Canada, Ottawa.

Vanderheiden, G.C. (1978) *Non-Vocal Communication Resource Book*. University Park Press, Baltimore.

Biofeedback training

Basmajian, J.V. (1981) Biofeedback in rehabilitation: a review of principles and practices. *Archives of Physical Medicine and Rehabilitation*, **62**, 469–475.

Herman, R. (1974) *Augmented Sensory Feedback Therapy for Children with Cerebral Palsy. Proposal*. Krusen Centre, Moss Rehabilitation Hospital, Philadelphia.

Orthotics

Anderson, M.H. (1965) *Upper Extremity Orthotics*. Charles C. Thomas, Springfield.

Brown, A.W.S. (1978) The electronic measurement of limb movement and function. In *Baclofen: Spasticity and Cerebral Pathology*. Cambridge Medical Publications.

Brown, A.W.S. (1981) A microprocessor based ultrasonic limb movement monitoring system. *Journal of Biomedical Engineering*, **3**(4), 275–280.

Harris, E.E. (1973) A new orthotics terminology. *Orthotics and Prosthetics*, **27**(2), 6–19.

Largent, P. & Waylett, J. (1975) Follow up study on upper extremity bracing of children with severe athetosis *American Journal of Occupational Therapy*, **26**, 341–348.

Morgan, M.H., Hewer, R.L. & Cooper, R. (1975) Intention tremor: a method of measurement. *Journal of Neurology, Neurosurgery and Psychiatry*, **38**(3), 253–258.

Taylor, A.G. & Rocca, L. (1982) An improved swivel walker for paraplegics. *Journal of Biomedical Engineering*, **4**(4), 325–327.

Microelectronics, microcomputers and information technology

An update by Andrew Brown, Deputy Technical Director of the Rehabilitation Engineering Unit, Chailey Heritage, Lewes, East Sussex.

There can be no doubt that recent technological advances will allow physically disabled people a measure of independence which would otherwise have been impossible. The areas of communication, mobility, education, employment, recreation and environmental control have already been significantly affected by the 'new technology'. In years to come, it is reasonable to assume that physically handicapped people will be able to compete on equal terms in open employment with the able bodied in many fields, and will also be able to enjoy the benefits of the leisure activities promised for all.

The well-established advances in computer-aided learning can be made available to the disabled person, as can the facilities of word processing, information handling, accountancy, book-keeping and stock control. Such things as global person-to-person satellite communication, electronic mail, armchair shopping and home banking facilities are also already provided. For those in research or in business, telephone access to computer data bases, library facilities and other information sources are readily available using any 'home computer' system. All of these combine to provide a variety of intellectually and financially rewarding opportunities for employment.

The cost and portability of self-contained microcomputer systems is improving rapidly, and it is now possible to provide a disabled person with a portable, battery powered unit, appropriately programmed to act purely as a matching device between him and other equipment. This means that he can, through his personalized input computer, operate another unmodified terminal or computer system running standard programs, and thus control other equipment which was not designed to accommodate his specific disability. This is the concept of a 'transparent' or 'surrogate keyboard', where the user's equipment can be used as a keyboard substitute for another computer system. Such equipment already exists in a variety of forms, but the potential for expanding it to provide a universal control interface between a physically disabled user and a wide range of other equipment including wheelchairs, telephones and environmental controllers requires further exploitation.

References

Perkins, W.J., ed. (1983) *High Technology Aids for the Disabled.* Butterworths, London.

Rosen, M.J., Goodenough-Trepagnier, C. (1982) Communication systems for the nonvocal motor handicapped: Practice and prospects. *Eng. Med. Biol. Mag.* **1**, (4): 31−33.

Chapter 8
Motor Learning Difficulties: 'Clumsy Children'

Ian McKinlay & Neil Gordon

Development of learning

Learning to control movement begins at birth and continues throughout life. Some skills are easier to acquire at one age than another but for humans these are optimum rather than critical periods. It is easier for most to learn to ride a bicycle or to play tennis in middle childhood than in the first few years of life or in adult middle age. The 5-year-old, unless exceptional, will show little initial improvement in spite of practice. The adult with aptitude may learn to become proficient with practice but is unlikely to become outstanding.

An infant in the first weeks of life can copy facial expression (e.g. protruding the tongue) if someone close to him pulls a face (Low, 1980) when the infant is in a receptive state. Neglected children, having no one to copy, do not acquire such experience. Many of the motor skills we learn are based on patterns of movement developed early in life. (Ritchie Russell in 1958 described this as a potential disadvantage as the furrows of habit become ruts, the guidelines become chains.)

The infant's brain is already programmed to organize walking and to deal with learning to speak. Neither of these is the result of sheer imitation, though the particular language learned and the accent with which it is spoken are strongly influenced by early experience. Writing, dressing, keyboard manipulation and ball games, on the other hand, are mainly learned. Predisposition to be good at these had not carried potent implications for reproduction or survival hitherto, and a great variety of ability is seen in the normal population.

Habits and skills

Whenever a skill is being acquired there must be an initial experience which is reinforced. This applies to motor skills especially and probably to speech also. Griffiths (1979) lists the components required as (i) receptor processes, by which information is transmitted to the brain, (ii) organiz-

ation and intention, or a plan of action based on environmental information received, (iii) effector processes by which the plan of action is
carried out, and (iv) feedback and flexibility by which the action is
monitored and adjusted to match intentions. It is the organization and
feedback which distinguish a skill from habit. The more a skill is practised
the more it is freed from organizational and feedback constraints. A habit
is described as an automatic and invariable response to an environmental
stimulus, while a skill is a response which is constantly related to environmental requirements. However, a skill may incorporate subroutines
which have become habitual. Previous knowledge enables us to make
sense of new information (Vass, 1979). High-knowledge individuals are
able to use the context of a subject to a greater degree during learning
than low-knowledge individuals.

So far as motor skills are concerned, a successful result may depend on
understanding the task required, visual perceptual ability, perception of
the position of body parts in space, balancing mechanisms, inhibition of
overflow movement, control of muscle tone, sequencing skills, eye–hand
or eye–foot control, and sufficient previous experience of the task or a
similar task. Motor planning and motor execution have been shown to
involve different, though adjacent parts of the brain (Ingvar, 1975;
Lassen *et al.*, 1978; Eccles, 1980). This may explain why some children
cannot work out how to perform a task initially, but later perform it well
when they have 'got the hang of it'. Other children know perfectly well
what they would like to do but cannot perform in the way they would
like. Learned motor skills can be transferred to novel groups of muscles.
A child who has learned to write 'C' with the right hand will also be able
to write it with the left big toe or the tip of the tongue. (A converse
process is sometimes used for children who have difficulty in learning to
write in school books. They can be taught the concept of letter formation
by writing on a blackboard making large shoulder and arm movements;
then they translate these to wrist and hand movements to write on
paper.)

Once a motor skill has been learned properly it remains, in spite of
lack of practice, for many years. We do not forget how to swim or to ride
a bicycle. Some children are thought to have a poor memory because they
seem to find difficulty in carrying over their teaching experience from day
to day. Over-learning may be required before the skill becomes robust
and persistent. If the child lacks the capacity to develop the skill through
immaturity, it may be best to teach something else for a while.

There is much to learn about how to teach motor skills. For example, it is not clear whether putting a description of an activity into words helps or hinders motor development by comparison with practical demonstration. In developing two-handed skills it is not known whether it is best to practise each hand's activities sequentially or alternately or together. The time-honoured process of breaking activities down into component parts may not facilitate learning by comparison with practising a whole activity, stressing individual aspects during teaching. Evaluative research for normal and remedial motor skill development might prove a fruitful area for co-operation between teachers, psychologists and therapists. (Indeed, there is a good case for exploring the possibility of devising some shared teaching in normal motor development for these groups.)

Brain development and learning disorders

An account of the relationship of current knowledge about brain development to learning disorders is given here because it can be helpful in offering explanations to parents and teachers.

Diverse pathological processes can disrupt a potentially intact nervous system. Disruption has different effects on the brain at each stage. In the first few weeks after conception, disorders lead to gross malformations of the nervous system and/or sense organs. In the next few weeks, disease processes can have extensive consequences because of the small size and immaturity of the structures involved and these may leave markers on other structures developing at the same time, e.g. face, ears, skin creases. At 7 or 8 weeks, anterior horn cells become connected to muscles, and active movement initiated from a spinal and brain stem level becomes possible. Then postural reflexes become organized, leading to an initially flexed posture, from 16 to 36 weeks an extended posture, then from 36 weeks onwards a semi-flexed posture to which are added later vestibular and proprioceptive reflexes. These do not involve the cerebral hemispheres and are seen in anencephalic and hydranencephalic foetuses who survive. Between 10 and 18 weeks of pregnancy there is a marked increase in the number of neurones. Noxious influences which interfere with this lead to mental handicap and severe forms of spastic cerebral palsy in survivors.

In the second half of pregnancy and early infancy the brain growth spurt reflects three major processes. Firstly, billions of interconnections grow between the many thousands of millions of nerve cells. Each nerve cell comes to receive fibres from other nerve cells at synapses numbering between hundreds and many thousands per nerve cell. It is likely that each synapse develops its own capacity for memory functions.

Reading aloud depends on adequate sensory input to the occipital cortex, connections between that and the temporal cortex where the language content is decoded, then transmission to part of the frontal brain concerned with the planning and co-ordination of the mechanisms of speech. Writing depends on links between the expressive language brain, the part of frontal brain involved in the planning and co-ordination of writing movements, and adequate mechanisms in the arm and hand whereby the writing can be performed. The performance of such activities is monitored by feedback of sound and visual input respectively. Deriving *meaning* from these activities involves much more widespread connections throughout the brain.

Neurones are arranged in cylindrical units or modules 200−300 μm in diameter on the surface of the brain (Eccles, 1980). Each module contains 1000−3000 cells, is linked to about 500 modules on the same side of the brain and about 50 modules on the opposite side.

The second process involved in the brain growth spurt is the proliferation of glial cells which come to outnumber neurones at least eightfold. They cushion neurones against mechanical insults, their processes act as the equivalent of extracellular space in the central nervous system, they are intimately involved in the metabolism of neurones, in directing and re-directing dendritic interconnections, in tissue repair, if required, and in myelinating nerve fibres.

Myelination is the third major process in later development of the nervous system. Myelin insulates nerve fibres and allows rapid conduction of electrical impulses in an enlarging brain, spinal cord and peripheral nervous system. Although effects of demyelination are clinically documented and some pathological processes and drug effects (e.g. methotrexate) are well described, the effects of variations in the natural rate of myelination and glial cell development are still poorly understood. This is also true of our knowledge of the brain's capacity to reorganize its interconnections in response to learning requirements or insults.

Why do children find it hard to learn to perform?

Children may fail to learn because of the way they are made, the way they feel, or the way they are taught at home and at school. Combinations of these commonly occur and interact. There has been a tendency for the 'nature versus nurture' debate to become polarized. It is preferable to clarify the mechanisms whereby biological and social class disadvantages operate, and to prevent either type of impairment becoming a handicap.

Genetic factors include mutation within the individual and inherited characteristics (Herman & Norrie, 1958; Bakwin, 1973; Finucci *et al.*, 1976). The nature of inherited learning difficulty is complex (Decker & De Fries, 1981) when closely analysed, and interacts with environmental influences. Maturational delay (Rodier, 1980; Connolly & Prechtl, 1981) needs to be considered, as do visual and hearing impairments. Amongst clumsy children there is an excess with squints, refractive errors, visual perception deficits (Hulme *et al.*, 1982), hearing deficits and immature vestibular mechanisms. It would not be surprising if distorted input and feedback led to impaired performance.

Accurate testing of vision and hearing are stressed as essential before inferences can be drawn about brain dysfunction or social factors (Fundudis *et al.*, 1979; Lassman *et al.*, 1980).

Inappropriate or insufficient teaching is difficult to investigate but does occur. Factors such as maternal age (Gillberg *et al.*, 1982), birth order and family size (Belmont *et al.*, 1976) and housing experiences (Essen *et al.*, 1978) are associated with educational failure. There is likely to be an interplay between genetic endowment and environmental factors (biological and social). A generous genetic potential may overcome the effects of brain insults or social misfortune but a lesser inheritance may be more easily lost. Social disadvantage *per se* is probably not a major factor (Drotar *et al.*, 1976; Gillberg & Rasmussen, 1982) but is associated with increased risk of illness, different learning experiences (Tizard & Hughes, 1984) and genetic factors.

Analysis of reasons for failure to learn requires a multidisciplinary approach for diagnosis and there is considerable potential for overcoming adverse influences.

Neurological dysfunction cannot be inferred solely from motor immaturity ('soft signs') but is more convincing with demonstrable structured abnormality (Anderson & Plewis, 1977; Minns *et al.*, 1977; O'Malley & Griffith, 1977; Galaburda, 1979), or functional abnormality associated with accepted neurological disorders such as hypothyroidism, epilepsy or lead poisoning (McFaul *et al.*, 1978; Stores, 1978; Smith *et al.*, 1983; Epir *et al.*, 1984).

Multifactorial aetiology of cerebral palsy syndromes has been well recognized (Hagberg, 1978). An important factor is 'fetal deprivation of supply' often compounded by perinatal asphyxia and, sometimes, hyperbilirubinaemia insufficient to cause kernicterus. Subnutrition, asphyxia and jaundice in susceptible individuals may also be relevant to learning disorders. There are certainly reliable animal models for this (Dobbing, 1970; Dobbing & Sands, 1971). Small-for-date babies have been shown to be predisposed to performance problems (Davies, 1976). Neonates who have suffered symptomatic asphyxia are liable to clumsiness, speech, language and behaviour problems (Brown, 1976). Cerebral irradiation for leukaemia in early childhood is known to be associated with memory, visual-motor and mathematical impairments (Eiser & Lansdown, 1977). Occipital ischaemia, for example after episodes of hypotension during cardiac surgery, can be followed by progressive recovery of visual acuity but more persistent visual perceptual deficit.

Accepting that these are special instances, they do illustrate the potential for diffuse and diverse processes to cause learning and performance deficits (see also McKinlay, 1980; Brown, 1981). They also indicate the heterogeneity of children with motor learning problems and clumsiness.

It is not justified to believe that risk factors are *causes* of disability. The concept of recovery from brain insults is important (Thomson *et al.*, 1977; Baum, 1977; Ounsted *et al.*, 1984). The brain withstands early focal insults quite well—hence the concept of plasticity (Bishop, 1980, 1981; Robinson, 1981). However, diffuse processes such as anoxic/ischaemic insult (Brown *et al.*, 1974) or malnutrition during the brain growth spurt (Lloyd-Still *et al.*, 1974; Brazelton *et al.*, 1977; *British Medical Journal*, 1978; Sibert *et al.*, 1978; Dobbing & Sands, 1981) are less well tolerated, presumably because potentially compensatory brain is also affected. Adult neurological experience has shown that reading, writing and spelling, though related, can be selectively impaired (Critchley, 1964; *British Medical Journal*, 1979; Benson, 1979; Eccles 1980). It is reasonable to suppose that these processes may fail to be acquired by children (Bradley & Bryant, 1978) because of failure or immaturity of development of appropriate connections in the brain.

Boys are more vulnerable than girls to insults to the nervous system (Ounsted & Taylor, 1972). The male brain matures more gradually than the female brain and remains susceptible to insult for a longer period (Taylor, 1969). This is one explanation for the male excess among children with neurodevelopmental and neuro-psychiatric disorders in population studies when the ratio is about 1.5:1. In clinic populations boys may outnumber girls by 4:1 because of boys' reactions to frustration and other people's expectations of boys. When brain damage does occur in girls, less common as that may be, the effects are often severe.

Medicine and children with learning disorders

Children with learning problems have been referred to doctors for many years, for many reasons and in many ways. There may be a screening system which involves school doctors (Bax & Whitmore, 1973). Secondary behaviour problems may come to the attention of child guidance and child psychiatry services. Parents may seek medical advice from family doctors or specialists because they are concerned about educational problems in their children and see doctors as experts, independent of the school system, who can ask questions on their child's behalf. However referral comes about, the doctor has a contribution to make (Gordon *et al.*, 1984; Robinson, 1984), should be aware of the nature of learning disorders and should know of ways to resolve the problem.

The children do not usually show features of neurological or psychiatric *diseases*, though these should be considered (e.g. muscular dystrophy, psychotic illness) especially if there is any suggestion of progression. Much more commonly the children show developmental immaturity or inconsistency. In the first instance the examination should be made by the family or school doctor. Referral to hospital specialists is not to be encouraged unless it is thought that the child shows more specific neurological or psychiatric abnormality.

History-taking

The doctor needs to be aware of the information in the history offered ('his writing is very untidy' or 'we don't think he has enough teaching') and the meaning of the consultation ('he's driving us round the bend and we don't know why'). The family may well attribute the child's difficulties to physical or psychosocial events so it is useful to ask 'What do you put his problems down to?' A family history of learning and performance abilities is interesting though probably not very accurate. Birth records do not always tally with the family's recollections, but there can be errors in either source. Birth weight is interesting in relation to birth weight of siblings. Recurrent ear infections, squint surgery, febrile convulsions, episodes of unconsciousness after head injury and other significant health details are recorded. Cause and effect are not often clear to the doctor, but discussion of the significance of the history is an important part of the explanation doctors and their colleagues can offer.

It may be necessary to ask an assistant to occupy the child elsewhere while the history—so often a catalogue of woe—is obtained. It can be informative in some ways to observe how parents denigrate a child in the child's presence, but it makes it more difficult to establish rapport with the child later. On the other hand, sensitive examination of the child in the parents' presence may demonstrate the child's difficulties to the parents, when everyday contact has dulled their objectivity. It is understandable that parents will expect children to perform uniformly and predictably. If they can be convinced that, though the child performs some tasks well he finds others are difficult, they may be helped to see the child afresh. It is not easy to help people to understand that inconsistency within an individual may be constitutional and not the consequence of known disease. But this is usually the case for children with learning problems or clumsiness.

Examination

During history-taking, attempts are made to involve the child in friendly, brief and uncritical ways. The examination begins with testing functions which can be expected to be intact (e.g. power) rather than those which are problematical. This allows rapport to develop and gives the child confidence to attempt more difficult tasks later. If the session is going well and the child performs happily, the parents gain confidence in the doctor's opinion. Usually sufficient neurological inference can be drawn from functional testing. A child who is having a good time will allow more formal testing, if required, especially if it is on the carpet or floor—where children are at home—rather than on a couch.

The functions tested will include the child's ability to balance, perform the Fog manoeuvres (Szatmari & Taylor, 1984), rapidly alternate hand movements and fine finger movements (Denckla, 1973), identify fingers touched with the eyes closed, distinguish right from left, demonstrate laterality for writing, catch and kick a ball, copy shapes, draw and write. Use of language and articulatory ability are listened to incidentally as the rest of the examination proceeds. Children with articulatory difficulties need to feel quite relaxed if an adequate sample of speech is to be assessed. A speech therapist could do this much more reliably and in more detail, but if enough speech is heard initially further assessment may not be needed. Throughout, the doctor adopts a style of curiosity and acceptance. The child who performs very awkwardly may be encouraged to know that the doctor understands and has found the child's efforts helpful.

The purpose of the examination is to develop some insight into the individual child's development which can be interpreted to the child, parents and school. There are all sorts of clumsiness, which is often task-specific, and learning disabilities. The child can emerge from the process as someone whose strengths and immaturities have been appreciated—not 'diagnosed' as showing 'the clumsy child syndrome', 'dysgraphia' or 'minimal brain dysfunction'.

Child development, child psychiatry and maladjustment

Children with learning and performance difficulties commonly show behavioural problems, restlessness, lack of concentration, anxiety, depression, isolation and even delusions. Families react to these in different ways. If the family is well balanced, they may perceive the problem in the context of disordered child development and will approach paediatric services asking for an explanation. If the family is already distressed by other factors, they may simply find the child to be exasperating and approach psychiatric or child guidance services. Those who work in child development services will tend to identify the child's developmental immaturities and play down the behavioural problems. Those who work in the psychiatric services will commonly come from a background of adult psychiatric training or behavioural management, and may find developmental immaturities difficult to assess. It would seem desirable for both services to work together for these children clinically and in staff education.

Children placed in educational facilities for the 'maladjusted' may well have language or performance difficulties as their primary disorder. To deal with them purely in terms of behavioural management or family therapy may ignore the fundamental issue. Learning and performance problems in such children are so frequent that they come to be accepted as 'features of maladjusted children' or 'typical of hyperactive children'. It is a common experience that when such children are offered appropriate education, they become more relaxed and self-confident, suggesting that the maladjustment is as much a feature of the educational system as of the child. Nonetheless, behavioural treatment of the child and discussion of the family's problems with the child's behaviour are important.

Occasionally, drug treatment may be helpful on a short-term basis. If the physical consequences of a child's anxiety are unpleasant, a β-adrenergic blocker such as propanolol may help the child to cope with stress. In the rare circumstance where a child is obligatorily hyperactive in all situations, a stimulant such as methylphenidate has been used. There may be short-term benefits, but long-term effects have yet to be proven.

If a child is clinically depressed, an anti-depressant drug such as amitryptiline may be tried. When sleep disturbance is troublesome the short-
term use of a night sedative such as chloral or a small dose of a benzodiazepine can be used in combination with a behavioural and educational
programme. Hangover effects on learning next day can be a disadvantage, so the balance between beneficial effects and side-effects needs to
be considered. Diets free of food additives, preservatives, colouring agents,
sugar, chocolate, oranges and even tap water have been advocated for
children described as 'hyperactive' by their parents. Trials seem to show
that diets which parents have faith in lead the parents to reinforce good
behaviour and ignore bad behaviour in the child with beneficial results.
Double-blind controlled trials have shown no benefit.

It would be desirable for developmental physicians to know more
about psychiatry and for child psychiatrists to understand more of child
development if the right balance is to be achieved in the health services
for children with learning, performance and behaviour problems.

Planning remediation for clumsy children

If athletes can be enabled to improve by training, it seems reasonable to
suggest that clumsy children can be helped—not to become athletes or
calligraphers but to overcome and compensate for difficulties. The starting point is to ask the child if help is wanted and if so in what way. There
is no future in imposing remedial activity on an unwilling child. Some
effort may be required to convince the child who lacks confidence that
help is possible.

If remedial teaching of motor skills by teachers (or therapists) is to be
effective, the teacher needs some structural basis for the treatment programme. The experienced teacher will develop that structure according to
the needs of individual children and the style of intervention with which
the teacher has most success.

Those interested in the details of therapy and remedial teaching must
refer to books specializing in these subjects (Gordon & McKinlay, 1980),
but it may help to discuss the principles that some of these workers
employ.

The physiotherapist, when available, can offer the clumsy child a great
deal of help, particularly among the younger age groups. First of all, an
assessment of physical activities will be carried out, the purpose of this
being explained to the child. It is carried out in the presence of the
parents. To start with, it may be necessary to see the child at frequent
intervals but, as time goes by, check-up and counselling sessions at 6−12

month intervals may be all that is required. The frequency of treatment sessions is dependent on the amount and efficiency of parent and teacher co-operation and upon the child's own ability to co-operate with them. Treatment is likely to start on an individual basis and may graduate to group therapy. Such treatment is taking place in an abnormal setting if this is done in a hospital department or a health centre, and as soon as possible the suggested routines should be incorporated into the child's normal school and home life after discussion with teachers and parents.

The long-term objectives of physical therapy for the clumsy child are to develop effective body and object control, with consequent improvements in learning social skills, self-concepts and self-esteem. This must start by giving the child experiences which will, through sensation and movements themselves, improve motor response and enhance perceptions. Improvement in gross motor skills can serve as a basis for more complex perceptual motor learning and the acquisition of fine motor skills. The programme is tailored for the individual needs of the child and should offer a rich, varied and controlled experience of activities, modified according to the results. Programmes of movement experience should incorporative activities which demand of the child differing amounts of control through time. Change of physical effort, direction, speed or stress in light and heavy movements are used within all the dimensions of movement. Tasks should be clearly explained and demonstrated. The child is initially assisted, advised and encouraged to perform. Observing the child's actions leads to further analysis of difficulties and to an assessment of improvements. Demands made by the therapist are adjusted to the results obtained. To begin with, tasks are simplified then gradually made more complex.

Lack of self-confidence among these children is often a major problem. By discussing the results of periodic assessments with the child, the parents and teachers, each can be helped to be realistic in their expectations. Following such ascertainments, it is possible to design necessary circumventions (for example, extended time in examinations, tape recorders, typewriters, velcro fasteners, slip-on shoes, or cross-country running instead of ball games).

Activities may be designed for such purposes as relaxation, the development of body awareness, body alignment, locomotion and balance, rhythm, temporal awareness, airborne activities and projectile skills. Other exercises will enhance manual dexterity, eye—hand co-ordination, eye—foot co-ordination, and body fitness, strength and endurance (Grimley, 1980).

The occupational therapist, if such a service is available, has a part to play in helping the clumsy child to acquire everyday skills. This particularly applies to manipulation. Teaching should be task-oriented. It does not seem to be adequate to hope for a 'halo' effect from a specific improvement in co-ordination. For example, it may be desirable to teach a child to use scissors. Provided the child is adequately supervised, sharp scissors are not particularly hazardous and their use decreases the frustration engendered by poor cutting blades. Scissors specially designed for left-handed people are available and should be provided when appropriate. The ability to thread laces is another example. This skill not only involves eye−hand co-ordination and manipulation but good motor-organization, and will need practice of graded tasks. A variety of toys and games can be used to develop perception, such as form boards and posting boxes for shape recognition among younger children, and 'Scrabble' or 'Lexicon' for the older child to practise sequencing. The occupational therapist may become involved in providing equipment to help with writing, from provision of a choice of writing implements or of a clipboard to hold the paper still, to the acquisition of a typewriter if the child wants this and can be taught to use it. Independence in self-care is of obvious importance, and help may be needed in activities such as eating and dressing. Practice may be needed in tying laces and fastening buckles or buttons. Parents often need advice on a suitable choice of clothing that avoids too many fasteners and is not too tight. If a child is slow at dressing he may lack practice because of the need for speed on school mornings. If this is so, and time cannot be allowed for the child to practise independence, then care must be taken to make the opportunity for him to undress at night, and to dress at weekends.

As the child is often under pressure from parents and teachers, the way he uses his free time may be of considerable importance. These children should be encouraged to follow up areas of particular interest, and suggestions may be made as to how these can be extended. It is often helpful to suggest that a child develops a skill that is unusual at that particular age as this may add prestige and increase confidence. Examples of such hobbies are horse riding, carpentry, baking, photography, gardening or amateur dramatics. The older child may choose an activity related to future employment (Bryant, 1980).

One of the major problems for clumsy children at school is the physical education class. There is the worry about changing clothes for this class and the almost inevitable failure in comparison with their peers. If the teacher recognizes that a child has a particular disability then the danger of ignoring him as being 'no good at games' may be avoided to some extent. Physical education provides an opportunity for him to learn requisite skills. This requires sophisticated class management, and help from parents, students or older pupils is worth considering. By teaching clearly and concisely and by progressing through the hierarchy of skills in a logical manner, the teacher will be able to give the clumsy child some of the support he requires without penalizing the rest of the class. The child will not want to be identified as clumsy, so the help he is given must not be too obvious. Equally, the class must not suffer from undue attention being paid to one member. The clumsy child must learn to adapt to the class just as they too must adapt to him and his problems. The activities in which the child is most likely to encounter difficulties in the physical education programme are pre-games and games activities, gymnastics and dance. Much can be done to develop co-ordination and help the child to acquire ball-handling skills and to introduce the element of competition gradually. When gymnastics and dance are introduced, emphasis can be laid on the importance of rhythm in the acquisition and execution of skills. Development of body awareness is the first stage in both dance and gymnastics. Gradually, complex skills can be built up from basic ones.

Of all the areas of physical education, swimming is the one most likely to offer the clumsy child a degree of success. General strength and co-ordination are developed in the water where the child cannot trip and can avoid many of the problems encountered on the sports field. If he can succeed, even in competitions, this may alter the child's whole outlook on life (Cooke, 1980).

The speech therapist is another member of the 'medical team' who may well be asked to help the child acquire motor skills, partly because articulation involves the co-ordination of complex movements and partly because of the overlap of disabilities which are likely to have a common aetiology. It must always be emphasized that parents, therapists and teachers must not work in isolation if the clumsy child is to benefit from all the effort involved. The doctor will play a larger part in the diagnosis and assessment of motor learning disorders than in their treatment, but can contribute to the team.

Advocacy can make sure that the child is receiving help from such experts as may be indicated or afforded, and enquiry can endeavour to find out if the treatment and education that is being given is beneficial. The field of learning disabilities in childhood is a most rewarding one, as the tendency is towards improvement, and it is a pleasure to partake in a small way in other people's successful accomplishments.

Though parents may be helpful allies in remedial processes, it is inevitable that too much time spent sharing a child's areas of difficulty will threaten relationships. There should be encouragement to parents to find activities both individually, and within the family, which can be shared with the child with mutual pleasure. Other children should not be neglected within the family or resentment will build up.

Parents confronted by a child who seems to be letting them down wonder if the child's problems are their fault. It is easy for parents to lose a sense of proportion about their child and to exaggerate their child's 'abnormality'. Reassurance that all parents of children with inconsistent performance find the situation difficult may be a relief. Studies of children with literacy problems have shown that emotional or behavioural consequences are not inevitable but become much more likely if the child has additional perceptual-motor difficulties (Bale, 1981). Overconcentration on the learning difficulty or clumsiness of the child may lead to neglect of other aspects of the child's experience of life (games, self-care skills, interest in pets or hobbies, ability to relate to people, and capacity for unassisted play). There may be problems or assets in these areas.

Teachers may need help to understand the child. Finding educational solutions for children and teachers may need involvement of other colleagues as described above, but usually the solutions can be found within the school.

One of the contributions doctors can make is to be involved in the in-service education of teachers, promoting an awareness of children with motor difficulties. More may be achieved by this than by developing a large case-load and trying to expand hospital-based remedial programmes.

The doctor can also participate in the design of research programmes to identify and help clumsy children, to understand how their difficulties have arisen, how a clumsy child affects the family and to clarify the prognosis.

Co-ordination tests

There is at present a gulf between the tests used by experimental psychologists (Pentland, 1982; Laszlo & Bairstow, 1980; Elliott & Connolly, 1984; Hulme *et al.*, 1984) and those in clinical or educational use (Bender, 1938; Gesell & Amatruda, 1947; Wechsler, 1949; Frostig *et al.*, 1963; Griffiths, 1970; Stott *et al.*, 1972; Bruininks, 1978; Gubbay, 1978). The research teams are seen by clinicians as idealistic and dependent on equipment. The clinicians are thought to be insufficiently precise by research workers. There is certainly a need to improve the validity and reliability of tests in clinical use and to derive local as much as national norms (Tew, 1979). Nothing but good can come of discussion between academic and service departments. At present, co-ordination testing lies in limbo between physical education teachers, psychologists and doctors.

Screening for clumsiness

Some studies have shown that co-ordination testing can have predictive value (Bax & Whitmore, 1973; McKinlay *et al.*, 1981) if the examination is sufficiently detailed or selection is strict. However, there is a dearth of evidence that screening benefits children or is cost-effective. If controlled studies can show benefit from early intervention this might alter our opinion that screening is not justified at present. It is desirable to collect good developmental data, however, preferably on a local basis, to assess the significance of motor immaturity demonstrated in a child who is in trouble by comparison with his peers.

Handwriting

The status of handwriting has fluctuated over centuries in the educational curriculum. At times it has been promoted to the point of boredom, while at other times it has been neglected. Few studies have been subjected to greater influences of fashion (Jarman, 1979) and the relative dearth of evaluative research is regrettable (Askov *et al.*, 1970; Peck *et al.*, 1980; Alston & Taylor, 1984).

Children normally learn to write with a pencil. Those who have difficulty in controlling a pencil have commonly been advised to use a thicker pencil or a pencil holder. Others have been advised to use a thinner pencil on the grounds that this may provide more sensory feedback. For the child with poor pencil control there is something to be said for providing a range of implements and allowing the child to make a choice. Motivation to use the pencil may be greater if the child has chosen it. Little is known about the strategies which enable individual children to write accurately. These are probably diverse and usually generated by the child, rather than taught. However, for those children who find it difficult to learn, a more formal and systematic approach is needed (Sassoon & Briem, 1984; Alston & Taylor, 1984).

If a child finds the mechanical process of writing difficult and tiring in spite of adequate teaching, it may be hard for that child to write neatly and at speed. Help in note-taking and in the planning of essays may be needed (Binns, 1978). As the volume of written work required increases, the child may find it harder to keep pace with educational demands in spite of an adequate understanding of the syllabus. Time extension for examinations may be justified. Exceptionally, the child may be taught to type. This may be necessary for examinations for some such children. For others typing may be useful to prepare neat job applications or important letters. Not all children with writing problems welcome the suggestion of typing, however, and it is not always possible to arrange for those who would benefit to receive appropriate teaching.

Conclusion

In spite of long-standing controversies about 'minimal brain dysfunction' and the significance of 'soft neurological signs', it is recognized that there are a number of children, perhaps 1 in 100, who show surprising, discrepant difficulty in everyday motor activities. There are many possible explanations and such children are a diverse group. Nonetheless, awareness of these children has increased among developmental paediatricians, therapists, psychologists, child psychiatrists and teachers. There are problems with methods of assessment of the children and means of helping them. Knowledge about the prognosis for clumsy children is very inadequate. Terminology is recognized to be unsatisfactory; 'clumsy' means different things to different people (Taylor & McKinlay, 1979). Some have been inclined to wash their hands of such troublesome issues in consequence. Nevertheless, involvement with children with motor learning difficulties is a growing and challenging area of developmental medicine, child psychiatry, therapy and education.

Development of hospital services is probably not the best way to proceed. A collaborative approach between the education and health authorities could lead to a better understanding of existing resources. More thought could be given to movement education in *infant* and *primary* schools. This will usually be supervised by the (non-specialist) class teacher. Assessment tools could be devised in discussion with both the physical education advisory service and therapists, both of whom have much to contribute as resources in devising programmes to develop postural and movement control. This needs to be an on-going advisory service, and in-service training is also desirable. In areas where the population is scattered, personal advisory services may need to be complemented by manuals for teachers. Involvement of parents and of older children in the physical education of young children has potential for mutual benefit, without costing money. There should be a support service for individual children who have exceptional difficulty 'fitting in'. Short courses of remedial movement and posture education, individually or in small groups, can be devised unobtrusively. The aim of such help should be agreed with the child and his parents.

For older children (of 12 years upwards) remedial physical programmes are often embarrassing and unnecessary. There should be a sufficient range of options available to allow all such pupils to enjoy a chosen physical activity. Although in the past PE teachers have tended to be sports coaches, there is now increasing interest in children with motor learning difficulties. Helping them has been found to be surprisingly rewarding. Hospital services should be reserved for those who, having been examined by the school doctor, may require more detailed investigation.

References

Alston, J. & Taylor, J. (1984) *The Handwriting File: Diagnosis and Remediation of Handwriting Difficulties*. Learning Development Aids, Wisbech, Cambs.

Anderson, E.M. & Plewis, I. (1977) Impairment of motor skill in children with spina bifida cystica and hydrocephalus: an exploratory study. *British Journal of Psychology*, **68**, 61–70.

Askov, E., Otto, W. & Askov, W. (1970) A decade of research in handwriting: progress and prospect. *Journal of Educational Research*, **64**, 100–111.

Bakwin, H. (1973) Reading disability in twins. *Developmental Medicine and Child Neurology*, **15**, 184–187.

Bale, P. (1981) Behaviour problems and their relationship to reading difficulty. *Journal of Research in Reading*, **4**, 123–135.

Baum, J.D. (1977) The continuum of caretaking casualty. *Developmental Medicine and Child Neurology*, **19**, 543–544.

Bax, M. & Whitmore, K. (1973) Neurodevelopmental screening in the school-entrant medical examination. *Lancet*, **ii**, 368–370.

Belmont, L., Stein, Z.A. & Wittes, J.T. (1976) Birth order, family size and school failure. *Developmental Medicine and Child Neurology*, **18**, 421–430.

Bender, L. (1938) *Visual Motor Gestalt Test and its Clinical Use*. American Orthopsychiatric Association, New York.

Benson, D.F. (1979) *Aphasia, Alexia and Agraphia*. Churchill Livingstone, Edinburgh.

Binns, R. (1978) *From Speech to Writing*. Scottish Curriculum Development Service, Moray House College of Education, Edinburgh.

Bishop, D.V.M. (1980) Handedness, clumsiness and cognitive ability. *Developmental Medicine and Child Neurology*, **22**, 569–579.

Bishop, D.V.M. (1981) Plasticity and specificity of language localisation in the developing brain. *Developmental Medicine and Child Neurology*, **23**, 251–255.

Bradley, L. & Bryant, P.E. (1978) Difficulties in auditory organisation as a possible cause of reading backwardness. *Nature*, **271**, 746–747.

Brazelton, T.B., Tronick, E., Lechtig, A., Lasky, R.E. & Klein, R.E. (1977) The behaviour of nutritionally deprived Guatemalan infants. *Developmental Medicine and Child Neurology*, **19**, 364–372.

British Medical Journal (1978) Nutrition and the brain. **i**, 1569–1570.

British Medical Journal (1979) Acquired cerebral disorders of reading. **ii**, 350–351.

Brown, J.K. (1976) Infants damaged during birth; perinatal asphyxia. In *Recent Advances in Paediatrics*, Vol. 5 (ed. D. Hull). Churchill Livingstone, Edinburgh.

Brown, J.K. (1981) Learning disorders: a paediatric neurologist's view. *Transactions of The College of Medicine of South Africa*, 49–104.

Brown, J.K., Puruis, R.J., Forfar, J.O. & Cockburn, F. (1974) Neurological aspects of perinatal asphyxia. *Developmental Medicine and Child Neurology*, **16**, 567–580.

Bruininks, R.H. (1978) *The Bruininks-Oseretsky Test of Motor Proficiency*. NFER, Windsor.

Bryant, M. (1980) Occupational therapy. In *Helping Clumsy Children* (eds N. Gordon and I. McKinlay). Churchill Livingstone, Edinburgh.

Connolly, K.J. & Prechtl, H.F.R., eds (1981) Maturation and development. *Clinics in Developmental Medicine*, **77/78**

Cooke, L. (1980) Physical education. In *Helping Clumsy Children* (eds N. Gordon and I. McKinlay). Churchill Livingstone, Edinburgh.

Critchley, M. (1964) *Developmental Dyslexia*. Heinemann, London.

Davies, P.A. (1976) Outlook for the low birthweight baby—then and now. *Archives of Disease in Childhood*, **51**, 817–819.

Decker, S.N. & De Fries, J.C. (1981) Cognitive ability profiles in families of reading-disabled children. *Developmental Medicine and Child Neurology*, **23**, 217–227.

Denckla, M.B. (1973) Development of speed in repetitive and successive finger movements in normal children. *Developmental Medicine and Child Neurology*, **15**, 635–645.

Dobbing, J. (1970) Undernutrition and the developing brain. In *Development Neurobiology* (ed. W.A. Heinrich). Charles C. Thomas, Springfield, Illinois.

Dobbing, J. & Sands, J. (1971) Vulnerability of developing brain. IX. The effect of nutritional growth retardation on the timing of the brain growth spurt. *Biology of the Neonate*, **19**, 363–378.

Dobbing, J. & Sands, J. (1981) Vulnerability of developing brain not explained by cell number/cell size hypotheses. *Early Human Development*, **5**, 227–231.

Drotar, D.D., Stern, R.C. & Polmar, S.H. (1976) Intellectual and social development following prolonged isolation. *Journal of Pediatrics*, **89**, 675–678.

Eccles, J.C. (1980) *The Human Psyche*. Springer, Berlin.

Eiser, C. & Lansdown, R. (1977) Retrospective study of intellectual development in children treated for acute lymphoblastic leukaemia. *Archives of Disease in Childhood*, **52**, 525–529.

Elliott, J.M. & Connolly, K.J. (1984) A classification of manipulative hand movements. *Developmental Medicine and Child Neurology*, **26**, 283–296.

Epir, S., Renda, Y. & Baser, N. (1984) Cognitive and behavioural characteristics of children with idiopathic epilepsy in a low-income area of Ankara, Turkey. *Developmental Medicine and Child Neurology*, **26**, 200–207.

Essen, J., Fogelman, K. & Head, J. (1978) Childhood housing experiences and school attainment. *Child: Care, Health and Development*, **4**, 41–58.

Finucci, J.M., Guthrie, J.T., Childs, A.I., Abbey, H. & Childs, B. (1976) The genetics of specific reading disability. *Annals of Human Genetics, London*, **40**, 1–23.

Frostig, M., Lefewen, W. & Whittlesey, J.R.B. (1963) *Developmental Test of Visual Perception*. Consulting Psychologists Press, California.

Fundudis, T., Kolvin, I. & Garside, R.T., eds (1979) *Speech Retarded and Deaf Children: their Psychological Development*. Academic Press, London.

Galaburda, A.M. & Kemper, T.L. (1979) Cytoarchitectonic abnormalities in developmental dyslexia: a case study. *Annals of Neurology*, **6**, 94–100.

Gesell, A. & Amatruda, C.S. (1947) *The Gesell Development Schedule*. Hoeber, New York.

Gillberg, C. & Rasmussen, P. (1982) Perceptual, motor and attentional deficits in seven-year-old children: background factors. *Developmental Medicine and Child Neurology*, **24**, 752–770.

Gillberg, C., Rasmussen, P. & Wahlstrom, J. (1982) Minor neurodevelopmental disorders in children born to older mothers. *Developmental Medicine and Child Neurology*, **24**, 437–447.

Gordon, N. & McKinlay, I., eds (1980) *Helping Clumsy Children*. Churchill Livingstone, Edinburgh.

Gordon, N., McKinlay, I. & Rosenbloom, L. (1984) Medical contribution to the management of dyslexia. *Archives of Disease in Childhood*, **59**, 588–590.

Griffiths, P. (1979) An approach to language therapy for children with specific language disability. *New Zealand Speech Therapists Journal*, **34**, 14–21.

Griffiths, R. (1970) *The Abilities of Young Children*. Child Development Research Centre, London.

Grimley, A. (1980) Physiotherapy. In *Helping Clumsy Children* (eds N. Gordon and I. McKinlay). Churchill Livingstone, Edinburgh.

Gubbay, S.S. (1978) The management of developmental apraxia. *Developmental Medicine and Child Neurology*, **20**, 643–646.

Hagberg, B. (1978) The epidemiological panorama of major neuropediatric handicaps in Sweden. *Clinics in Developmental Medicine*, **67**, 'The Care of the Handicapped Child'. (eds Bax, M. & Apley, J.) S.I.M.P., Heinemann, London.

Herman, K. & Norrie, E. (1958) Is congenital word-blindness a hereditary type of Gerstmann's syndrome? *Psychiatria et Neurologia*, Basel, **136**, 59–73.

Hulme, C., Smart, A. & Moran, G. (1982) Visual perceptual deficits in clumsy children. *Neuropsychologia*, **20**, 475–481.

Hulme, C., Smart, A., Moran, G. & McKinlay, I. (1984) Visual, kinaesthetic and cross-modal judgments of length by clumsy children: a comparison with young normal children. *Child: Care, Health and Development*, **10**, 117–125.

Ingvar, D.H. (1975) Patterns of brain activity revealed by measurements of regional cerebral blood flow. In *Brain Work* (eds D.H. Ingvar and N.A. Lassen). Munksgaard, Copenhagen.

Jarman, C. (1979) *The Development of Handwriting Skills*. Blackwells, Oxford.

Lassen, N.A., Ingvar, D.H. & Skinjoj, E. (1978) Patterns of activity in the human cerebral cortex graphically displayed. *Scientific American*, **239**, 50–59.

Lassman, F.M., Fisch, R.O., Vatter, D.K. & La Benz, E.S. (1980) *Early Correlates of Speech, Language and Hearing*. PSG Publishing Company, Littleton, Mass.

Laszlo, J.I. & Bairstow, P.J. (1980) The measurement of kinaesthetic sensitivity in children and adults. *Developmental Medicine and Child Neurology*, **22**, 454–464.

Lloyd-Still, J.D., Hurwitz, I., Wolff, P.H. & Schwachman, H. (1974) Intellectual development after severe malnutrition in infancy. *Pediatrics*, **54**, 306–311.

Low, N.L. (1980) A hypothesis why 'early intervention' in cerebral palsy might be useful. *Brain and Development*, **2**, 133.

McFaul, R., Dorner, S., Brett, E.M. & Grant, D.B. (1978) Neurological abnormalities in patients treated for hypothyroidism in early life. *Archives of Disease in Childhood*, **53**, 611–619.

McKinlay, I. (1980) In *Helping Clumsy Children* (eds N. Gordon and I. McKinlay). Churchill Livingstone, Edinburgh.

McKinlay, I., England, A., Nash, S., Sands, J., Chesham, I. & Dobbing, J. (1981) The predictive value of co-ordination testing. *Neuropediatrics*, **12**, Supplement, 426.

Minns, R.A., Sobkowiak, C.A., Skardoutsou, A., Diuick, K., Elton, R.A., Brown, J.K. & Forfar, J.O. (1977) Upper limb function in spina bifida. *Zeitschrift für Kinderchirurgie*, **22**, 493–506.

O'Malley, P.J. & Griffiths, J.F. (1977) Perceptuomotor dysfunction in the child with hemiplegia. *Developmental Medicine and Child Neurology*, **19**, 172–178.

Ounsted, M., Moar, V.A., Cockburn, J. & Redman, C.W.G. (1984) Factors associated with the intellectual ability of children born to women with high risk pregnancies. *British Medical Journal*, **288**, 1038–1041.

Ounsted, C. & Taylor, D.C. (1972) *Gender Differences; their Ontogeny and Significance*. Churchill Livingstone, Edinburgh.

Peck, M., Askov, E.N. & Fairchild, S.H. (1980) Another decade of research in handwriting: progress and prospect in the 1970s. *Journal of Educational Research*, **73**, 283–298.

Pentland, A.P. (1982) Maximum likelihood estimation: the best PEST. *Perception and Psychophysics*, **28**, 377–379.

Robinson, R.J. (1984) The doctor and the child with learning problems. *British Medical Journal*, **288**, 1937–1938.

Robinson, R.O. (1981) Equal recovery in child and adult brain? *Developmental Medicine and Child Neurology*, **23**, 379–383.

Rodier, P.M. (1980) Chronology of neuron development: animal studies and their clinical implications. *Developmental Medicine and Child Neurology*, **22**, 525–545.

Russell, W.R. (1958) The physiology of memory. *Proceedings of the Royal Society of Medicine*, **51**, 9.

Sassoon, R. & Briem, G.S.E. (1984) *Teach Yourself Handwriting*. Hodder and Stoughton, London.

Shaffer, D., Schonfield, I., O'Conner, P.A., Stokman, C., Trautman, P., Schafer, S., Ng, S. (1985) Neurological soft signs: their relationship to psychiatric disorder and intelligence in childhood and adolescence. *Archives of General Psychiatry*, **42**, 342–351.

Sibert, J.R., Jadhov, M. & Infaraj, S.G. (1978) Maternal and fetal nutrition in South India. *British Medical Journal*, **1**, 1517–1518.

Smith, M., Delves, T., Lansdown, R., Clayton, B. & Graham, P. (1983) The effects of lead exposure on urban children: the Institute of Child Health/Southampton Study. *Developmental Medicine and Child Neurology*, **25**, Supplement 47.

Stores, G. (1978) School-children with epilepsy at risk for learning and behaviour problems. *Developmental Medicine and Child Neurology*, **20**, 502–508.

Stott, D.H., Moye, F.A. & Henderson, S.E. (1972) *Test of Motor Impairment*. NFER, Windsor.

Szatmari, P. & Taylor, D.C. (1984) Overflow movements and behaviour problems: scoring and using a modification of Fog's tests. *Developmental Medicine and Child Neurology*, **26**, 297–310.

Taylor, D.C. (1981) The influence of sexual differentiation on growth development and disease. In *The Scientific Foundations of Paediatrics* (eds J.A. Davis and J. Dobbing), 2nd edn. Heinemann, London.

Taylor, D.C. & McKinlay, I.A. (1979) What kind of thing is 'being clumsy'? *Child: Care, Health and Development*, **5**, 167–175.

Tew, B. (1979) Differences between Welsh and Canadian children on parts of the test of motor impairment. *Child: Care, Health and Development*, **5**, 135–141.

Thomson, A.J., Searle, M. & Russell, G. (1977) Quality of survival after severe birth asphyxia. *Archives of Disease in Childhood*, **52**, 620–626.

Tizard, B. & Hughes, M. (1984) *Young Children Learning: Talking and Thinking at Home and at School*. Fontana, London.

Vass, J.F. (1979) Organisation, structure and memory; three perspectives. In *Memory Organisation and Structure* (ed. C.R. Puff). Academic Press, New York.

Wechsler, D. (1949) *The Wechsler Intelligence Scale for Children*. The Psychological Corporation, New York.

Chapter 9
Children with Delayed Development of Speech and Language

Ena Davies & Neil Gordon

Introduction

Disorders of speech and language in childhood are relatively common and a number of medical specialists will have to work closely with speech therapists, psychologists and social workers if these children are to be given the help they need. It is estimated that in the United Kingdom there are 400,000 children and adults with speech and language disorders, of whom 200,000 are severely communicatively handicapped. Many children with neurological disorders are 'at risk' of developmental or acquired language impairment. Among the doctors involved will be paediatricians, paediatric neurologists, audiologists, ENT specialists and child psychiatrists. The importance of the medical contribution is emphasized by the fact that up to a third of children attending a hospital-based speech clinic were found to have medical conditions associated with their speech defects (Ingram, 1969; Bax *et al.*, 1980; Lassman *et al.*, 1980; Robinson, 1982). It has been shown that problems of this kind are common enough; in one study the speech of 14.4% of boys and 9.7% of girls was not fully intelligible on school entry, and at this time the speech of 1.8% of boys and 0.9% of girls was largely unintelligible (Peckham, 1973). The fact that relatively few children have such disorders on leaving school is no argument against accurate assessment and treatment, for if this is omitted there will be an inevitable price to pay. There will be an almost certain failure to reach a full potential due to the amount of emotional and intellectual energy devoted to trying to overcome the disability unaided.

A communication problem will threaten relationships with parents and teachers, and perhaps set up a style of relationship that persists after speech has improved. It is also common to observe that speech is worse in emotionally charged situations, which is especially frustrating for the child. A Newcastle study (Fundudis *et al.*, 1979) has also shown that children whose speech disorders have resolved by the age of 7 or 8, commonly still have difficulties with literacy.

This has been confirmed in the follow-up of the 1958 cohort in the

National Child Development Study. Fogelman's data (unpublished) show that the children commonly have difficulties with literacy whether or not their speech has improved. In this study, 16% of 1000 children at the age of 7 were described as unintelligible according to their doctors and teachers. They were more numerous, had more problems and showed less improvement than children with hearing loss. Boys outnumbered girls by 2 to 1. There were over three times as many poor readers or non-readers as in the general population (81% versus 26%). More than half had persisting speech problems at the age of 16, and even those who had improved showed no advantage in literacy over those who had not. More than a third of those whose problems persisted between the ages of 7 and 11 were not receiving speech therapy. Only a quarter of those whose speech had improved had received speech therapy. Six of the 54 with persisting problems at the age of 16 were considered maladjusted and four were attending Borstal (punitive) institutions.

It may be interesting to assess the effects of the role of the speech therapist as an adviser to remedial teachers for such children. Quite apart from remedial speech therapy, which may or may not be effective for particular children, there is a need for someone who understands speech and language problems to act as an advocate and interpreter for the child. Mentally handicapped children are especially prone to behaviour disorders if they have additional speech or language impairment.

A distinction must be made between the production of words and the meaning they convey. As with so many skills, those who perfect them are usually selective in their use. Shakespeare can convey in a sentence the same wealth of meaning that others will only manage in several pages, and then in an inferior manner. On the other hand, among those who are mentally handicapped it is not uncommon to find a child who can produce a large number of words if encouraged to learn these by rote memory, but they do not have real meaning to the child and are soon forgotten. A certain degree of complexity in cerebral structure will be necessary if spoken language is to develop, and if there is a marked lack of neurones or inter-connections, resulting in a severe degree of mental handicap, this development may be impossible. Other means of communication will have to be developed.

Even in such severe disorders the situation is a complex one. It has, for example, been shown that once children have been labelled as mentally handicapped people's attitudes will change, and mothers in particular will talk in a restricted manner to them (Cashdan, 1969). Although care must be taken that speech is meaningful to the child, it can be over-simplified, thus depriving him of the wider experience on which children depend to increase their vocabulary.

Physically handicapped children are often severely deprived in terms of the experience that is so essential for the formation of concepts and then the elaboration of language. A normal child of 3 or 4 will be constantly on the move, exploring the environment and gaining experience, which emphasizes the importance of trying as far as possible to bring the world to the child who cannot move normally. Otherwise his world can be very restricted, perhaps consisting of one or two rooms at home and the classroom at school.

Inevitably, a child who is deaf will suffer from delayed and sometimes deviant language development, with impairment of the main input channel. Children with severe peripheral deafness as their only handicap still have difficulties with abstract thought, even if successfully treated from an early age. One reason for this may be the difficulty in explaining to such children ideas rather than facts. Recently, more attention has been paid to intermittent deafness in early childhood due to recurrent otitis media, and the effect this may have on the spoken language and even reading ability. Although there is evidence of such a communication, there is also considerable controversy over recommendations for treatment (Paradise, 1980; Zincus *et al.*, 1978).

Severe emotional disturbances in early life can affect language development, although it is difficult to be certain of the effects of lack of experience at this age. Rutter (1980) concludes that children's intellectual development is sensitive to environmental changes in both earlier and later childhood, but whether the former have more effect is uncertain. They may do, but if so it is only a relative difference and not a qualitative distinction due to a sharply defined critical period of development in the first 5 years. Delayed language development is a conspicuous feature of 'autism'. Boucher (1976) has reviewed some of the theories suggesting that language disorders have a central role in the genesis of the autistic syndrome. The evidence did not support a form of receptive executive developmental dysphasia, or a dysphasia combined with visual impairments causing failure to develop visual language systems. The language disorder did not seem to be the specific result of an impairment of symbolizing processes or of the acquisition of concepts or conceptual thinking either. It may well be that autism is a generalized cognitive abnormality with wide-ranging effects, of which language impairment is only one, though obviously an important one. Boucher rightly points out that if this is so it is misleading to speak of the language disability as the fundamental feature of autism, however conspicuous or handicapping it may be. This concept has implications for management, since therapeutic techniques have to take into account the child's cognitive and social emotional impairments, as well as the language difficulties.

Acquired disorders of language development in childhood present special problems, at least if the child is affected before the age of 10. Not only will there be the results of the damage in terms of loss of function, but also an interference with the continuing development of language function. This is well illustrated in Charles Dickens' description of Laura Bridgman's early life. He met her in 1842 and wrote a clear account of how she was helped after becoming blind and deaf (Gordon, 1969). It not only emphasizes how advanced communication can be without the use of speech, but also that expressive speech is the final stage of language development and how complex must be the cerebral integration that occurs before the child uses words. If Laura Bridgman and Helen Keller had not started to use words to communicate before their illnesses it is most unlikely that they would have accomplished what they did. It may help parents to realize this, and that the first word a child says with meaning is the beginning of the last stage of language development. It emphasizes the importance of speaking to normal children in as meaningful a way as possible without asking much in return for long periods. In language acquisition, as opposed to disordered language learning when there is a specific disorder of development, the emphasis is on meaning and language use, and not on structure (Griffiths, 1979).

When the development of language function appears to be delayed to a much greater degree than other aspects of development, and in the absence of secondary causes such as those discussed, it can be regarded as a specific disorder. The majority of children with such disorders, as with any other disability, will improve and, if given a certain amount of help and understanding in their early years, will overcome their disability if they have average intelligence. As the severity of the disability increases, sounds other than those of language may lack meaning, and the term congenital auditory imperception has been used to describe such children (Worster-Drought, 1943). Fortunately rare, the auditory agnosia can be even more profound. Then the child may not respond to sound of any kind and the abnormal auditory response may be thought to be due to peripheral deafness. The diagnosis may be particularly difficult, because a number of causes (such as anoxia at birth) can damage the auditory nuclei in the brain stem as well as causing more widespread brain damage. Central and peripheral deafness will coexist. Diagnostic techniques, in-

cluding auditory evoked potentials, can often help to analyse these problems; this is necessary if the child is to receive the educational help most
suited to his needs.

Even when the auditory agnosia is severe the abnormal response can
alter as the child grows older. The child will begin to react to sounds, and
this may be the result of the necessary association being made between
different parts of the cortex so that meaning can be given to the electrical
stimuli coming from the peripheral auditory receptors.

Ingram (1969) has emphasized the great variety of speech and
language disorders that can affect children: disorders of voicing; of
respiratory co-ordination; of speech sound production due to neurological
abnormalities, or structural abnormalities of the organs of articulation, or
occurring in association with other diseases and adverse environmental
factors; and finally, developmental speech disorders of a specific type.
A child quite often suffers from two or more of these conditions; for
example, it is not uncommon for a child with the spastic form of cerebral
palsy to have a marked degree of malocclusion of the teeth and an
inadequate nasal airway. If physical and language disabilities coexist, the
impairment may be compounded. When effective treatment is possible
for even one of such disorders, the improvement in the child's speech can
sometimes be considerable.

Although the speech therapist obviously plays a key role in the
management of the child with disorders of speech and language, it is still
as a member of 'the team' including the parents and the teachers. The
work of the speech therapist must be widely based: from taking the
disabled child out of the home and school and into the community to gain
experience of the outside world, to the treatment of the stammerer, and
the complex task of treating the young child who has lost speech after a
head injury. As soon as concern is expressed about a child's development
of speech and language, there must be an involvement of the 'medical
team', not necessarily in treatment as such, but certainly in assessment
and advice to parents and teachers.

Communication is the most fundamental of all human abilities. It is
the way in which we transmit and receive thoughts, ideas and feelings,
through body language (eye contact, signals, gestures, facial expression),
made audible through speech and recorded in writing.

Articulate speech is unique to mankind, and the manner of speaking
unique to each individual. It is estimated that speech represents only 35%
of the total communication process (Mehrabian, 1972). The remaining
65% is dependent upon non-verbal expression. Yet enormous importance

is attached to speech: parents wait anxiously for their child's first intelligible utterances, and anxiety increases if there is any significant delay in spoken language. Within the first 5–7 years of life the average child will acquire mastery over communication skills that will provide the basis for social interaction, control of environment, development of intellect and imagination, and equip the growing child to meet the educational challenges ahead.

The miracle of language is that anyone learns to speak intelligibly. It is only when the process is disrupted by some developmental or acquired disorder that the commonplace miracle is revealed.

Pre-linguistic behaviour

At a pre-linguistic level primitive reflexes govern behaviour (Gesell, 1945): grasping, sucking, swallowing, locating the teat for feeding (initially by tactile sensation, later by smell). The baby will be startled by loud sounds, will jump and draw breath, raising the arms above the head. These are but a few of the early reflexes that may, if they persist, have a detrimental effect on speech production.

The speech musculature is primarily designed for feeding. It is only at a later stage in the infant's development that it becomes modified and adapted for speech, echoing phylogenetic development.

Speech-related reflexes

The sucking reflex can be stimulated in embryo as early as the 20th week of prenatal existence, when amniotic fluid may be swallowed in a rehearsal for life (Gesell, 1945). The lips protrude, the tongue tip rises to the teeth ridge in order to depress the teat. The sucking reflex is closely allied to the 'rooting' reflex—lip rounding and preparatory sucking movements stimulated by pressure to the cheek or oral area. 'Rooting' by tactile stimulation is usually superseded by the emergence of the sense of smell as a means of location at about 3–4 weeks of age. The grasp reflex is complementary to sucking, dramatically demonstrated in animals where the young cling to the mother whilst suckling. The grasp reflex is strong enough to support the baby's weight, but unlike the mature palmar grasp, the thumb is held adducted across the palm. Both sucking and grasp reflexes become modified as the baby matures. By the 5th, 6th, or 7th month, chewing becomes established as the teeth begin to erupt and solids are increasingly introduced into the diet. The tongue now retracts for swallowing rather than thrusting forward, and lip closure is gradually achieved, replacing the open-mouthed messiness associated with early attempts at spoon feeding.

Many early phonemes are produced in association with feeding: the dental sounds *t*, *d*, *n* and *l*, as the tongue tip contacts the teeth ridge; the labial sounds *p*, *b* and *m*, as lip closure is achieved; and the sounds of contentment *k*, *g* and *ng*, as the tongue lolls against the soft palate when the baby lies at rest. Babbling emerges as a precursor to speech (Menyuk, 1974), but the ability to articulate is of little purpose without the vehicle of language for effective communication.

Prerequisites for language acquisition

Language acquisition is dependent upon multisensory input: auditory, visual, tactile, kinaesthetic, and to a lesser extent the sensation of taste and smell.

However, the *manner* in which language is perceived by the action, reaction and interaction of the cells in the cerebral cortex continues to be a fascinating area of debate. How the child acquires the labels, the functions and the categories of objects, and is then able to select according to size, shape and colour, and to relate in time and space, is a challenge to all who work in the area of childhood language. It is not within the scope of this chapter to enter into the debate, or evaluate the theories, but it may be relevant, in terms of management, to be aware of current trends.

The language debate

The old dictum that 'comprehension precedes production' is viewed by many researchers as an over-simplification of the nature of understanding and the manner of production. In her book, *Children's Minds*, Donaldson (1978) poses two questions that during the last two decades have produced widely variant responses to the debate on cognitive versus linguistic development. 'Does the child understand the words he hears in the sense that they are in his vocabulary' (i.e. by meaning), or does he understand the words in their *context* (linguistic or non-linguistic).

The cognitivist school led by Piaget and his colleagues maintains that knowledge is acquired by and through action. Piaget (1968) regards the baby as a living organism that adapts to the environment by assimilation (reacting) and accommodation (taking action). Language, according to Piaget, does not create intelligent thought, rather it is a vehicle for thought, a system of signs, an ability to represent absent objects or events.

Luria (1961), however, regards language as a tool for the development of intellectual processes, following clearly defined developmental stages. Chomsky (1972) revolutionized thinking in the 1960s by postulating an innate ability to develop language—a 'language acquisition device'.

Bruner (1975) switched attention to the function of language rather than its structure. He stressed that linguistic concepts are realized *in action*, reinforced in the mother–child interaction. Snow (1977), summarizing her paper on 'The development of conversation between mothers and babies', suggests another avenue for research—'the extent to which the nature of the interaction between mothers and infants in the first years of life contributes to the speech and nature of later language acquisition'.

Schlesinger (1977) discussing the role of cognitive development and linguistic input concludes that 'it is not *either* cognitive development *or* linguistic input which determines linguistic growth but an interaction between these factors.' This pragmatic view is shared by Yoder & Calculator (1981), who advocate 'an approach that perceives language *not as an isolated repertoire of sounds that can be trained, then combined into words, then re-combined to produce grammatical strings*' but 'as a medium of interaction between persons, which is conditioned by the various contexts in which persons operate'. This philosophy has important implications for therapy, particularly for the more severely handicapped child, shifting the emphasis from exclusive concentration on phonetic, phonological, semantic or syntactic remediation, to the broader perspective of 'communication'. This does not devalue specific intervention programmes for children for whom these are appropriate, but places them within the wider context of the communicative needs of the child. Yoder sums it up eloquently: 'From a communication standpoint social interaction provides the child with a *reason* to *communicate*, cognitive interaction assures the child will have *something* to *say*, and linguistic interaction provides the child with a *means* of *saying it*.' [The italics are those of the authors.]

Identifying the problems

The child with a neurological impairment is likely to be 'at risk' of some disorder of communication. Dependent upon the site and degree of damage, the child may experience difficulties with reception, decoding, encoding or production of language.

Reception may be distorted by hearing loss; total or partial deafness can distort language acquisition and disrupt expressive ability (Moores, 1974). Visual defects may affect acuity and/or perception, delaying development of language skills (Fraiberg, 1977). Tactile and kinaesthetic input may be impaired, making discrimination of objects by size, shape and texture difficult or impossible. Taste and smell may also be affected by damage to sensory input.

The *dysphasic* child may hear without understanding the language of his environment. He may see without knowing the people and objects around him, and produce speech that is unintelligible to him and to his listeners. The damage may be, and often is, selective, enabling the child to compensate through intact sensory pathways, unlike the mentally handicapped child who, despite intact receptors, may be unable to compensate because poor innate endowment affects his overall ability to interpret what he sees, hears and feels.

The *dysarthric* child is often unable to co-ordinate the movements of tongue, lips and palate even for the basic functions of chewing, sucking and swallowing, and this frustrates all attempts at intelligible speech. Co-ordination of breathing and voicing may be at a primitive level, close to the limits for life, incapable of adaptation for the higher functions of speech. Breathing may be shallow and irregular, and the movements of the diaphragm may be out of phase with the expansion of the chest cavity by the upward and outward movement of the ribs.

The synchronous vibration of the vocal cords necessary for voice production is often thwarted by *hyper-tonicity* (producing voicing with a 'strangulated' quality, initially loud then fading to a whisper) or by *hypo-tonicity* (when there is insufficient muscle tone to sustain audible voicing). The movements of the tongue may be affected by the persistence of the sucking reflex—extension of the jaw, producing extension of the tongue followed by the all-or-nothing response of head extension, arching of the back and extension of the limbs. This is a pattern that will distort both feeding and speech.

The *dyspraxic* child may be able to perform the functions of chewing, sucking and swallowing, including the emotional responses of laughing, smiling and crying, and yet because of oral dyspraxia be unable to protrude the tongue to order, open or close the lips or stretch them. Dyspraxia may also affect the child's ability to imitate the movements required for the production of speech sounds—an articulatory dyspraxia that may exist alone or together with oral dyspraxia. The inability to locate or imitate movements in space may extend to volitional control over arms and/or legs.

Stammering may affect expressive speech in those children who are also unable to co-ordinate breathing, voicing and articulating. Children with neurological disorders are not exempt from speech and language problems of psychological origin, the desire to communicate inhibited by emotional problems.

There is no register of communicatively disordered people, unlike the 'deaf' or the 'blind' population, partly because the speech and language disorder is often a secondary symptom of some primary diagnosis. The origins may be *congenital* (e.g. deafness, cerebral palsy, mental handicap, autism, developmental language delay or cranio-facial abnormalities) or *acquired* (e.g. trauma, infection, vascular, post-epileptic).

Assessment

'The team approach'
The speech therapist is a member of the multidisciplinary team involved in the management of the child with neurological problems and of those who relate to the child. The composition of the team may vary according to the child's needs, age and placement. The paediatrician may co-ordinate the primary team drawing on resources of audiology, ophthalmology, psychology, physiotherapy, occupational therapy and speech therapy. Nursing and dietary advice may also be relevant, and the expertise of the rehabilitation engineer for the more severely physically handicapped child is often necessary.

The co-ordinating role may change as the child enters school and educational needs take precedence.

The constant core member of the team should be the parent(s) or care-givers, acting in consultation with professional support, and any decisions will have to be considered within the context of the family.

Assessment procedures
Assessment may be informal (through trained observation), formal (through standardized tests), or on-going (through evaluation of the child's progress).

It is difficult to define the intuitive knowledge which grows from experience, but the value of such informed observation cannot be over-emphasized. The child's behaviour, his frustration or apathy, the span of auditory and/or visual attention, and non-verbal signals are all important aspects of informal assessment. The 'look in the eye' or the 'spark of recognition' may be interpreted by the observer who has time to attend to this silent communication. It may also be misleading for parents and occasionally professionals, who become convinced that the child understands all that is being said. The child too is receiving non-verbal clues from his environment, and to a question demanding a 'yes' or 'no' response has a 50% chance of being correct.

Standardized testing provides an objective analysis of the child's abilities and disabilities. It also provides a yardstick for evaluating progress. The more frequently used tests for evaluating language comprehension include the Reynell Developmental Language Scales (Reynell, 1977), Carrow's test (Carrow, 1973) and the Illinois Test of Psycholinguistic Abilities (Kirk *et al.*, 1968).

Assessment of expressive language skills may be undertaken using the expressive language scales of the above tests, and vocabulary measured by the Peabody Picture vocabulary test or the English Picture Vocabulary Test. The lexicon is likely to be depressed because of limited experience.

Specific articulatory or phonological problems may be identified by standardized tests, e.g. the Edinburgh Articulation Test (Anthony *et al.*, 1971), or by non-standardized assessment of the child's idiosyncratic use of the speech sounds in his/her repertoire. The important distinction to be made is between those children who are unable to imitate and produce specific speech sounds (articulatory), and those who, despite being able to produce the entire repertoire of speech sounds, make inconsistent errors of articulatory substitutions and omissions in connected speech (phonological).

Profiles identifying dysarthric or dyspraxic features, similar to those for adults (Goodglass & Kaplan, 1972; Enderby, 1981), have been devised to evaluate efficiency of treatment programmes. Analysis of spoken output may be recorded as profiles, e.g. language, assessment, remediation and screening procedures (Crystal *et al.*, 1976), and prosody profiles (PROP) or phonological profiles (PROPH) (Crystal, 1982). A 'communication inventory' devised by Coggins & Carpenter (1981) provides a baseline to evaluate the level of functional communication.

The above overview of assessment procedures is by no means exhaustive, but may be useful in providing guidelines for therapeutic intervention. The primary goal of assessment is to provide qualitative and quantitative analysis of the communicative problems, leading to their remediation. Müller *et al.* (1981) evaluate the efficiency of assessment tools in their practical handbook, *Language Assessment for Remediation.*

Tests that examine cognitive and linguistic development, analyse phonology and record syntactical features, provide guidelines for speech therapy when taken into consideration with the results of tests and observations by other members of the multidisciplinary team.

The majority of tests are based on developmental 'norms'. The enormous fluctuations in so-called normal development are comparable with attempts to describe a 'typical' Dane, Norwegian or Italian. There are certain distinguishable features just as with average stages of development, but there are considerable variations within those defined stages. For the handicapped child the yardstick of 'normal' development is often inappropriate because of the deprivation of experiences, lack of manual dexterity and poor expressive ability.

Standardization procedures for tests may also vary considerably, often modelled on the responses of children within one geographical area and of similar socio-economic background. Scores will also be subject to variation because of the way in which the test is administered. Despite rules for administration, some professionals will unintentionally provide more non-verbal clues by their posture, directed eye gaze or speech emphasis.

The child too will be an unknown quantity, subject to changes of mood, attention, alertness, drug therapy or test situation. On-going assessment incorporates both informal and formal approaches, and discussion with the multidisciplinary team will ensure that the child's changing needs will be met.

As with assessment, most intervention procedures follow a developmental model (Cooper *et al.*, 1978). However, there are some notable exceptions to this approach (e.g. Peto) who consider it inappropriate to follow normal developmental guidelines when dealing with an irreversible neuropathology.

It is essential therefore, that the speech therapist has a good understanding of the stages of language acquisition as a guideline for assessment and as a basis for evaluation of treatment and progress.

Language intervention to help the handicapped child

If, as is suggested, language is acquired through action, the neurologically handicapped child is at an immediate and obvious disadvantage. The inability to explore the environment, to experience through sight, sound, touch, taste and smell, limits the child's knowledge of the world. The inability to co-ordinate movements of breathing, phonation and articulation will deprive the child of auditory and kinaesthetic feedback of speech.

'Language should be helped during development at the normal developmental stage' (Cooper *et al.*, 1978). On that premise the use of the parent as the therapist is all-important to ensure that the child's world is brought within his reach throughout his waking day. Handling, positioning, seating and mobility are equally as important to language acquisition as they are in establishing feeding skills. Each situation can be used as a learning experience if the mother or care-giver is attuned to the needs of the child and is given guidelines for management. These may be informal or structured (as with the Portage programme), providing a practical developmental approach for parents of those children who may be at risk of delay.

'A developmental programme for children with early language handicaps' is outlined in *Helping Language Development* (Cooper *et al.*, 1978) and the theoretical framework provides a practical model for intervention.

The development of attention control is fundamental to the development of visual perception and verbal comprehension.

Visual attention may be difficult for the baby with little volitional control over head movement. Positioning is important to enable the child to focus visual attention with the minimum of physical effort until some modicum of head control is achieved. Initially, the mother may need to support the child's head in order to gain eye contact—the natural face to face position adopted by mothers when talking to their non-handicapped babies. Vocalization and verbalization are increased when eye contact is maintained (Snow, 1977), and can be stimulated in the ritual interactive games of 'Ride-a-cock horse', 'Peek-a-boo' or 'Pat-a-cake'.

Whether the child is in his cot, pram, chair or play-pen, play materials should be easily accessible and within his range of vision. Mobiles suspended above the cot to attract visual attention; colourful wall friezes at the child's eye level; toys of differing shapes, colours and textures strung across the cot or pram, within reach of an outstretched hand, are all useful. Toys that provide different tactile experiences may also incorporate a range of different sounds, linking visual with auditory attention.

Auditory attention may also be difficult for the neurologically handicapped child. The incidence of hearing loss, although decreasing because of improved perinatal care, is still greater than in the normal population. Early screening is important to ensure that there is no significant loss. Poor head control may also disrupt auditory attention as the child may be unable to turn in order to locate sound. Recognition and association of environmental sounds can be encouraged by the mother: the rattle of the spoon in the cup preparatory to feeding, or the swish of water in preparation for bath time. Suggestions for improving auditory and visual skills are outlined in the two practical books, *Let Me Speak* (Jeffree & McConkey, 1976) and *Let Me Play* (Jefree *et al.*, 1977).

Visual perception and verbal comprehension, in turn, provide the bases for the development of concept formation, symbolic understanding and visuo-motor skills.

Whereas the non-handicapped child may develop an awareness of the permanence of objects by exploring the environment, the handicapped child's ability to represent absent objects and abstract language will be restricted. A programme based on matching objects, classifying by colour, shape and category, quantifying according to size and number, and determining similarities and differences, provides a structured and graded approach for parents under professional guidance. The physically handicapped child may need additional help to locate objects in space, and a combined therapeutic approach may be used to improve spatial perception and stimulate language development in action. The protective extension of the arms and hands achieved when the child is rocked in a prone position over a large inflated ball or foam roll will improve hand–eye co-ordination for the development of visuo-motor skills. A box of objects of differing sizes, shapes and textures can be placed within reach of the outstretched hands and the child can be encouraged to dip in for games of matching, categorizing or quantifying. Concepts of 'in', 'on', 'under', 'over' can be learned in action in physiotherapy, the event reinforced in language by the speech therapist, and the concept applied in functional tasks by the occupational therapist.

Cooper *et al.* (1978) trace the development of symbolic understanding from the earliest stages of object recognition, to recognition of miniature representations in play materials, two-dimensional representations (pictures, line drawings, symbols), to the understanding of written labels in preparation for the acquisition of reading and writing skills. Gestures are also considered at this developmental level. This is useful for both teachers and therapists in the preparation of pre-speech and pre-reading communication programmes. It helps avoid the pitfalls of inappropriate selection of aids, e.g. the aid based on traditional orthography for the child who has not progressed beyond the earliest stages of symbolic understanding. The structure also provides a developmental approach to reading, a stage which some children with neurological disorders may never achieve because of deficient association between auditory comprehension and the auditory and visual processes (see later this chapter).

Expressive language is dependent upon the co-ordinated motor functions of breathing, voicing and articulation. Phonation is better controlled when the child is relaxed and can be facilitated by sighing on outgoing air. The therapist may need to apply some pressure to the sternum to assist phonation. Motivation to improve volume and duration of voicing can be stimulated by toys that are activated by sound, e.g. a sound-activated monkey, a teddy bear with eyes that glow, or a worm that wiggles out of an apple in response to sound input. The volume control can be adjusted so that even minimal attempts at phonation are rewarded as the toy is activated. Laryngeal tone can be improved by the techniques of proprioceptive neuromuscular facilitation (PNF).

Articulation therapy is valuable as part of an integrated approach, with the dysarthric or dyspraxic child. Exclusive concentration on tongue, lip and palate exercises is to little or no avail if the child has nothing to communicate. However, tongue and lip exercises are beneficial when used selectively to improve muscle tone for gross movement or fine co-ordination for articulation.

The use of lollipops to motivate tongue extension, or vermicelli around the lips to increase mobility of the tongue tip are incentives for the young child. There are, however, no English speech sounds made by the total extension of the tongue, nor by the licking action of the tongue tip, yet these exercises have gained almost a ritual place in therapy. Although they provide a useful method of assessing the range of tongue movement, this form of intervention would be contraindicated for the severely handicapped child in whom tongue extension would trigger the all-or-nothing response of head extension, back arching and extension of all four limbs reminiscent of embryonic behaviour.

Proprioceptive neuromuscular facilitation (PNF) techniques may be used to improve strength and symmetry of tongue action. Using dental gauze to hold the tongue tip, the therapist can assist movement and placement of the tongue. The child may be asked to push the tongue forward against resistance provided by the therapist, or attempt to retract the tongue whilst the tip is firmly held. Symmetry of movement can be improved by applying pressure alternately to the unaffected side, then to the weaker side to improve tone. Lip movements can also be facilitated by exercises using alternately stretch then flexion, so that lip closure for articulation and swallowing is improved. These exercises can be supplemented by games incorporating sucking and blowing (e.g. blow football), and linked with improving action for drinking through a polythene tube.

The labial sounds *p*, *b*, *m* and *w*, and the lip rounding necessary for the production of *sh*, *ch* and *j* may induce flexor spasm unless the child's head is supported to prevent the chin dropping forward on to the chest in response to the lip flexion.

Conversely, the sibilant sounds *s* and *z* and the fricatives *f* and *v* are primarily extensor sounds, as are the vowels *ee* and *i* (as in ink). Total extension of the jaw for the production of *ah* may also trigger an extensor spasm.

The dental sounds of *t*, *d*, *n* and *l* can be assisted by the therapist using a dental gauze to grasp the tongue tip to elevate it to contact the alveolar ridge.

The production of the velar consonants *k*, *g* and *ng* can be helped by applying firm pressure upwards and backwards to the base of the tongue to make contact with the soft palate. This is more easily achieved if the head is slightly extended.

The random movements of the tongue that distort the articulation of dysarthric children can be reduced by holding the jaw to provide stability.

In contrast, the child with a phonological disorder will benefit from a programme concentrating on visual, auditory, semantic and kinaesthetic feedback of the sounds in his repertoire. The development of self-monitoring is an important aspect of self-correction.

Palatal dysfunction is a common symptom amongst children with neurological disorders, occurring either in isolation or in conjunction with other problems of co-ordination. Nasal speech can also result from a submucous cleft. There may be relatively little to see on examination, although a wide, grooved or bifid uvula is a suggestive finding. Sometimes transillumination of the palate with a nasopharyngoscope is a help in diagnosis. Plastic surgery is likely to be needed, especially if the soft palate is affected.

The spastic child may be unable to elevate the palate to produce an adequate seal. Persistent problems may be alleviated by the use of a palatal training device (a small acrylic plate similar to that used for dentures) with a loop extended to contact the soft palate. The modification of tongue action which occurs in some patients has proved effective in reducing hyper-nasality and dribbling (Ellis & Flack, 1979). The visual speech aid which can be used in conjunction with the palatal trainer provides a visual monitor for palatal closure, and the lip sensor developed by the same team provides an audible reminder for lip closure. A palato-graph (Hardcastle, 1974) using electrodes embedded in an acrylic plate provides an effective means of monitoring tongue placement and contact. The pattern of movement is projected on to a visual display unit (VDU) so that the child can imitate the correct model presented by the therapist. This has important implications for therapy because the child learns to correct his own pattern rather than by assisted movement.

For the dyspraxic child this new technology of electropalatography has yet to be fully exploited. The mastery of routines through repetition, so that they become automatic, may be reinforced by the visual cueing provided by the VDU. The use of visual or rhythmic cues, on the premise of tapping right hemisphere language abilities, is a technique used in the management of children and adults with dyspraxia and/or dysphasia (Sparks, 1981). Starting with phonemes, the child progresses to single syllable—consonant—vowel imitation, moving to polysyllabic utterances, then to simple sentences, using rhythm and accentuated intonation patterns to facilitate imitation.

Retrieval is a major problem for these children, who may respond to immediate cueing techniques but have difficulty in retaining the pattern or engram of the articulatory movements. The importance of short intensive periods of treatment is emphasized for these children. Repetitive drills, to establish routines using visual, phonemic, semantic or contextual cues, are an essential feature of management of dyspraxia. Cues should be gradually withdrawn so that the child develops self-cueing strategies. Because of the repetitive nature of treatment, children with similar problems may prefer the competition of group therapy.

Group therapy has been effectively used with cerebral palsied children within the concept of Peto Conductive Education (Cotton, 1975). On the principle of rhythm, repetition and statement of intention, specific programmes are included in the daily educational programme. The child verbalizes each activity, which is graded into its component parts, e.g. 'I put on my sock', 'One, two, three, four, five'. The Peto approach is based on the principle of achieving independence through the development of these 'subroutines'. Unlike the majority of developmentally based programmes, Peto Conductive Education is based on the premise of an irreversible neuropathology that cannot be resolved by a developmental approach.

Group therapy may also be a consideration for the dysfluent child, for whom the concentration on speech exacerbates stuttering. Fluency programmes (e.g. Monterey Fluency Programme; Ryan, 1979) and approaches that utilize rhythm or prolonged speech are often better applied within a supportive group, than in isolation. The generalization of use of these techniques is also improved if first rehearsed within the familiar group.

Intervention for children with specific disorders of language development
The majority of children with specific disorders of language development can be helped within the normal school, but sometimes only in a special class with the teacher and the speech therapist working together in the classroom. There will be a few children so severely affected that the expert help with both assessment and treatment can only be provided in a special school devoted to the needs of children with disorders of language development.

The management of the child with a specific disorder of language development, with no other handicap, presents special problems, particularly for teaching language. Griffiths (1979), in discussing language therapy for children, makes the point that if children fail to learn language structure in the home environment, even under optimum conditions, there seems little justification for supposing that an attempt to duplicate this process in an educational setting is going to be any more successful. McNeil (1974) suggests that just as linguists and phoneticians have to become conscious of the language processes of syntax and phonology, so do children who have specific difficulties with language development. Teaching this skill, then, has to start with the learning of individual sounds and words.

For the majority of children, the acquisition of the mother tongue may well be a question of hearing the auditory symbols in a meaningful situation, with the brain at a stage of development capable of integrating the sensory input into the complex structure of a lexicon. If this method is not successful, as with any other skills, it may be necessary to break down the language structure into its component parts so that these can be made conscious and practised. Skills are built up of 'subroutines'. The more these are practised, the more automatic they become, freed from the restraints of organization, intention and feedback. Then these units, no longer having to be monitored, can be detached from the context in which they were learnt, discarded if proved inefficient, or used as the building blocks of more complex actions. The finite set of rules that constitute language function can be regarded as 'subroutines' which can be presented to the child to practise until they become so habitual that the child can use them at will to generate an infinite set of sentences (Griffiths, 1979). Obviously there must be close co-operation between the speech therapist and class teacher in the education of children with specific disorders of language development, whatever method is used.

Integration of the handicapped child into the wider group of the classroom or local school is advocated by the Education Act of 1981.

Children with language disorders may be more isolated by their inability to communicate than those who may be in a wheelchair but are articulate. Children suffering from speech and language disorders are also 'at risk' of delay in the acquisition of reading and writing skills, their defective feedback impairing the development of these language-related skills. Vygotsky (1962) suggests a time lag of 6–7 years between the acquisition of speech and the development of writing skills in 'normal' children. What of the speech- and language-disordered children who may not have these foundations on which to build?

A number of approaches to teaching language that have been advocated in the past, such as the Association Method (McGinnis, 1963), have used a phonic approach, which seems illogical as this is the input channel mainly affected. It seems better to use the unaffected visual pathways as much as possible, as in the method devised by Lea (1965). In this scheme, the parts of speech are differentiated by colour: nouns in red, verbs in yellow, adjectives in green, prepositions and conjunctions in blue, and adverbs in brown.

Words can be respresented by lines of appropriate colour and the lines built into patterns to show what is required to describe pictures or events. The red lines of nouns are cut by a small vertical line if preceded by the indefinite article and the yellow lines of verbs are cut by a small vertical line when preceded by 'is' or 'are'. Nouns are taught first as whole words in association with objects, beginning with an actual object and then with many different objects of the same type so that the full concept of what is represented by the particular symbol is demonstrated. Every time a word is written, it is reinforced not only by other visual associations but by the sound of the word as well. With the teaching of sentence structure, the present tense is introduced first, then the past and finally the future. Often these children can write and read to a greater extent than they can speak.

Speech supplements

'A reason to communicate ... a means of saying it' (Yoder & Calculator, 1981). Despite conventional therapy, many severely handicapped children remain 'locked in' by their inability to speak but 'during the past few years there has been considerable work on developing non-speech (non-vocal) communication modes or systems' (Kiernan *et al.*, 1982). Based on reports in the literature, it would be difficult to conceive of a child or adult so severely impaired that there would be no non-speech communication system that he or she could use'. This preface to the book *Communication for the Speechless* by Franklin Silverman (1980) voices the hope of many children and adults who by reason of their physical handicap may be speechless, yet given the right supplement or augmentative, may become effective communicators. The phrase 'alternative systems of communication' has crept into the vocabulary of therapists and educators during the past 10 years. Implicit within the term *alternative* is the suggestion of *failure*, either on the part of the child to develop effective oral communication, or on the part of the therapist or clinician who has failed to achieve for their client the ultimate goal of speech. It may also reflect the reluctance on the part of some professionals to introduce supplementary modes of communication, regarding this form of intervention as a 'last resort'.

Reservations, often based upon concerns that such systems inhibit language development, suppress functional speech and limit intellectual functioning, are apparently unfounded. Silverman (1980) tables the 'impact of non-speech modes on the ability to communicate'. In most, if not all of the examples cited, a significant improvement in communicative ability is recorded. Improvement in vocalization and verbalization is reported, together with improved social interaction and reduction of frustration. These improvements are not restricted to one particular system but apply to manual, visual and technological techniques (Table 2:1 Silverman, 1980).

Fristoe & Lloyd (1977) presented 16 points related to the effectiveness of supplements or augmentatives to speech. A common denominator to all forms of non-speech intervention is (i) the removal of pressure for speech, and (ii) the circumvention of problems of auditory short-term memory and auditory processing.

The struggle to produce intelligible speech in an effort to conform with 'normality' is often an intolerable burden for severely handicapped youngsters. We, as effective communicators, accept the discrepancies of spoken languages and dialects in the verbal world. Perhaps we should show more tolerance in accepting the different modes of communication used by those deprived of articulated speech, and cease to regard these modes as 'second best' alternatives.

As Harris (1980) put it: 'Rather than being an alternative to speech, non-vocal techniques should be viewed as augmentative or supplementary techniques which are used to enhance communication by complementing whatever vocal skills the individual may possess.'

Many children with neurological disorders may depend on visual or graphic systems as their only means of expression, and it is hardly surprising that spelling is often defective; and semantic and syntactic problems are recorded in their output. The choice of system may be determined by their level of educational attainment and many technological aids presuppose an ability to read and spell.

Historical background of alternative methods of communication

Gesture is a natural complement to speech, used effectively to expand meaning when the command of spoken language is limited in either the speaker or the listener. The use of gesture increases according to one's expectations of the listener's ability to understand, either because of the barriers of spoken language, limited mental ability, impaired hearing or poor expressive ability.

Perhaps the oldest gestural system is that of American Indian Hand Talk, developed as a code by the nomadic tribes of North America to transcend the problems of the multiplicity of spoken languages. In its modern, modified form, Amer-Ind has been used as an effective means of communication by severely handicapped children and adults. Concepts such as eating, drinking, washing etc. are signalled in action and can be extended by the addition of further concepts (e.g. eating + morning = breakfast). The system has been informally coded to retain the universality of the ancient hand talk. In practical terms, this is an advantage in that it restricts idiosyncratic variations, ensuring that dialectic variations do not creep in to obscure meaning.

Skelly (1979) summarizes the application of the system thus: 'The American Indian Code's low symbolic level, ease of acquisition, flexibility, speed, lack of grammatical structure and rules, and use of concrete, demonstrable referents which enable the viewer to interpret without formal instruction, make it adaptable to the use of many patients who are unable to speak.'

The use of Amer-Ind in Britain has been primarily with adults with acquired neurological damage, and its potential as an expressive medium for children at a pre-symbolic level of development has yet to be fully explored.

Manual signing systems

Much of the pioneering work into speech supplements has been undertaken in the field of manual communication systems developed by deaf people as 'natural' languages to meet their specific needs. These systems are almost as variable as spoken languages stemming from different origins and incorporating many regional 'dialects'.

Controversy still exists between those educators who are confirmed 'oralists' in approach, believing that the deaf child has to conform to a 'hearing' society and those who support signing to complement poor verbal skills, or include manual signing as part of a 'total communication' programme. Yet researchers (Moores, 1974; Wilbur, 1976) concur that 'the use of manual communication with deaf children beginning at a very early age can have positive effects upon linguistic, academic and psychological development.' May not the same philosophy be true for other 'speechless' children?

Systems developed to fulfil a specific need, e.g. manual signing, have become adopted and adapted by teachers and therapists to meet the needs of other speech handicapped children. British Sign Language (BSL) and Irish Sign Language are the two manual communication systems which predominate in the United Kingdom. Criticism has been levelled at the classification of these systems as 'languages' because they do not abide by linguistic rules, but they provide a speedy and effective way of communicating, supplemented by finger spelling and gesture.

It was because of the reservations concerning linguistic concepts in manual signing that Sir Richard Paget in collaboration with Pierre Gorman devised a systematic sign system modelled upon the grammatical and syntactical rules of spoken English. The Paget Gorman Systematic Sign System provided a logical, conceptually based sign system incorporating past, present and future tenses, plural markers etc., so that the young deaf child could see spoken language in action. This system too has proved a valuable tool for children with language impairment other than that caused by deafness.

The Makaton vocabulary has been widely adopted in the United Kingdom by workers in the field of mental handicap. The structured vocabulary devised by Margaret Walker for the mentally handicapped patients in her care is supplemented by British Sign Language. The vocabulary is graded in complexity and is taught by relating the signs to pictures or objects in order to improve comprehension and stimulate expression.

The major advantage of using gestural or signing supplements is that they are unaided. In fluent use some signing systems have the speed and spontaneity of spoken language, and signing, like speech, is transitory in nature.

The major disadvantage is that the 'listener' must know the code to promote effective two-way communication.

Gestural and signing systems may be appropriate for some children with neurological disorders, but for those with poor hand function and short visual and kinaesthetic memory, signing may not be a feasible supplement.

Visual systems

Visual systems range from pictorial representations to symbolic representations and traditional orthography.

Picture boards have long been used as an expressive medium for severely handicapped children (McDonald & Shultz, 1973). Pictures or photographs presented on a display can provide the child with a functional vocabulary within arm's length. The content will be limited by space, and the complexity of representing verbs, prepositions and adjectives in pictorial form will restrict the user to the developmental level of 'one word' utterance. A symbolic approach utilizing manipulable symbols, plastic discs or tokens to represent required objects, has proved effective for an action−reaction exchange to stimulate communication in severely handicapped children.

Pictographic symbols, e.g. Blissymbolics (Silverman *et al.*, 1978; McDonald, 1980; McNaughton, 1985), have also provided a breakthrough to communication for children unable to read or spell, yet able to express their 'internalized' language through pictures indicated on a symbol display. Blissymbols are *conceptually* based pictorial representations and are accompanied by the written word so that the 'receiver' may interpret the message. The constant visual reinforcement of symbol and word provides a bridge towards reading, the rationale behind the Rebus approach where pictorial representations depict the *word* rather than the concept.

Alphabet boards have been the traditional communication tools of literate speechless individuals, but the rate is often painfully slow as each letter is laboriously spelled out. Whereas instructors using systems that are conceptually based report improvements in vocalization and verbalization, this is not observed with the phonic level of approach. Word boards speed up the communicative process, but the selection of vocabulary and its presentation is an important consideration. Scanning a word board can present problems for those unfamiliar with the display, nor do single words afford the same flexibility as signs or symbols which convey wider concepts.

Technology has broadened the horizons for clinicians and has pro-vided even the more severely handicapped with the tools to communicate (see Chapter 7).

Keyboards with hardcopy print-out (e.g. Canon Communicator, Sharp Memowriter) or incorporating a visual display (Elkomi II, Lightwriter) enable the user to monitor output.

Communicators using pictorial, symbolic or word displays (Possum, Chailey Communicator, splink) using light-emitting diodes (LEDs) or infra-red signals are effective as educational and communication aids. Microprocessors have facilitated communication at the touch of a finger, expanding the storage and retrieval of information which can be printed (Micro-writer, Autocom), used as environmental control or converted into synthesized speech (Handivoice, Blisstalk). Computer programs for physically and/or mentally handicapped children are reaping the rewards of increased output from children previously unable to work without supervision. The potential is enormous, but the responsibility for selec-tion is even greater, for the inappropriate choice may add to the frus-tration and disappointment of the user and family.

Selection criteria

Technological aids may be self selective, based on availability, portability, maintenance and cost, but there are many aids, inappropriately selected, that lurk in the back of storerooms.

The criteria for the selection of any supplement should also be applied to the provision of an aid, *viz.* (i) psycholinguistic skills, (ii) cognition, (iii) motor skills, (iv) communication needs, short- and long-term prog-nosis, (v) social/emotional behaviour, (vi) history and (vii) time and support. (Items i—vi from *Handivoice Seminar Manual*, 1979.)

Systems are not competitive nor mutually exclusive. One system may be more appropriate to the developmental level of the handicapped child than another. Like medicine, the choice should be prescriptive, catering for individual needs. However, the choice is all too often idiosyncratic, dependent upon the level of knowledge and confidence of instructors who are likely to employ the system with which they are most familiar. Some authorities have adopted one system or approach to the detriment of those children for whom the choice may be inappropriate. 'Although there are arguments in favour of planned diversity, unplanned diversity seems undesirable' (Kiernan *et al.*, 1982).

Specific medical problems

From time to time a child will present with a problem of language development, but underlying this will be a well-defined neurological disorder. For example, occasionally and unexpectedly a chromosome abnormality will be found, particularly a sex chromosome aneuploidy (Garvey & Mutton, 1973). Also, diseases such as Duchenne muscular dystrophy can present in unusual ways. The boy may be noted to be clumsy in his movements and to be delayed in development, especially of language; and if a widely based differential diagnosis is not considered, the primary disorder may not be identified, with inevitable loss of the parents' confidence in the advice they are being given, and an early opportunity for genetic counselling will be missed.

The link between a language disorder and the neurological condition may be a much closer one, as in the acquired epileptic aphasia syndrome. There are a number of progressive diseases affecting the brain and resulting in dementia and epilepsy, but in this syndrome no definite cause has been found, although some form of 'encephalitis' has been suspected. It was first described by Landau & Kleffner (1957). Typically, a previously normal child becomes aphasic between the ages of 3 and 9 years without other neurological abnormalities or known brain pathology. At about the same time, most of these children develop generalized or partial seizures and all of them have abnormal EEGs with asymmetrical paroxysmal activity, mainly over the post-central areas. The onset of the condition may be sudden or gradual and its course is very variable. Recovery can occur after quite a short period, but some children remain with a permanent impairment of language function. Worster-Drought (1971) emphasized that a receptive aphasia was the central feature of the syndrome and that intelligence can be well preserved.

It seems possible that the epilepsy may cause a disruption of language function at a critical stage of development, but why this should only occur in certain children without other evidence of brain damage is unexplained. Perhaps the epileptic activity prevents the necessary connections being established at a subcortical level. Anti-epileptic drugs are worth trying but there is no definite evidence that they benefit the disorder of language (O'Donohoe, 1979). It has been suggested that the ketogenic diet may be of benefit.

Reading retardation or dyslexia

The World Federation of Neurology has defined specific developmental dyslexia as 'a disorder manifested by difficulty in learning to read despite conventional instruction, adequate intelligence, and socio-cultural opportunity. It is dependent upon fundamental cognitive disabilities which are frequently of constitutional origin.' The choice of terms used (reading retardation, dyslexia, word blindness, etc.) does not seem to be fundamental to the issue that there are a number of children with reading, writing and spelling difficulties who are in need of help, and are often not getting it. The management of these children will be considered in Chapter 10, but it may be of help to consider certain aspects of the subject in relation to language development, and the possible role of the speech therapist.

A number of workers in this field have claimed that children with specific reading retardation can be classified into several main groups of disorders (Boder, 1973; Ingram, 1960; Ingram *et al.*, 1970). By far the largest group is the audiophonic one and the trend has been to regard 'developmental dyslexia' as a disorder of language development. There is no doubt that children who have difficulties in acquiring spoken language are, after overcoming these, at risk of finding reading and spelling a problem when they start school. However, a much smaller group of children with a severe perceptual disability do occasionally seem to have problems of recognizing the shapes and relationship of letters, at least when they start to learn to read.

Studying children with 'dyslexia', Pavlidis (1979) has found that, compared with a normal control group without reading difficulties and a group of slow readers, the children with 'dyslexia' had obvious defects of eye movements. The normal readers moved their eyes in an orderly way from left to right and their eye movements had a consistent size, duration and pattern, while those with dyslexia showed erratic eye movements in a random fashion. A particular difference between normals and children with 'dyslexia' was in their regressive movements, which were much more frequent in the latter group and were also irregular and often bigger than the preceding forward saccade. Unlike normal readers, these children sometimes went far back to fixate on words in a manner in which the normal and backward readers did not. It was considered that the differences were sufficient to be the basis of a diagnostic test of specific developmental dyslexia. It seems unlikely that the findings are specific or the cause of dyslexia, but as the affected children also have other difficulties in sequential tracking and in maintaining fixation, it is more probable that the malfunctioning of the eye movement control system and the dyslexia share a common cause: a central, non-modality specific, sequential disability. If so, there are obvious implications for remedial teaching.

The problems of other children sometimes do not fit into any such classification, for example a failure of visual recognition of a very specific type. There has been no difficulty with spoken language or with acquiring motor skills. Words can be spelled verbally without difficulty but when written down they are often incorrect with a failure to recognize mistakes.

Once the development of perceptual motor and language functions has reached a certain stage of complexity, the child can acquire the skills of reading and writing. Backwardness in learning to read can be due to a variety of causes, from loss of schooling through illness, to myopia, and may be one of many symptoms of a generalized retardation of development. Among children with specific developmental dyslexia, Boder (1973) found that in the group she studied 67% had a deficit in symbol–sound integration (dysphonetic group). These children had difficulty in developing the phonetic word analysis and synthesis skills that affect the development of language. Children in this group recognize words globally and are unable to sound out and blend component letters and syllables of a word. Reading is easier in context when guesses at words can be made from minimal clues. Spelling is by sight, not by ear, and words are only spelt correctly when they can be visualized. Ten per cent of the children in this study had an obvious difficulty in perceiving letters and whole words as configurations (dyseidetic group). They had a good auditory memory and could recite letters well. They were poor spellers but their errors were not bizarre. Twenty-three per cent of the children had difficulties in reading both by sight and by ear.

Those who are involved in helping children with problems related to speech and language in their younger years must surely notify the education authorities that these children are at risk of difficulties with reading and spelling. Remediation will be discussed in Chapter 10, but a number of people involved in treating disorders of language can contribute to the help that children with difficulties in reading, spelling and writing so often need.

A diagnostic test using the identification of these abnormal patterns of reading and spelling has now been published (Boder & Jarrico, 1982).

Summary

An eclectic approach to management of speech and language disorders, based on formal and informal assessment procedures, is proposed. Early intervention to alleviate speech-related problems is advocated. Intervention to stimulate language development and improve expressive ability is suggested, together with speech supplements and augmentatives, appropriately selected to meet the individual needs of the speech- and language-disordered child.

In the case of the young child with delayed language development, there must be increased collaboration between the speech therapist, the primary school teacher and the nursery nurse. If these professionals can devise a teaching programme to include the teaching of language, it is likely to be more effective than therapy by the speech therapist in isolation. Communication between experts is obviously a problem, especially with limited resources and time, but an increased use of written material may be of benefit. Also, it must never be forgotten that most parents can make a major contribution to helping their child. The exact form of their contribution may well be the subject for further research, but it does seem illogical not to include them as members of the team trying to help a particular child. How often does one hear a parent say that their child has seen a speech therapist, or the speech therapist has changed some months ago, and no further meeting has been arranged. This is particularly true in services to schools; and teachers can make the same complaint.

More research is also needed, both on the effectiveness of speech therapy for various speech and language disorders in childhood, and on its method of application. Is individual or group therapy best? Is intensive therapy more beneficial for certain disorders than regular treatment sessions at intervals over long periods of time?

In an era when expenditure has to be increasingly justified, it will become essential to decide if the right policy is for every authority to provide special classes, particularly for the younger child with delayed language development whatever the cause. As with any disability, there are a few children who are so severely handicapped that even this special provision is inadequate, and it may be that on a national basis there is justification for residential schools. Not only can these provide special teaching impossible in any other environment, but they can also be centres of excellence and research.

More follow-up studies are needed after such children have left school. To what extent do their disabilities remain, even if modified, and what provisions are necessary to help the young adult? It may be considered unrealistic to suggest any expansion of services at this time, but not if it can be shown that this is a false economy and that in the long run the community, as well as the individual, will be the loser if help is not given.

References

Anthony, A., Bogle, D., Ingram, T.T.S. & McIsaac, M.W. (1971) *The Edinburgh Articulation Test.* Churchill Livingstone, Edinburgh.

Bax, M., Hart, H. & Jenkins, S. (1980) Assessment of speech and language development in the young child. *Paediatrics,* **66,** 350–354.

Boder, E. (1973) Developmental dyslexia: a diagnostic approach based on three typical reading-spelling patterns. *Developmental Medicine and Child Neurology,* **15,** 663–687.

Boder, E. & Jarrico, S. (1982) *The Boder Test of Reading-Spelling Patterns.* Grune & Stratton, New York.

Boucher, J. (1976) Is autism primarily a language disorder? *British Journal of Disorders of Communication,* **2,** 135–143.

Braine, M.D.S. (1971) On two types of models of the internalisation of grammars. In *The Ontogenesis of Grammar* (ed. M. D. L. Slobin). New York, Academic Press.

Bruner, J.S. (1975) The ontogenesis of speech acts. *Journal of Child Language,* **2**(1), 1–19.

Carrow, E. (1973) *Test for Auditory Comprehension of Language.* Teaching Resources Corporation, Boston.

Cashdan, A. (1969) The role of movement in language learning. *Clinics in Developmental Medicine,* **33.** S.I.M.P., Heinemann, London.

Chomsky, N. (1972) *Language and Mind.* Harcourt Brace Jovanovich, New York.

Coggins & Carpenter (1981) Communicative intention inventory. *Journal of Applied Psycholinguistics,* **2,** 235–252.

Cooper, J., Moodley, M. & Reynell, J. (1978) *Helping Language Development. A Developmental Programme for Children with Early Language Handicaps.* Edward Arnold, London.

Cotton, E. (1975) *Conductive Education and Cerebral Palsy.* The Spastics Society, London.

Crystal, D. (1982) *Profile in Linguistic Disability.* Edward Arnold, London.

Crystal, D., Fletcher, P. & Gorman, M. (1976) *The Grammatical Analysis of Language Disability.* Edward Arnold, London.

Donaldson, M. (1978) *Children's Minds.* William Collins, Glasgow.

Ellis R.E. & Flack, F.C. (1979) *Palato-Glossal Malfunction.* (Monograph) College of Speech Therapists, London.

Enderby, P. (1981) Frenchay Dysarthria Assessment, Bristol.

Fraiberg, S. (1977) *Comparative Studies of Blind and Sighted Infants.* Basic Books, New York.

Fristoe, M. & Lloyd, L.L. (1977) Manual communication for the retarded: a resource list. *Mental Retardation,* **15,** 18–21.

Fundudis, T., Kalvin, I. & Garside, R.F. (1979) *Speech Retarded and Deaf Children, their Psychological Development.* Academic Press, London.

Garvey, M. & Mutton, D.E. (1973) Sex chromosome aberrations and speech development. *Archives of Disease in Childhood,* **48,** 937–941.

Gesell, A. (1945) *The Embryology of Behaviour.* Harper, New York.

Goodglass, H. & Kaplan, E. (1972) *The Assessment of Aphasia and Related Disorders.* Lea and Febiger, Philadelphia.

Gordon, N. (1969) A history of Laura Bridgman—from American notes by Charles Dickens. *British Journal of Disorders of Communication,* **4,** 107–116.

Griffiths, P. (1979) An approach to language therapy for children with specific language disability. *New Zealand Speech Therapist Journal,* **34,** 14–21.

Hardcastle, W.J. (1974) Instrumental investigations of lingual activity during speech. *Phonetica*, **29**, 129–157.

Harris, D. (1980) Enhancing the development of communication interaction in non-vocal severely physically handicapped children. In *Proceedings of International Project on Communication Aids for Speech Impaired*. London.

Ingram, T.T.S. (1960) Paediatric aspects of specific developmental dysphasia, dyslexia and dysgraphia. *Cerebral Palsy Bulletin*, **2**, 254–277.

Ingram, T.T.S. (1969) Disorders of speech in childhood. *British Journal of Hospital Medicine*, **4**, 1608–1625.

Ingram, T.T.S., Mason, A.W. & Blackburn, I. (1970) A retrospective study of 82 children with reading disability. *Developmental Medicine and Child Neurology*, **12**, 271–281.

Jeffree, D.M. & McConkey, R. (1976) *Let Me Speak*. Souvenir Press, London.

Jeffree, D.M., McConkey, R. & Hewson, S. (1977) *Let Me Play*. Souvenir Press, London.

Kiernan, C., Reid, B. & Jones, L. (1982) *Signs and Symbols*. Heinemann, London.

Kirk, S.A., McCarthy, J.J. & Kirk, W.F. (1968) *Examiner's Manual, Illinois Test of Psycholinguistic Abilities* (revised edn). University of Illinois Press.

Landau, W.M. & Kleffner, F.R. (1957) Syndrome of acquired aphasia with convulsive disorder in children. *Neurology*, **7**, 523–530.

Lassman, F.M., Fisch, R.O., Vetter, D.K. & La Benz, E.S. (1980) *Early Correlates of Speech Language and Hearing*. PSG Publishing, Littleton, Mass.

Lea, J. (1965) A language scheme for children suffering from receptive aphasia *Speech Pathology and Therapy*, **8**, 58–68.

Luria, A.R. (1961) *The Role of Speech in the Regulation of Normal and Abnormal Behaviour*. Pergamon Press, Oxford.

McDonald, E.T. (1980) *Teaching and Using Blissymbolics*. Blissymbolics Communication Institute, Toronto.

McDonald, E.T. & Schultz, A.R. (1973) Communication boards for cerebral palsied children. *Journal of Speech and Hearing Disorders*, **38**, 73.

McGinnis, M.A. (1963) *Aphasic Children*. Alexander Graham Bell Association for the Deaf, Washington.

McNaughton, S. (1985) *Communicating with Blissymbols*. Blissymbolic Communication Institute, Toronto.

McNeil, D. (1974) How to resolve two paradoxes and escape a dilemma. In *The Growth of Competence* (eds K. Connolly and J. Bruner). Academic Press, London.

Mehrabian, A. (1972) *Non-Verbal Communication*. University of Chicago Press, Chicago.

Menyuk, P. (1974) Early development of receptive language: from babbling to words. In *Language Perspectives, Acquisition, Retardation and Intervention* (eds L. Lyle and R.L. Schiefelbusch). University Park Press, Baltimore.

Moores, D. (1974) Non-vocal systems of verbal behaviour. In *Language Perspectives, Acquisition, Retardation and Intervention* (eds L. Lyle and R.L. Schiefelbusch). University Park Press, Baltimore.

Müller, D.J., Munro, S.M. & Code, C. (1981) *Language Assessment for Remediation*. Croom Helm, London.

O'Donohoe, N.V. (1979) *Epilepsies of Childhood*. Butterworths, London.

Paradise, J.L. (1980) Otitis media in infants and children. *Pediatrics*, **65**, 917–943.

Pavlidis, G.T. (1979) How can dyslexia be objectively diagnosed? *Reading*, **13**, 3–15.

Peckham, C.S. (1973) Speech defects in a national sample of children aged seven years. *British Journal of Disorders of Communication*, **8**, 2–8.

Piaget, J. (1968) *Six Psychological Studies*, Chapter on 'Language and thought from the genetic point of view'. University of London Press, London.

Reynell, J. (1977) *Manual for the Reynell Developmental Language Scales* (revised). NFER, Windsor.

Robinson, R.J. (1982) The child who is slow to talk. *British Medical Journal*, **285**, 671–672.

Rutter, M. (1980) The long term effects of early experience. *Developmental Medicine and Child Neurology*, **22**, 800–815.

Ryan, B.P. (1979) Stuttering therapy in a framework of operant conditioning and programmed learning. In *Controversies about Stuttering Therapy* (ed. H. Gregory). University Park Press, Baltimore.

Schlesinger, I.M. (1977) The role of cognitive development and linguistic output in language acquisition. *Journal of Child Language*, **4**(2), 153–170.

Silverman, F. (1980) *Communication for the Speechless*. Prentice-Hall, Englewood Cliffs, New Jersey.

Silverman, H., McNaughton, S. & Kates, B. (1978) *A Handbook of Blissymbolics*. Blissymbolics Communication Institute, Toronto.

Skelly, M. (1979) *Amer-Ind Gestural Code*. Elsevier, New York.

Snow, C.E. (1977) The development of conversation between mothers and babies *Journal of Child Language*, **4**(2), 1–22.

Sparks, R.W. (1981) Melodic intonation therapy. In *Language Intervention Strategies in Adult Aphasia* (ed. R. Chapey). Williams and Wilkins, Baltimore.

Vygotsky, L.S. (1962) *Thought and Language*. MIT Press, Cambridge, Mass.

Wilbur, R.B. (1976) The linguistics of manual languages and manual systems. In *Communication Assessment and Intervention Strategies* (ed. L. Lyle). University Park Press, Baltimore.

Worster-Drought, C. (1943) Congenital auditory imperception (congenital word-deafness) and its relation to the idioglossia and allied speech defects. *Medical Press and Circular*, **210**(5460), 411–420.

Worster-Drought, C. (1971) An unusual form of acquired aphasia in children. *Developmental Medicine and Child Neurology*, **13**, 563–571.

Yoder, D. & Calculator, L. (1981) Some perspectives on intervention strategies for persons with developmental disorders. *Journal of Autism and Developmental Disorders*, **2**(1), 107–124.

Zincus, P.W., Gottlieb, M.I. & Shapiro, M. (1978) Developmental and psychoeducational sequelae of chronic otitis media. *American Journal of Diseases of Children*, **132**, 1100–1104.

Chapter 10
Remedial Teaching for Literacy

Audrey Leatherbarrow

Introduction

Reading as a skill for all did not become an issue in the United Kingdom until 1870 when compulsory full-time education was made law. Given the opportunity, most children learn to read and write. The majority of the population become effective readers and proficient writers who take literacy for granted. However, there are people who experience difficulty and who never master reading and writing. (Clark, 1970; Vernon, 1971). Despite the influence of television, we still live in a culture dominated by print, and for an adult to be illiterate is a handicap.

There has been a longstanding interest in children who are incompetent in reading (Clark, 1970; Rutter *et al.*, 1970). All of these children, of adequate intelligence, unexpectedly failed to learn to read, write or spell. Both Farnham-Diggory (1978) and Hulme (1981) provide reviews of the literature concerning such children.

These children worry parents and teachers, for a child who cannot read cannot become an independent learner. The difficulties experienced are out of proportion to their abilities in other areas of the school curriculum. As a result, the children may feel that their difficulties are insurmountable and some may develop emotional problems (Leach & Raybould, 1977; Galloway & Goodwin, 1979; Sturge, 1982).

Researchers into reading problems have described separate categories of difficulty, showing that it is not a homogenous condition. Although terminology varies according to the author, there does seem to be agreement about the categories of dysfunction, e.g. auditory, visual or mixed difficulties (Myklebust, 1965; Ingram *et al.*, 1970; Clay, 1972; Boder, 1973).

In recent years, doctors and teachers have used a number of screening procedures to identify children likely to show learning problems in spite of average general ability. Although Rennie (1980) and Wedell & Lindsay (1980) found screening to be ineffective, class teachers have been prompted by screening procedures to analyse the achievements of young

children and to modify their teaching methods according to progress
(Department of Education and Science, 1975; Ainscow & Tweddle,
1979).

Alberman (1973) maintains that superior predictors of learning disability are family size, position of the child within the family, and low
socio-economic conditions. These factors, she claims, surpass birth weight
and abnormal neurological signs in early infancy. Neurologically impaired
children who have literacy problems are likely to run into difficulty
earlier, are more likely to experience failure and frustration and to
present greater management problems to parents and teachers. That
retarded readers exist is not in dispute. The question is, once identified
and provided with remedial treatment, do they 'get better'?

Research into the effects of remedial teaching is not encouraging. In a
thorough review of remedial educational research design and results
available up to 1961, together with the results of a good original study,
Collins (1961) was unable to find evidence that remedial teaching was
effective in the long term. In 1976, Yule could find no further convincing
evidence of the success of remedial teaching. He examined the issues with
which remedial education is concerned and suggested that an important
question is the level of reading ability deemed necessary to function in
society. The 1940s level of 9 years he maintains is not sufficient at the
present time. Hewison (1982) in a recent review agreed with Yule and
suggested new solutions, including greater parental involvement.

Standards are arbitrary. As Jansen (1979) points out, the required
level of reading varies according to the demands made of individuals in
an increasingly literate society. Reading failure is a relative condition
(Downing, 1977). As normal reading instruction is upgraded, these
targets become a further challenge to weak readers.

It is generally agreed that a reading age of 17 years is needed to
complete income tax forms, read quality newspapers and follow instructions on certain packaged goods. This target is unrealistic for many
retarded readers, but a reading age of at least 12 years should be aimed
for, so that young people may be able to read popular newspapers and
social language, i.e. signs and notices in streets, supermarkets, railway
stations, etc.

The progress that is made in a remedial group is not usually maintained once the child is discharged to his normal class. However, Cashdan
et al. (1967) have shown that where remedial help is continued over a
long term, progress continues. At the conclusion of their research into
three groups of retarded junior school boys, Cashdan & Pumfrey (1969)

pointed to the need for a continuous programme of remedial help as an integral part of the whole school curriculum. Unfortunately, this type of help is often limited or not available throughout the education system, particularly after the age of 10 or 11.

Remedial provision varies greatly. Teaching may take place within the child's school in the shape of a remedial class or withdrawal group. Alternatively the school may be visited by a peripatetic teacher. Some authorities require the child in need of remedial help to visit a reading centre once or twice weekly; or specialized instruction may be given at Child Development Centres which may be part of a hospital service.

The peripatetic remedial teacher has a splendid opportunity to seek the co-operation of the class teacher in making provision for a severely retarded reader. Remedial teachers based in reading centres or hospital units often work as part of a team, including a psychologist and a doctor, who can provide skilled diagnosis, assessment and remediation for reading retarded children. The psychologist's information gives a guide to the general level of an individual's cognitive ability and the evenness of performance in different tasks. The doctor, usually with the help of other colleagues, can contribute information about vision, hearing and co-ordination. Such teams also provide an advisory service for teachers in schools. They can build up a library of reading materials at child level and books at teacher level which could be available for non-specialists to browse through and discuss with the remedial expert.

There is current dispute concerning the effectiveness of diagnostic teaching with methods geared to strengths and weaknesses (Hewison, 1982). However, knowledge of the factors underlying literacy helps teachers to approach their pupils with understanding and flexibility (Vernon, 1971). The resourcefulness demanded of a teacher faced by a child who makes slow progress is enhanced by knowledge of alternative strategies.

Remedial teaching

Remedial teaching has two main functions. Firstly, it is an attempt to compensate for the effects of a learning problem, finding the most effective strategies, giving more intensive help, learning to advise parents and class teachers on how best to help the child. Secondly, it offers the child the experience of appropriate learning and planned success. As class teaching is necessarily directed to the mainstream, the child with a learning problem may struggle with written work, even though the oral content is interesting. If the learning problem is the result of a developmental lag, inappropriate teaching, lack of motivation, or an undiagnosed visual or hearing deficit, rapid progress may follow intervention. Some children have very persistent difficulties, however, and will be at a disadvantage in later years when so much learning depends on fluent literacy. Both the child and those involved with him may need to be imaginative if the frustrations and drudgery of academic work are not going to become overwhelming. The child or adolescent may opt out with a sense of hostility to school and parents, and with a lack of self-respect.

Assessment

It is important to realize (Finucci *et al.*, 1982) that some supposed learning difficulties, if judged by reading age and IQ, are statistical artefacts. Standards of literacy vary greatly from place to place, being lowest in inner city areas. Thus national norms may not be appropriate, and schools need to be prepared for the children who live in their catchment area, not the children they would like to be there. A third of inner city 7-year-old children in some cities may not have started to read yet. The following discussion refers to assessment of all children who are finding it unusually or unexpectedly difficult to read.

The first step is to ascertain the present level of attainment in reading and spelling. As both Pumfrey (1971) and Farnham-Diggory (1978) point out, present diagnostic procedures for assessment of underlying skills, although not perfect, nevertheless form an important basis on which a remedial programme may be planned.

A useful instrument to aid the teacher in diagnosis is the Aston Index (Newton & Thompson, 1976) designed for use with children aged between 5 and 14 years. It samples visual, auditory and general intellectual ability broadly relevant to reading, writing and spelling.

After the test items are scored, an individual profile may be plotted. Although no two profiles are ever identical, a child's difficulties may be described as general intellectual, linguistic, auditory, visual or mixed. The type of difficulty suggests the kinds of remedial techniques to be used.

Once a reading programme has been planned and put into operation, it should be regularly monitored, the child's reaction to it assessed, and if necessary a new programme drawn up and implemented. If a child fails in a particular area, the teacher should try to diagnose what it is about that particular task the child finds difficult, and, if possible, present the same learning in a different way.

In summary, what is required is an initial diagnosis using selected available tests, and continual monitoring of the child's response to the various elements of learning, with adjustment of the reading programme if necessary.

Teaching strategies

As yet, it is not possible to state with any degree of certainty how a child learns. Learning and teaching are extremely complex processes. Some of these will be discussed under the section on classroom management. There is more to remediation than requiring the child to perform tasks designed to give him practice and ultimate competence in the basic skills under consideration. For example, the level of interest in the content of books will affect the incentive to learn. Children will also be more motivated to learn how to write down their own ideas rather than imposed ideas.

However, for the present, the child's difficulties will be treated as though they were neutral, and the procedures described will be those necessary to improve the specific deficits of the child. Broadly, teaching is directed to the strong channel, either visual or auditory, whilst trying to improve the weak modality in a general context of language development.

Visual difficulties

Children with poor visual recall and sequencing find a whole word approach to reading extremely difficult. They cannot look at words and recognize them instantly, as they have difficulty in remembering word configurations. Thus, it would be inappropriate to teach via a 'look and say' approach, as it would take them a long time to acquire even a limited sight vocabulary.

Those children whose strength is in the auditory area find it easier to learn from a structured phonic approach. A start is usually made with single sound/symbol associations, using these to build up regular three letter words, e.g. *fat, pen, big*. Next, initial two letter blends are introduced. These may be used to make new words, e.g. *blot, drip, pram*. Then consonant diagraphs *ch, sh, th, wh* are taught, to add more phonic knowledge and the capacity to form new words.

In this careful, systematic fashion, phonic knowledge is built up. Spelling rules may be introduced gradually and so, step by step, the child acquires a means of spelling and reading words. As well as using pencil and paper, variety and reinforcement are introduced through writing on a chalkboard, using plastic letters to build up words, and tracing over sand paper letters. Generalizing from one word to other words in a 'family' is not difficult for this group of children, e.g. *at*, *bat*, *cat*, *fat*, *hat* etc. Phonic analysis and synthesis is one way to independent reading, but a problem is encountered when irregular words appear. This may be dealt with by teaching other word identification techniques, e.g. semantic clues (word meaning, sentence meaning, general meaning of the prose) and syntactic clues (expected word order of the English language). These children who rely heavily on phonics may become unrhythmical, staccato readers. They need to be helped to read at speaking pace, by practice in reading phrases. In spelling, irregular words are often best learned in the following manner, which is a modified form of a spelling procedure outlined by Bradley (1981).

1 Write the word.
2 Name each letter as it is written.
3 Say the word.
4 Repeat two or three times.
5 Cover the word and write from memory.
6 Practise daily for a week.

At the end of each week, spellings learned in this way must be checked.

One way of helping to improve visual memory for irregular words is to use a series of slides with irregularly spelled words on a sound/slide machine or a slide carousel projector. The slide is exposed for 5 seconds and then removed from the screen. Several words of increasing length may be shown to the child in this manner. After each exposure, the child is required to write the word he has just seen. Checking reveals the number of letters he has difficulty in remembering.

Some of these children have difficulties with letter formation and need the additional support of language to enable them to remember where to start to write a letter. They often confuse certain letters, *b—d*, *u—n*, *w—m*, *p—q*, *p—b*. Teaching correct letter formation goes some way to eliminating this problem. In practice it is very difficult to eradicate *b—d* confusion and they should be taught separately. Some teachers ask the child with established confusion to write *b e d* and learn in that way. Others use one of the letters if it should occur in the child's name, e.g. Ro*b*ert, Bar*b*ara, E*d*ward, Lin*d*a. I find the most effective way of avoiding confusion is to ask the child to remember to check *b*s and *d*s using the following method (Fig. 10.1). The child says the letters of the alphabet with his hands outstretched—a quick glance at a word and back to his hand shows whether or not the *b* or *d* is written correctly.

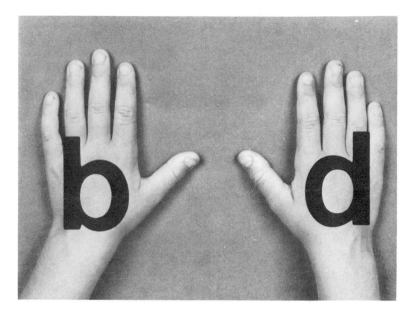

Fig. 10.1. Palm down, the left hand, with the thumb at 90° to the fingers, looks like a *b*. The right hand, with thumb at 90° to the fingers, looks like a *d*.

(Another technique is to point out that in saying and writing a *b* the lips and pen make a line initially, whereas the initial lip and pen shape is round for a *d*. Also, a lower case *b* fits inside a capital *B*. [Ed.])

Auditory difficulties

The group of children with auditory difficulties often have associated language problems. Auditory memory and auditory sequencing present the major difficulties. Although the children understand speech, they often have difficulty in making themselves understood. They find it difficult to relate a story in sequence. Giving information is a problem, as they often forget what they are saying or are unable to find the word they need. Polysyllabic words may present difficulties and the order of the syllables may be confused, e.g. *obversatory* for *observatory*. Some children have association problems (similar to paraphasia). They may find the correct category of word, e.g. dog, but choose *corgi* for *collie*. Difficulty is also experienced in repeating a series of numbers, days of the week or months of the year. Short vowel sounds, as in *bag, beg, big, bog, bug*, are difficult for this group to discriminate. It is often more productive to introduce long vowel sounds initially, as they are easier to discriminate, e.g. *oo, ee, ai*. End blends present a particular problem, *ng, nt, nd, nch, mp,* so that *sting* may be written *stig, sand—sad, lunch—luch.* Often these children make errors in pronunciation which leads them to make spelling errors; is for his, fin for thin, vish for *fish, thun for fun.* Children with auditory difficulties are often unable to detect or supply a rhyming word, or are convinced that dissimilar words rhyme. Galt's games of rhyming pairs and rhyming snap are useful for this problem. The rhyming difficulty is apparent when one tries to teach words in 'family' groups of *an, ban, can, Dan, fan* etc. Even after using plastic letters to build up the group of words, the children find it difficult to generalize. They fail to detect that all the words have certain letters in common. Each word appears unique. However, retaining the last letters and changing the word by changing the first letter only, is a helpful concrete demonstration.

Teaching initially consists of a Language Experience Approach, in concert with a reading scheme which uses a 'look and say' approach, e.g. Reid's 'Link-Up' Books.

The Language Experience Approach uses the child's speech patterns, which he finds easier to remember and read than those of an author. After dictating a sentence, reading it and copying it from the teacher's writing, the child covers the sentence and tries to write it from memory. The child is often successful at this and from this base, using his own language, a start is made in both reading and spelling. The words that are often easiest to learn are the ones which carry most meaning for the child, e.g. Easter eggs, swimming. A store of words that have been learned are kept by the child and used in a variety of games and activities. The child can see that he is making progress as his store of words grows.

So the process of reading, writing and spelling begins. But progress is slow, as teaching must be geared to the learner's pace and new knowledge is best introduced when previous knowledge has been internalized, i.e. can be recalled at will. Frequent revision is essential.

Auditory and visual difficulties
This group of children are the most difficult to teach as they have no strong channel which can be used. Usually, one channel is slightly better developed than the other and this is preferred when teaching. Thus, strategies for visual or auditory difficulties may be used as appropriate. Initially, one would start by using the child's own interests and language patterns. Reading, writing and spelling would be learned simultaneously.

With one particularly difficult child, the words of a 'pop' song were used to make a start. The child could sing the song from memory. He showed amazement and pleasure when he was able to read the words of the song which had been written for him.

Learning to spell is very difficult for this group of children. Fernald's (1943) method, even though it is initially very slow, is often useful.

Classroom management

Classroom management of children with severe reading difficulties merits consideration of the following points.

1 After a period of failure the child needs to have confidence re-established. Frequent reassurance about present and future progress in reading and writing is given. It is often helpful to take the child into one's confidence regarding the individual strengths and weaknesses brought to the reading task and to explain why particular techniques are being used.

2 Reduce the pressure on the child and try to create a learning environment which will give the security needed to make a fresh start in reading.

3 By praise and encouragement the child is helped to feel liked and valued, as after years of failure, he may have a poor self-image.

4 Time should be spent in talking and listening to the child to discover interests that can be used in the reading programme (Ashton-Warner, 1963; Bradley, 1980).

5 Work should start at or slightly below the level the child has achieved. By doing this teaching will be efficient. The child should be able to cope with the work and find initial success.

6 The child should be allowed to work at his own rate, no matter how slow this is initially. Output should be encouraged in spite of errors or small quantity at first, so long as the child has been seen to try.

7 Exercises need to be repeated in different ways so that interest is maintained whilst one aspect of learning is firmly established. Then new learning may be introduced.

8 A variety of materials should be used, appropriate to the stage of learning. Preferably these should be new to the child, e.g. reading games, reading kits, spelling kits, television reading programmes for schools or synchrofax machine plus reading books that are appropriate to the reading and interest level.

9 A variety of activities should be used at each session, including talking, listening, reading (visual to verbal), writing to dictation (verbal to visuo-motor), motor activities, visual sequencing activities, and auditory

sequencing activities. Painting, drawing and construction toys are also useful from the point of view of practising eye—hand co-ordination activities to improve fine motor skills.

10   There should be no long tiring work sessions as these can be unproductive, resulting in the child's concentration lapsing. A varied sequence of activities can help the child to work longer, and in this way attention can be maintained and the concentration span increased.

11   Children do not necessarily learn at a constant rate; there are spurts and plateaus when new learning is assimilated and consolidated. When a plateau is reached, there is a need to consolidate past learning and wait before introducing a new element.

12   Progress can be evaluated in co-operation with the child, who will then be aware of improvement.

13   Many children have difficulty in letter formation and some use space poorly, so that words may run into each other. They are not written in discrete clusters. One way of helping children to relearn the above skills is to introduce cursive writing. This often motivates a child to write when previously he was reluctant to do so. This may be because cursive writing appears to be thought of as a 'grown-up' skill by many children. Teaching cursive writing provides an opportunity for the teacher to emphasize letter formation, use of space and use of punctuation. Also, words are seen as whole units instead of sequences of letters.

14   There is a need to help the children to develop the ability to organize thoughts and plan a piece of written work. Ideas for this may be found in works by Binns (1978), Britten (1975) and Rosen & Rosen (1973).

15   Miscue analysis is a useful technique to employ when hearing children read. By noting the errors or miscues that children make, a teacher may record and later analyse the errors, using these to form a diagnostic hypothesis for future teaching (Goodman & Goodman, 1978; Clark, 1977; Pumfrey, 1976). These errors may be collected under the following headings: semantic, syntactic, phonic and graphic. Analysis of the miscues reveals to the teacher the strategies for word identification being used by the reader. This in turn reveals the teaching the child needs. Reading aloud, however, is only one part of the process. Most of the reading that people do in the course of their lives involves silent reading. In order to ascertain the level of understanding of a piece of prose, cloze procedure may be used (Moyle, 1976). Children are asked to fill in missing words (about 1:10) in a paragraph. Thus, by the use of miscue analysis and cloze procedure, as complete a picture as possible may be gained of a reader's facility when dealing with written language.

16 Reading to children of any age can form part of the daily session. This can stimulate a child's imagination, increase his knowledge of literature and may encourage him to read more independently.

17 Time may be set aside for children to read books of their own choice. A surprising number of children are able to read books that are of particular interest to them, even when these have a high readability level.

18 Although the child spends many thousands of hours in the classroom (Rutter *et al.*, 1979), this is only part of the child's life. Relationships and activities outside school will often be of greater importance. It is difficult to learn when hungry, frightened or preoccupied, but it is possible for a classroom to be warm, enriching and accepting.

19 One must never forget that one is dealing with a thinking, feeling person, not simply a set of learning difficulties! Whilst trying to remedy the problems, one must not lose sight of the whole child and his unique personality.

Management by parents

In general, parents are not educational experts; many feel uncomfortable visiting school and find it difficult to know what their children should be capable of. If the school does not complain and the child likes going to school, many parents will be satisfied. Other parents, perhaps ambitious, perhaps unrealistic, impose prolonged, often unhappy, sessions of homework which can impair both family relationships and attitudes to learning. Lack of contact between parents, who may both be working during school hours, and teachers, who receive little training for parent counselling, results in frequent misunderstanding, especially when the child has problems. The parents view the school as complaining about something that is the teacher's responsibility, while the teachers see the parents as uninterested and unsupportive. Yet a great deal can be achieved by a combined approach.

It is true that assessment and remedial facilities vary enormously from school to school. Secondary schools may not see remedial literacy as a responsibility, except for slow learners in a remedial class perhaps. In such a class, the child does not receive the interesting content of mainstream subject teaching. If the child is clever enough to understand mainstream class ideas, but not to deal with the written material, the dilemma can be acute. Copying from the blackboard is generally an overused technique which is a particular drawback for these children. An expert on literacy, to act as an advocate and liaise with subject teachers, and supportive parents are needed if a secondary school is to provide an appropriate education for clever children with learning difficulties. If a school does not have such an educational expert, it may be necessary for the parents to find help outside school or find another school with more remedial facilities, in spite of the social disadvantages such a change many imply.

Parents from an early stage should be urged to support the work of the teacher in undertaking activities with the child at home. These may include games to develop auditory memory, auditory sequencing, visual memory, visual sequencing or sound—symbol correspondences. Working together in this way for short periods and with teaching advice can develop the parent—child relationship. It may give the parent insight into the child's difficulties, enabling the parent to be understanding and more sympathetic to the child.

The parent's task is a difficult one, as they must endeavour to encourage and elicit the best the child can do, at the same time keeping their expectations within realistic limits. Parents should try not to become over-demanding or set impossible goals which the child cannot reach and which can only result in the child becoming discouraged. Comparison with siblings is unhelpful. Parents should see their respective children as unique individuals who can only develop in their own particular way.

If a child withdraws into a fantasy world, parents can help by gently but firmly emphasizing the real world, knowing as they do, that the real world can at times be painful for their child. If parents read well, they can do much to interest the child in books by reading to him. If the child is more interested in facts than fiction, again the parents can help by reading the wanted factual information. Thus, information is provided which peers are able to achieve independently. Tizard *et al.*, (1982) have shown the beneficial effects of parents regularly listening to their children read and this is to be encouraged. However, it must be stressed that the parents of reading-retarded children will need to be extremely patient and tactful if this is to be an enjoyable activity for both participants.

The things the child can do well should be encouraged. He may be good at swimming or dancing, fishing or cooking. One boy who had the utmost difficulty with writing and spelling, won medals for modern dancing and certificates for swimming.

As adults, we may abandon the learning of skills and activities at which we do not excel. Indeed, we probably prejudge the extent of our likely achievement in a new area before submitting ourselves to the challenge. In this way, we avoid failure and our self-esteem is not lowered. Children cannot avoid learning to read and thus may daily face failure in what is recognized as being an important skill. A cheerful, positive and supportive attitude from parent to child is the one to strive for. Praise and encouragement achieve far more than blame and criticism.

Case studies

The following case studies show Jennifer who has visual difficulties and Adam who has mixed difficulties.

CASE Jennifer (born 6 June 1971) was delivered postmaturely by caesarean section. She weighed 8 lb. 5 oz. and was the third child in the family.

In 1979, aged 8, Jennifer had had several operations on her eyes and was described by a paediatrician as having a congenital abnormality of the ocular muscles, mild congenital heart disease and co-ordination difficulties.

The same year, this girl was assessed by a clinical psychologist at the request of her school, as she was having difficulty in learning to read, write and spell. The results showed that intellectual functioning was within the average range. She produced a verbal score of 96, performance score of 92, full scale IQ 93 on the Wechsler Intelligence Scale for Children.

As her school felt unable to provide for her learning difficulty, Jennifer started to attend a hospital Child Development Centre for extra tuition.

Jennifer is a friendly, relaxed, cheeful and co-operative girl who is highly motivated to learn, hardworking and willing to practise reading and spelling in her own time.

Although orally fluent, Jennifer was initially unable to write very much. On her first day in class, after trying to write a story, she finally sighed and said 'Can't write much. I get it jumbled up!' (See Fig. 10.2)

After assessment using the Aston Index, it was found that Jennifer had stronger auditory than visual skills. Some letters were confused, e.g. *b–d, v–f, f–t, u–n*, and many letters were incorrectly formed. She needed language to direct the formation of letters, so that she knew where to start a given letter and which direction to follow. A variety of equipment was used to reinforce learning of correct letter formation, including a phonic alphabet, sand-paper letters, plastic letters and worksheets on a synchrofax machine.

Initially, reading was slow, hesitant and staccato. Word identification strategies—semantic, syntactic and phonic—had to be taught. Reading books slightly below readability level were used to ensure immediate success in reading. Gradually, reading improved and it is now, after 1 year's teaching, swift and fluent.

Auditory sequencing skills were built up from repetition of common sequences e.g. days; months; the alphabet; learning short poems and rhymes, and sequential games, plus directing attention to the order of sounds in words.

Visual sequencing skills were improved by various techniques, one of which

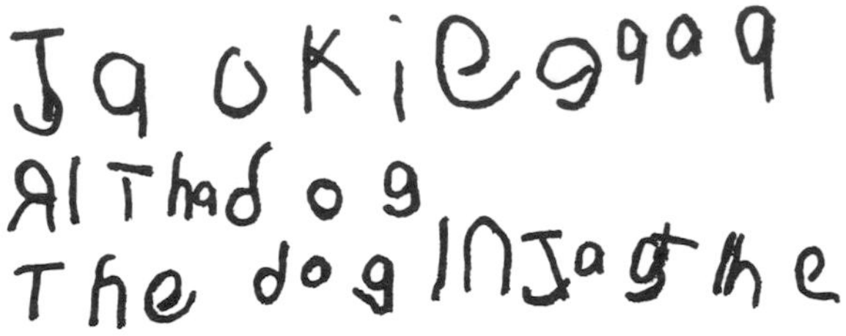

Jq oKie g9a9
Al Thad o g
The dog INJag the

Fig. 10.2. Writing by Jennifer. When asked to write this, she said, 'Can't write much.
I get it jumbled up. *The dog into the* ... Didn't know what to write.'

was showing three pictures for a few seconds, removing and shuffling them. The
child's task is to produce the original sequence. This activity may be undertaken
using longer sequences as the child becomes more proficient at the task. It was
noted that Jennifer found the task easier when using the added support of
language rather than when using visual input alone.

Establishing phoneme—grapheme relationships was a slow process, but after
3 months Jennifer was able to write simple sentences within the limits of the
teaching she had received. After 1 year, this girl had increased her reading age
by 3 years and her spelling age by 2 years.

As she made progress, Jennifer developed in self-confidence. She is proud of
her success in reading and spelling and is a cheerful child despite her handicaps.

	June 1980	June 1981
Reading age	6.7 years	9.4 years
Spelling age	5.7 years	7.6 years
Calendar age	9.0 years	10.0 years

CASE   Adam (born 14 December 1968) was the fourth child born to his parents
after a normal pregnancy and delivery. He walked at 12 months of age, but
speech was late to emerge, not beginning until after he was 3 and being quite
limited when he first went to school. About this time Adam began to stammer.

He had marked co-ordination problems. He had difficulty in eating and drinking tidily, dressing himself, tying shoe laces and fastening buckles. He was also
poor at jigsaws. He was reported by his parents to be an impatient child who was
prone to temper tantrums.

Adam was referred when aged 10 years 6 months because of his profound
difficulties in learning to read and write, even after some years of extra remedial
help within his own school. It is interesting to note that Adam's father and two of
his sisters have difficulty with literacy.

Adam was noted to have an immobile face with an open mouth but showed no other formal neurological abnormalities. His muscles were poorly developed, he had some impairment of fine finger movements, did not know left from right, had a poor sense of rhythm and an inaccurate knowledge of the position of his arms in space.

After testing by a clinical psychologist using the Wechsler Intelligence Scale for Children, the results were: verbal scale IQ 84, performance scale IQ 87, full scale IQ 86. He was referred to a special class for assessment and teaching.

He presented as a timid, anxious but co-operative boy. The results of the Aston Index were not encouraging as Adam had low level scores in both visual and auditory items. He presented quite a challenge to the teacher, as he had the added disabilities of being distractable and lacking in concentration. Adam had only managed to learn 13 letters of the alphabet by the age of 11. He was unable to relate a story in sequence, had an articulatory defect and a slight stammer which became more pronounced when he was excited. Speech therapy was arranged to help alleviate this problem.

Adam could not reproduce a tapped rhythm, nor could he detect a rhyming word. In class Adam interacted very little with the other children who behaved in a friendly way towards him. He appeared to live in a fantasy world and related stories that could not have happened. He maintained that he had played football for a famous First Division football club, that he had driven a bronze coloured Rolls Royce and that he kept a 'real live, 3 inch high man' in his bedroom.

Teaching concentrated on a visual approach to reading, as this was Adam's stronger channel. Words from his reading book were written on one card by the teacher and on a second card by Adam. Thus, he built up his own store of 'known' words which were used for various activities.

A parallel approach of a language experience kind was also used. At each session, the previous stories were read, so that in this way, Adam became familiar with many words. Some of these, which were of high interest to him, were used to teach spelling.

On admission to the classroom, Adam was unable to hold a word in his auditory memory and respond with the correct initial, medial or final sound. He needed the added support of visual presentation of the word to overcome this difficulty as his auditory channel was so weak.

In his first few weeks in class, Adam either omitted vowels from words or included a vowel in the desperate hope that it was the correct one, as he knew by this time that all words in the English language contain at least one vowel per syllable.

Without the help he received Adam might still be at the stage he was on admission to the classroom: that of spelling words in a bizarre fashion. His spelling mistakes became phonic, which was a vast improvement as it showed that he was beginning to understand phoneme–grapheme relationships and sequencing. Moreover, phonic mistakes are more readily understood by the reader than the bizarre spellings that Adam used to write, e.g. *boap* for *in*, *haot* for *yet*, *foef* for *good*, *heae* for *with*.

Slowly, Adam made progress in reading and writing. Concentration improved, as did motivation to learn. He still lives in a fantasy world but perhaps further success in reading and spelling will help Adam to face reality more readily.

He will need a great deal of praise, understanding, encouragement and not least structured teaching fitted to his needs over a long period of time, if he is ever to become literate. Fortunately, his family's expectations of him are realistic and he is therefore relieved of some of the pressures with which some children have to contend.

After 6 months' teaching, Adam's reading age had improved by 4 months and his spelling age by 13 months.

Reading age	6.7 years	6.11 years
Spelling age	5.3 years	6.4 years
Calendar age	12.1 years	12.7 years

References and further reading

Ainscow, M. & Tweddle, D.A. (1979) *Preventing Classroom Failure. An Objectives Approach.* John Wiley, Chichester.

Alberman, E. (1973) The early prediction of learning disorders. *Developmental Medicine and Child Neurology,* **15,** 202−204.

Alston, J. & Taylor, J. (1984) *The Handwriting File.* LDA, Wisbech, Cambs.

Ashton-Warner, S. (1963) *Teacher.* Secker and Warburg, London.

Binns, R. (1978) *From Speech to Writing.* Scottish Curriculum Development Service, Moray House College of Education, Edinburgh.

Boder, E. (1973) Developmental dyslexia: a diagnostic approach based on three atypical reading-spelling patterns. *Developmental Medicine and Child Neurology,* **15,** 663−687.

Bradley, L. (1980) *Assessing Reading Difficulties, A Diagnostic and Remedial Approach,* pp. 28−29 Macmillan, London.

Britten, J. (1975) *Developing Writing Abilities,* pp. 11−18. Macmillan, London.

Carroll, H.C.M. (1972) The remedial teaching of reading: an evaluation. *Remedial Education,* **7,** 10−15.

Cashdan, A. & Pumfrey, P.D. (1969) Some effects of the remedial teaching of reading. *Educational Research,* **11,** 138−142.

Cashdan, A., Pumfrey, P.D. & Lunzer, E.A. (1967) A survey of children receiving remedial teaching in reading. *Bulletin of the British Psychological Society,* **67,** 17A.

Cashdan, A., Pumphrey, P.D. & Lunzer, E.A. (1971) Children receiving remedial teaching in reading. *Educational Research,* **13,** 98−105.

Clark, M.M. (1970) *Reading Difficulties in Schools.* Penguin Books, Harmondsworth.

Clark, M.M. (1977) Reading considered in a language context. In *Reading: Problems and Practices* (eds J.F. Reid and H. Donaldson), pp. 67−73. Ward Lock, London.

Clay, M.M. (1972) *The Patterning of Complex Behaviour,* pp. 160−161. Heinemann, London.

Collins, J.E. (1961) *The Effects of Remedial Education.* (Educational Monograph 4) University of Birmingham Institute of Education.

Curr, W. & Gourlay, H. (1953) An experimental evaluation of remedial education.

British Journal of Educational Psychology, **23**, 45–55.

Department of Education and Science (1975) *A Language for Life* (*The Bullock Report*). HMSO, London.

Downing, J. (1977) How society creates reading disability. *Elementary School Journal*, **17**, 274–279.

Durnham, J. (1960) The effects of remedial education on young children's reading ability and attitude to reading. *British Journal of Educational Psychology*, **30**, 173–175.

Farnham-Diggory, S. (1978) *Learning Disabilities*, pp. 22–42. Fontana, London.

Fernald, G.M. (1943) *Remedial Techniques in Basic School Subjects*. McGraw-Hill, New York.

Finucci, J.M., Isaacs, S.D., Whitehouse, C.C. & Childs, B. (1982) Empirical validation of reading and spelling quotients. *Developmental Medicine and Child Neurology*, **24**, 733–744.

Galloway, D.M. & Goodwin, C. (1979) *Educating Slow-Learners and Maladjusted Children*. Longman, London.

Goodman, K.S. & Goodman, Y.M. (1978) Learning about psycholinguistic processes by analysing and reading. In *Reading from Process to Practice* (eds L.J. Chapman and P. Czerniewska), pp. 126–146. Routledge and Kegan Paul, London.

Hewison, J. (1982) The current status of remedial intervention for children with reading problems. *Developmental Medicine and Child Neurology*, **24**, 183–186.

Hillmann, H.M. & Snowdon, R.L. (1960) Part-time classes for young backward readers. *British Journal of Educational Psychology*, **30**, 168–172.

Hulme, C. (1981) *Reading Retardation and Multisensory Teaching*, pp. 1–54. Routledge and Kegan Paul, London.

Ingram, T.T.S., Mason, A.W. & Blackburn, I. (1970) A retrospective study of 82 children with reading disability. *Developmental Medicine and Child Neurology*, **12**, 271–281.

Jansen, M. (1973) Denmark. In *Comparative Reading* (ed. J. Downing), pp. 285–307. Macmillan, New York.

Kellmer Pringle, M.L. (1961) The long term effects of remedial treatment: a follow-up enquiry based on the case study approach. *Educ. Res.* **4**, 62.

Leach, D.J. & Raybould, E.C. (1977) *Learning and Behaviour Difficulties in Schools*. Open Books, London.

Lovell, K., Byrne, C. & Richardson, B. (1963) A further study of the educational progress of children who had been given remedial education. *British Journal of Educational Psychology*, **33**, 3–9.

Lovell, K., Gray, E.A. & Oliver, D.E. (1964) A further study of some cognitive and other disabilities in backward readers of average non-verbal reasoning scores. *British Journal of Educational Psychology*, **34**, 275.

Lovell, K., Shapton, D. & Warren, N.S. (1964) A study of some cognitive and other disabilities in backward readers of average intelligence as assessed by a non-verbal test. *British Journal of Educational Psychology*, **34**, 58.

Lytton, H. (1967) Follow-up of an experiment in selection for remedial education. *British Journal of Educational Psychology*, **37**, 1.

Moyle, D. (1976) *The Teaching of Reading*, 4th edn. Ward Lock, London.

Myklebust, H.R. (1965) *Development and Disorders of Written Language: Picture Story Language Test*. Grune and Stratton, New York.

Newton, M. & Thomson, P. (1976) *The Aston Index*. LDA, Wisbech, Cambs.

Pumfrey, P.D. (1971) Children with reading difficulties. In *Literacy at all Levels* (ed. V. Southgate), pp. 140–160. Ward Lock, London.

Pumfrey, P.D. (1976) *Reading: Tests and Assessment Techniques.* Hodder and Stoughton, London.

Rennie, E.F.N. (1980) The West Riding screening, six years on. *Educational Research*, **23**, 47–50.

Rosen, H. & Rosen, C. (1973) *Language of Primary School Children.* Penguin, Harmondsworth.

Rutter, M., Graham, P. & Yule, W. (1970) A Neuropsychiatric Study in Childhood, pp. 35–36. (Little Club Clinics in Developmental Medicine, Spastics Society), Heinemann, London.

Rutter, M., Maughan, B., Mortimore, P. & Ouston, J. (1979) *Fifteen Thousand Hours.* Open Books, London.

Shearer, E. (1967) The long term effects of remedial education. *Educational Research*, **9**, 219–222.

Sturge, C. (1982) Reading retardation and anti-social behaviour. *Journal of Child Psychology and Psychiatry*, **23**, 21–31.

Tizard, J., Schofield, W.N. & Hewison, J. (1982) Collaboration between teachers and parents in assisting children's reading. *British Journal of Educational Psychology*, **52**, 1–15.

Tobin, D. & Pumphrey, P.D. (1976) Some long term effects of the remedial teaching of reading. *Educational Review*, **29**, 1–12.

Vernon, M.D. (1971) *Reading and its Difficulties.* Cambridge University Press, Cambridge.

Vincent, D., Green, L., Francis, J. & Powney, J. (1983) *A Review of Reading Tests.* NFER Nelson, Windsor.

Wedell, K. & Lindsay, G.A. (1980) Early identification procedures: what have we learned? *Remedial Education*, **15**(3), 130–135.

Yule, W. (1976) Issues and problems in remedial education. *Developmental Medicine and Child Neurology*, **18**, 674–682.

An update—further studies on parental involvement and teaching methods

In recent years there has been a move to involve parents in the education of their children. Brighouse (1982) suggests that rather than blaming each other for a child's underachievement, parents and teachers should co-operate to help children progress.

Encouraging news from research concerned with 'Paired-reading' programmes has emerged, although these have varied as to procedure (Morgan & Lyon, 1979; Bush, 1983; Belcher, 1984; Spalding, 1984; Bradley & Bryant, 1985)

It has been suggested that simply involving parents is not enough; they need training and ongoing advice from a specialist teacher to guide them (Spalding, 1984) However, having an interested parent listen to him read, may well motivate the child to further achievement.

The Education Act 1981, which came into operation in April 1983, encourages the fullest involvement of parents as partners, working alongside the professionals to ensure that the special educational needs of learning-disabled children are met. The Act emphasizes the need for all teachers to be proficient in the identification of learning-disabled children, and suggests that where possible, every effort should be made to cater for these children within mainstream school. Perhaps this will encourage a new approach to remedial education in secondary schools with a continuous programme of help available from 11 to 16 years of age, as Cashdan and Pumfrey (1969) had suggested some years earlier.

Teaching methods

Discussion continues concerning appropriate methods of teaching retarded readers. Gittelman and Feingold (1983) showed that an intensive four-month teaching programme produced significant changes in reading ability. However, Blau and Loveless (1983) maintain that in the initial stages of remediation, tactile methods produce better results than other approaches with reading-retarded children.

The concepts of reading retardation

The usefulness of the concept of reading retardation has been questioned by Van Der Wissel and Zegers (1985) They reviewed the Isle of Wight study and argued that the distinction found between retarded and dull readers, based on same I.Q. related aspects, should be abandoned. These Dutch authors suggest that the 'hump' in the distribution of underachievement scores may be due to the ceiling effect of the reading test used; this does not support the notion that the two groups fail because of different causes.

Neither Yule (1985), co-author of the Isle of Wight study, nor Frith (1985) dispute these conclusions. However, both contend that a group of children may exist whose reading is qualitatively different from other groups.

Yule (1985) hopes that the differences between the groups may further our understanding of aetiological factors. Frith (1985), in a cogently argued article, maintains that the concept of unexpected reading failure need not be abandoned as a consequence of criticisms from the Dutch authors. She suggests a need to discover the strategies used in a reading performance, and states that studies which analyse the underlying reasons for success or failure in literacy acquisition are the ones that may provide evidence for qualitatively different types of reading failure.

References

Belcher, M. (1984) Parents can be major assets in teaching reading. *Remedial Education*, **19** (4) 162–164.

Blau, H. & Loveless, E.J. (1983) If they can speak, why can't they read? And spell? They may now. *Reading*, **17** (1) 23–29.

Bradley, L. & Bryant, P. (1985) *Rhyme and Reason in Reading and Spelling*. International Academy for Research in Learning Disorder Monograph Series, Number 1. The University of Michigan Press, Ann Arbor.

Brighouse, T. (1982) A LEA perspective on underachievement. *Secondary Education Journal*. **12**, (3) 2–23.

Bush, A. (1983) Can pupils reading be improved by involving their parents? *Remedial Education*, **18**, (4) 167–170.

Frith, U. (1985) The usefulness of the concept of unexpected reading failure. Comments on reading retardation revisited. *British Journal of Developmental Psychology*, **3**, Pt 1, 15–17.

Gittelman, R. & Feingold I. (1983) Children with reading disorders, 1 Efficacy of reading remediation. *Journal of Child Psychology and Psychiatry*, **24**, 167–191.

Morgan, R.T.T. & Lyon, E. (1979) Paired reading, a preliminary report on a technique for parental tuition of reading-retarded children. *Journal of Child Psychology and Psychiatry*, **20**, 151–160.

Spalding, B. *et al.* (1983) if you want to improve your reading ask your mum—an attempt to involve parents in the reading process at secondary age level. *Remedial Education*, **19** (4) 157–161.

Van Der Wissel, A. & Zegers, F.E. (1985) Reading retardation revisited. *British Journal of Developmental Psychology*, **3**, 3–9.

Yule, W. (1985) Comments on Van Der Wissel and Zegers: Reading retardation revisited. *British Journal of Developmental Psychology*, **3**, 11–13.

Chapter 11
Children with Epilepsy

Jean Aicardi & Jean-Jacques Chevrie

Seizure disorders constitute a major area of child neurology since 3–7% of *all* children experience one or more epileptic seizures before the age of 5 years. They pose specific problems as the types of fits observed, the outcome of the epileptic syndromes encountered, the causes and the handling of anti-epileptic drugs differ considerably from those in adults.

Definitions and classification of epileptic seizures and epilepsies

Definitions
Epileptic seizures are attacks of cerebral origin due to an excessive, hypersynchronous activity of neuronal populations. This abnormal neuronal activity is manifested clinically by abrupt changes in consciousness, behaviour, motor activity, autonomic disturbances, etc. Isolated epileptic seizures can occur in non-epileptic persons under certain stresses, especially in young children and infants. Such provoked epileptic seizures are termed occasional, and are always expressed clinically by tonic or clonic muscle contractions. They are thus properly called convulsions. Epilepsy is a chronic condition in which a propensity to recurring seizures exists on the basis of structural (lesional) or physiological (cryptogenic) abnormalities of the brain.

Classification
Epileptic seizures, whether or not they are part of a chronic epilepsy, can be classified according to various criteria. The classification most widely used is that proposed by the International League Against Epilepsy in 1971 and revised in 1981 (Gastaut, 1970; Commission on Classification, 1981). This classification is shown in Table 11.1. As there is still much controversy concerning the 1981 revision and since many published works have used the 1971 version, the latter is indicated in the table, with mention of the modifications made in 1981. Those modifications are mainly as follows. (i) Partial complex seizures are now defined by the

Table 11.1 Classification of epileptic seizures, simplified from the 1969 and 1981 international classifications (Gastaut, 1970; Commission of Classification, 1981)

I *Generalized seizures*

 Tonic-clonic seizures (grand mal) and variants (purely tonic or clonic seizures)
 Absence attacks:*
  simple (alteration of consciousness only)
  complex (also include motor, tonic or automatic components)
 Myoclonic seizures (massive or bilateral synchronous myoclonic jerks)
 Atonic seizure (astatic, drop attacks)
 Infantile spasms†

II *Partial seizures‡*

 With simple symptoms (motor, sensory, autonomic, psychic)
 With complex symptoms

III *Unilateral seizures§*

IV *Unclassified seizures*

---

 *Absence attacks are also classified as typical or petit mal absences if the EEG shows the classical 3 Hz rhythmic discharge, and atypical when the EEG discharge is slower or irregular.
 †Removed from the 1981 revision since it is regarded as a syndrome, not a seizure type.
 ‡Classification of the partial seizures has been revised in 1981 (see text).
 §Deleted from the 1981 revision and considered as partial motor seizures.
 Partial seizures can evolve from simple to complex and/or may become generalized.

existence of an impairment of awareness or responsiveness, while they were previously defined by the occurrence of manifestations expressing the involvement of organized high-level activities. (ii) Simple partial seizures now include any type of psychic phenomena, provided awareness is maintained (e.g. illusions or hallucinations). (iii) Unilateral seizures are no longer separated from partial seizures. Lateralized seizures in children may be unassociated with any demonstrable structural abnormality of the brain and may occur in the same circumstances (e.g. fever) as generalized seizures. They are apt to be prolonged and are one of the most common forms of status epilepticus in children under 5 years of age. (iv) Infantile spasms are now excluded from the classification of seizures as they are thought to constitute an epileptic syndrome.

There is no accepted system of classification of the *epilepsies*, as opposed to the epileptic seizures. For therapeutic purposes, a simple classification scheme will be used in this chapter, although its short-comings are obvious. In this scheme, an epilepsy is classified according to

Table 11.2 Principal types of epilepsy and main appropriate drugs (in order of preference)*

Generalized convulsive epilepsies	Carbamazepine, valproate, phenytoin, phenobarbitone, primidone, benzodiazepines†, (valproate is particularly indicated in primary forms, carbamazepine in secondary types)
Primary (cryptogenic)	
Secondary (due to one or several brain lesions)	
Partial epilepsies	
With simple seizures	
Benign partial epilepsy	Carbamazepine
Other types	Carbamazepine and others
With complex seizures	id.
Absence epilepsy (pure petit mal)	Valproate, ethosuximide, benzodiazepines†, diones, Diamox
Myoclonic epilepsies‡	
Lennox-Gastaut syndrome (and related)	Valproate, benzodiazepine†, all other drugs (ACTH and corticosteroids rarely indicated)
Infantile spasms (West's syndrome)	ACTH or corticosteroids, valproate, benzodiazepines†

*Association of two (rarely more) drugs may be indicated (see text).
†Clonazepam, clobazam, nitrazepam, diazepam (seldom for long-term treatment)
‡Applies exclusively to epilepsies characterized by myoclonic jerks and 3 Hz spike waves, not synonymous with Lennox-Gastaut syndrome (Aicardi, 1982)

the exclusive or predominant type of its seizures. Some emphasis is also given to the suspected aetiological factors, thus separating, in some forms, primary and secondary subtypes, as this distinction has prognostic and therapeutic value. This simplified classification is displayed in Table 11.2. It should be noted that the various types considered do not have the same significance. Some (e.g. partial benign epilepsy, petit mal, primary generalized epilepsy of adolescents) are well-defined and easily recognizable. Others (e.g. many of the generalized convulsive and partial epilepsies) constitute heterogeneous groups with various causes and outcomes. The distinction drawn between myoclonic epilepsy and the Lennox-Gastaut syndrome has been detailed elsewhere (Aicardi, 1982, 1985). Although this distinction is open to criticism, it has practical value since myoclonic epilepsy, in the restricted sense used, has a significantly less severe prognosis than the Lennox-Gastaut syndrome, and different treatment.

Assessment and investigation

Most patients with occasional seizures have febrile convulsions, the assessment and management of which are described below. In occasional seizures unassociated with fever, routine investigations include: blood sugar, calcium, magnesium and electrolyte determination, since changes in any of these may be a cause and therapy in such patients should be directed against the causal disorder. According to the clinical circumstances, special attention should be given to particular problems, e.g. hyponatraemia or hypoglycaemia in post-operative patients or those with chronic CNS disorders. Patients with recurrent seizures (epilepsy) require a combined neurological and electroencephalographic assessment. This can usually be done on an out-patient basis, as a careful history and neurological examination and a routine EEG record are all that is necessary in the vast majority of children. Sleep records are often very useful and are usually easily obtained in infants and young children. Only very few patients (those with very frequent seizures or with associated signs) will require hospitalization for intensive monitoring and observation.

The initial assessment has two objectives. The first one is to confirm the epileptic nature of the fit. This is mainly a clinical problem which is easy in many patients (e.g. those with clonic or partial seizures), but more difficult in some (e.g. those with purely tonic or atonic fits). It is extremely important to enquire about precipitating factors, since syncopes or anoxic seizures are almost always provoked by emotional or physical triggers. When in doubt, some workers (Stephenson, 1980) advocate compression of the eyeballs, with appropriate precautions, to try to reproduce the spontaneous anoxic attacks of the patient.

The second aim of the initial assessment is to type the epilepsy, an essential step for the selection of therapy. In addition to identification of the type of seizures, proper classification of an epilepsy demands knowledge of such factors as the relation of fits to the sleep cycle, or to other possible triggering events such as watching television, startling at sudden noises, etc. Whenever a suspicion of absences arises, the patient should be asked to hyperventilate for 3–4 minutes as this manœuvre is without danger if the child is seated. It will provoke an absence in virtually all children with untreated petit mal, and also elicits many partial complex seizures, helping to classify the type of epilepsy.

The EEG is of help both in the diagnosis and in the typing of an epilepsy, provided it is recalled that a normal tracing does not exclude the diagnosis and that an abnormal and even a paroxysmal tracing can be associated with non-epileptic fits. Some EEG patterns are distinctive, for example the 3 Hz rhythmic spike-wave discharge of petit mal or the chaotic pattern of hypsarrhythmia. Other patterns, such as focal lower Rolandic spikes, are extremely useful in confirming a diagnosis of benign partial epilepsy but they occur also very commonly in normal children of 6–14 years of age (Cavazzuti *et al.*, 1980; Petersen *et al.*, 1975). As a general rule, over-interpretation of the EEG should be avoided, especially in children in whom the normal range of variation is extremely large. In particular, rhythmic, often notched, slow waves induced by hyperventilation or by drowsiness should not be mistakenly interpreted as abnormal. Likewise, parietal humps of stage II sleep are not to be confused with spike-wave formations, and a paroxysmal response to intermittent photic stimulation may occur in about 8–10% of non-epileptic children (Petersen *et al.*, 1975).

Further investigations are not indicated if the patient can be confidently assigned to one of the non-lesional epileptic syndromes listed in Table 11.2 (i.e. primary generalized epilepsy of adolescents, benign partial epilepsy, petit mal), even though non-progressive brain damage, or even brain tumours, may exceptionally mimic them. In children with refractory epilepsies due to probable focal or multifocal lesions, or in those with generalized seizures whose primary or secondary character is unclear, we usually obtain a CT scan with enhancement, not only to exclude a cerebral tumour, which is in fact a rare occurrence, but also to gather information of possible prognostic value on the nature and extent of brain lesions, if any. The exact cost-effectiveness of CT scans, however, remains to be evaluated, and it is often negative in the presence of temporal lobe lesions, such as insular sclerosis and hamartomas. In such cases nuclear magnetic resonance imaging will probably be of considerable interest. Other laboratory investigations are of little help. The isotope brain scan is now obsolete. Angiography and pneumoencephalography are no longer indicated in the presence of a normal CT scan. The former may be used if the CT scan suggests the possibility of a vascular malformation.

Some basic assessment of the intellectual and behavioural problems of the patient ought to be performed by the physician himself. There is much evidence that a number of children with epilepsy have cognitive and behavioural difficulties (Holdsworth & Whitmore, 1974; Rutter *et al.*, 1970; Stores & Hart, 1976). Recent work (Stores, 1978, 1983) has shown that these difficulties are not usually mentioned at referral nor complained of by the parents, only to be revealed later by more thorough investigation. Thus, at least a rough assessment of basic cognitive function, general intelligence and school record, and an evaluation by questioning and direct observation of the behaviour at home and at school and in relation to other children or playmates, should be done at the first visit. Likewise, a general evaluation of the family, from a social as well as a psychological point of view, is in order. In particular, their reliability as witnesses and as dispensers of treatment should be judged. Their attitudes towards the child (anxiety, overprotection) and their ability to cope with the problems of the child and family should be appreciated, as well as their general level of understanding and ideas about their child's disorder.

More formal psychological assessment is often highly desirable, though it depends on available facilities. It is imperative whenever there is school deterioration or serious behaviour change. Although routine tests are generally used, some specific functions, such as reading, powers of concentration, fatiguability, persistence and memory, may be particularly important to evaluate in children with epilepsy (Stores, 1971, 1973). An initial testing, especially in these particular areas, will be useful as a baseline to assess subsequent progress and the possible effects of drugs. It often discovers unsuspected deficits in specialized functions which should be taken into account in the global management of the child.

Psychiatric assessment is not routinely indicated in the great majority of epileptic patients. However, some forms of epilepsy, such as West and Lennox-Gastaut syndromes, may be associated with considerable dysfunction which will require special skill. Such may also be the case when the family is psychologically unable to face adequately the many problems raised by epilepsy. Investigation of the social problems associated with epilepsy is essential. Some families will require the evaluation and assistance of a social worker with regard to school problems, finances, transportation and housing arrangements. This may also lead to a better knowledge of the family attitudes, as well as conditions of living.

Treatment of the seizures

Control of the seizures is obviously a major aim of therapy. This objective, however important, does not justify attempts at obtaining control at any price. The drawbacks of persisting seizures may be less severe than those associated with drug toxicity, the more so as excessive dosages do not necessarily improve seizure control, and may have the opposite effect. Complete suppression of fits is obtainable in a majority of the childhood epilepsies. A significant proportion of these, moreover, tend to remit spontaneously before adulthood; another reason to avoid excessive drug treatments whose effects on a growing brain are far from fully understood.

Anti-epileptic drugs

Anti-epileptic drugs are the standard form of therapy today. The main available anticonvulsant drugs are listed in Table 11.3, which also indicates some of their pharmacokinetic properties.

Pharmacokinetics

For any anti-epileptic drug to act, it must be absorbed from the digestive tract (or a parenteral site) into the blood stream, then distributed throughout the body, especially to the brain. In the blood, drugs are variously bound to albumin. This bound fraction (Table 11.3) is in equilibrium with the unbound or free fraction, the latter being able to cross biological membranes and, therefore, to reach the brain receptors. The theory of drug action postulates that the anticonvulsant action of an anti-epileptic drug is determined by its concentration at the receptor sites. This concentration, in turn, is proportional to the plasma concentration (in fact the free fraction) provided the drug is not irreversibly bound to the receptors and is active itself rather than through active metabolites (Brodie & Hogben, 1957). The rationale for the determination of the blood levels of drugs, a practice that is central to clinical pharmacology, is that the probability of obtaining a given therapeutic effect from a certain plasma concentration is much greater than the probability of achieving a given plasma concentration from a given dose (Pippenger, 1980). A satisfactory correlation between plasma and brain concentrations has been shown for phenobarbitone, phenytoin, primidone, carbamazepine and its epoxide. The correlation is much less satisfactory for sodium valproate, which is found in the brain only at low concentration and the therapeutic effects of which are only roughly related to blood level. Diazepam, on the contrary, is immediately taken up and markedly concentrated in the brain, but is secondarily redistributed to other tissues, with possible loss of anticonvulsive effects. The time for blood and brain levels to equilibrate is usually from a few minutes to 30–45 minutes (Wilder & Bruni, 1981), an important consideration in the treatment of status epilepticus.

The blood levels of anticonvulsant drugs are dependent on a number of absorption, distribution and elimination variables (Pippenger, 1980). The sources of variation are both intrinsic and extraneous ones. Intrinsic sources include genetic factors (e.g. fast and slow metabolizers for

Table 11.3 Main pharmacokinetic data and usual dosages of major anticonvulsant drugs in infants and children

Drug	Time to peak serum level* (hours)	% Protein bound*	Half-life (hours)		'Therapeutic' range µg/ml (µmol/l)	Usual dosage/day
Phenobarbitone	2–8	50	Neonates Children Adults	> 100 30–70 50–120	10–30 (45–130)	3–5 mg/kg < 5 years 2–3 mg/kg > 5 years
Phenytoin	2–8	90	Neonates Children Adults	> 100 8–30 24–60	10–20 (40–80)	8–10 mg/kg < 2 years 4–6 mg/kg > 2 years
Carbamazepine	6–15	70–80		8–19† 20–40	5–12 (20–50) epoxide: 0.5–5.5 µg/ml	6–12 mg/kg‡ 15–20 mg/kg
Primidone	1–5	< 10		5–10	5–10§ (23–46)	15–25 mg/kg
Ethosuximide	2–7	0	Children Adults	30 60–100	40–100 (300–750)	25–30 mg/kg
Sodium valproate	1–3 (plain) 5–8 (enteric-coated)	90		8–15	50–100 (350–700)	20–30 mg/kg‡ 30–60 mg/kg
Clonazepam	1–3	80		20–50	0.025–0.075 (0.08–0.24)	0.1–0.2 mg/kg

* Average values in adults. In infants absorption is faster while protein binding is low.

† Upper line = values on chronic therapy. Lower line = values after single dose administration.

‡ Upper line = dosage on monotherapy. Lower line = dosage on chronic polytherapy.

§ Uncertain significance. Monitoring of phenobarbitone produced by metabolism is often used.

phenytoin), duration of administration with drugs that induce their own metabolism (e.g. carbamazepine) and, especially, *age*. In general, the variations of elimination (especially in metabolism) are more marked than those of absorption. Elimination rates, with prolonged half-lives, are very slow in neonates, then increase, often suddenly, after a few weeks so that the half-lives now become very short. Thereafter, the high rates tend to persist, although at a lower level throughout childhood, adult levels being reached fairly suddenly at some time during the pre-pubertal period (Morselli, 1977; Pippenger, 1980). This course explains the necessity for higher doses to obtain the same blood levels in young patients, as well as the difficulty in adjusting dosages in young infants and adolescents, with the double hazard of toxic effects or loss of control. Extraneous sources of variation are mainly represented by drug interactions. These are capable of modifying considerably the blood levels by enzyme induction or interference with excretion (Perucca & Richens, 1980). Thus, sodium valproate increases the levels of phenobarbitone by an average of 30%, carbamazepine and valproate can be used in much smaller dosages (respectively 10–15 and 20–25 mg/kg) as a monotherapy than when combined with other drugs (Johannessen, 1981) because their metabolism is not accelerated by induction. Therapeutic interaction can also increase the free (active) fraction of a drug without changing the total blood level which is the one that is measured routinely: this may occur with sodium valproate which displaces phenytoin from its binding sites so that its action is increased in spite of unchanged measured levels. This is one argument in favour of the determination of free levels which is, unfortunately, technically difficult.

Measurement of drugs in saliva or tears has been advocated as a substitute (Rylance & Morland, 1981). Thus, the concept of therapeutic range of anti-epileptic drugs is a complex one and should be interpreted intelligently (Vajda & Aicardi, 1983). The concept is that there is a range of blood levels below which control is infrequent and above which toxic effects are likely. In fact, the therapeutic range is too narrow and probably applies only to severe epilepsies. 'Infratherapeutic' levels are frequently effective, and 'supratherapeutic' levels are at times necessary for control. Furthermore, the significance of the range is even less clear with drugs, such as carbamazepine or valproate, whose blood levels show marked daily fluctuations. As a consequence, no change of therapy should ever be decided on to obtain 'therapeutic' levels if clinical control is satisfactory.

Table 11.4. Toxicity and main side-effects of the major anti-epileptic drugs

Drug	Severe toxicity	Side-effects	Comments
Phenobarbitone	Lyell syndrome (toxic epidermal necrosis)	**Hyperkinesis and alterations in sleep pattern**: rashes; drowsiness; rickets; folate deficiency; adverse effects on memory and learning?	Withdrawal may precipitate fits A potent enzymatic inducer
Phenytoin	Encephalopathy Pseudo-lymphoma and malignant lymphoma Lupus erythematosus Hepatic disease	**Acute cerebellovestibular dysfunction, diplopia, nystagmus** (dose-related); dyskinesia; neuropathy; **gum hypertrophy**; **rashes; hirsutism; acne**; coarse facial features; folate deficiency; rickets; IgA deficiency; hyperglycaemia; adverse effects on cognitive function?	Low therapeutic ratio Interference with other anti-epileptic drugs (VPA, PB, CBZ, etc.) Enzymatic inducer Overdosage can produce tonic fits
Carbamazepine	Aplastic anaemia Hepatic disease Lupus-like syndrome	**Diplopia; ataxia; dyskinesia; rashes; neutropenia**; eosinophilia; water intoxication; cardiac slowing	Should not be used with macrolide antibiotics and MAO inhibitors Enzymatic inducer
Sodium valproate	Hepatic disease Pancreatitis Stupor (in association with other drugs)	**Nausea and vomiting; weight gain** (esp. adolescent females); **tremor**; thrombocytopenia (dose-related); enuresis	Hyperammonaemia is frequent Transaminases at times slightly raised Interaction with PB and PHT

Ethosuximide	**Gastric distress: nausea; vomiting;** rashes; neutropenia; eosinophilia; drowsiness; psychotic syndrome?	Aplastic anaemia	
Trimethadione	Blurred vision in bright light; drowsiness; vertigo; neutropenia; eosinophilia	*Aplastic anaemia* *Nephrotic syndrome*	
Benzodiazepines	**Somnolence;** hypotonia; ataxia; **salivary and bronchial hypersecretion:** irritability and hyperkiresis (with clonazepam)	*Respiratory depression* (i.v. route) Bronchial hypersecretion in babies especially if brain damaged, and drooling bronchorrhoea and chest infections among older children	Not to be combined with phenobarbitone (i.v. route) May induce tonic status in certain forms of epilepsy Withdrawal may precipitate seizures
Primidone	**Drowsiness;** rashes; ataxia; anaemia	Stupor with over-dosage	Withdrawal may precipitate seizures Not to be associated with phenobarbitone
ACTH and steroids	**Cushingoid facies hypertension; fluid retention glycosuria; osteoporosis; disturbed behaviour**	*Infections*	

Serious toxicity is rare with any drug (with the exception of infections on steroids or ACTH). The less rare ones are in *italics*. The most common side-effects are in **bold**.

Side-effects of anticonvulsant drugs

Numerous unwanted effects of the anti-epileptic drugs have been described (Bruni & Wilder, 1979; Eadie, 1980; Reynolds, 1975; Schmidt, 1982; Oxley *et al.*, 1983) and are listed in Table 11.4. Some of them develop acutely, the commonest being drowsiness and ataxia which can be produced by most drugs. High levels of phenytoin may give rise to a vestibulo-cerebellar syndrome, often with diplopia, which is fully reversible on reducing dosage. Diplopia is also common with excess carbamazepine. Rashes are common and are usually regarded as an indication to discontinue the causative drug. Changes in blood counts may result from various mechanisms, including folate deficiency (Eadie, 1980). Rare idiosyncratic reactions, such as aplastic anaemia (often in relation to the diones and methoin) or hepatic disease (in particular with valproate), obviously indicate immediate discontinuation of therapy. More insidiously, developing side-effects may raise difficult diagnostic problems. The commonest ones are the aggressiveness and hyperkinesia induced by phenobarbitone, which severely limit its use in children, and the effects on skin and mucous membranes (gum hypertrophy, hypertrichosis, acne, coarsening of facial features) observed with phenytoin.

Immunological disturbances may occasionally occur. The diagnosis of lupus erythematosus and of lymphoma should never be accepted in treated epileptics without due consideration to an induced disorder. Effects of long-term treatment on bone (rickets), peripheral nerve function and endocrine functions may need special surveillance. Possible effects of anticonvulsant drugs on the development of cognitive functions are a major source of concern. Preliminary reports suggest that long-term treatment with phenytoin may be associated with a reduction in IQ and with memory problems (Trimble *et al.*, 1980). This indicates that it may well be better not to use phenytoin, and to limit as much as possible the duration and dosages of drugs of any type, since all long-term side-effects are certainly not known. In our present state of knowledge an order of preference can be established among the major anti-epileptic drugs with regard to side-effects. Carbamazepine and sodium valproate come first, followed by phenytoin, phenobarbitone, primidone and benzodiazepines. The diones and methoin are very little used nowadays.

Principles of drug therapy

A correct choice of drug, according to the type of seizure or, if possible, type of epileptic syndrome, is essential (see Table 11.2). Several drugs are often equally effective (e.g. carbamazepine, phenytoin, primidone, valproate in grand mal seizures) in a particular syndrome. The drug with the least toxicity (especially on long-term cognitive functions) and that is easiest to handle is then indicated.

A correct dosage is relatively easy to establish during periods of stable metabolism but is often very difficult to reach, necessitating frequent monitoring at critical ages, especially in early infancy. Most drugs should be started in small doses and slowly increased to improve the initial tolerance and avoid rejection by patients of effective drugs. Giving the drug in as few doses as possible improves compliance and avoids the embarrassment of taking pills at school. Two doses a day are almost always possible, even with drugs of short half-life such as carbamazepine and valproate. These may occasionally be given three times a day, to improve tolerance by diminishing the height of the peaks of concentration. With phenobarbitone, a single dose at bedtime is usually adequate.

The use of a single drug (monotherapy) is highly commendable, as it is simpler for the patient and excludes the risks of drug interactions. Considerable evidence (Reynolds & Shorvon, 1981; Richens, 1976) indicates that monotherapy is adequate for the majority of the common epilepsies (primary generalized epilepsy in adolescents, petit mal, benign partial epilepsy). The most severe forms are less likely to respond to a single drug but the evidence that they will do so with polytherapy is meagre. In any case, two drugs should never be used from the start. If the first drug in adequate amounts clearly fails, a second drug should be gradually added. Some physicians push the doses of the first drug up to the appearance of toxic signs (and 'supratherapeutic' blood levels) before resorting to a second drug. This may be permissible with the less toxic drugs, e.g. carbamazepine, but is probably best avoided except in the most severe cases.

If the patient responds to a two-drug regime, it is advisable to withdraw the first drug progressively, unless a clear recurrence of fits forces a resumption. In patients with epilepsies that are difficult to control, it is wise not to change the treatment, however illogical it may seem, if the response is adequate. Generally, associations of more than two drugs are not recommended and should be discouraged. There is evidence, though not complete, that reduction of polytherapy may not only increase the patients' alertness, but also reduce fit frequency (Reynolds & Shorvon, 1981; Viani *et al.*, 1977). When using an association of drugs, certain rules should be respected. (i) The dosage of each drug should be correct, taking into account the likely interactions such as that of valproate with phenobarbitone. Since interactions may make the total blood levels difficult to interpret, close clinical supervision is essential to detect toxicity. (ii) Associations of drugs that have similar toxicity or produce the same type of behavioural disturbances (e.g. clonazepam and phenobarbitone) are best avoided. (iii) The same applies to combinations such as primidone and phenobarbitone which are, at least in part, additions rather than associations, since primidone is largely metabolized to phenobarbitone.

Regular supervision of therapy is essential in a disorder that lasts for years, especially in childhood when the disease, the metabolism of drugs and the patient's reactions are constantly changing. Frequent reviews permit readjustment of therapy, encourage compliance and provide psychological support. EEG supervision is only occasionally needed, since there is no necessary parallelism between EEG changes and frequency of fits, and since drugs can modify the records (e.g. carbamazepine may produce marked slowing). Clinical supervision is normally on an outpatient basis, unless a rapid change in treatment is contemplated or a marked increase in seizure frequency or signs of toxicity occur. Blood counts, urine examination, tests of hepatic function are usually recommended with certain drugs (ethosuximide, carbamazepine, diones, methoin, sodium valproate): there is no evidence that such tests are of any value in preventing severe toxicity, while the mildly abnormal results they may give are responsible for many an unwise interruption of therapy.

Monitoring of the blood levels of drugs has become an important part of management, and is indeed very useful if determinations are correctly indicated and interpreted. Blood level measurements have well-defined indications. (i) When the patient's compliance is in doubt: this may be difficult to evaluate, since one or two tablets of a short half-life drug before the visit may produce significant blood levels; conversely, low blood levels may result from metabolic induction with normal doses. (ii) When control is not obtained with an apparently correct dose or when previously established control is lost: this may result from an insufficient dose or an abnormal metabolism, and may require a change of dosage. (iii) When unwanted or toxic effects are suspected, especially in infants, in whom they are difficult to diagnose. (iv) When polytherapy is used, even though the results may be difficult to evaluate due to drug interactions. (v) When other diseases or treatments known to interfere with the metabolism of anticonvulsants are present. (vi) When drugs of unpredictable metabolism, especially phenytoin, are employed. (vii) Some advocate a systematic determination at initiation of treatment (after a steady state has probably been reached). On the other hand, blood level determinations of valproate or carbamazepine are of uncertain value as the levels fluctuate widely and may not be well-correlated with the therapeutic effect (Vajda & Aicardi, 1983).

The timing of sampling for blood levels is important. Samples should not be obtained before steady state is obtained (3 weeks after starting treatment) depending on the half-life of the drug used. Daily fluctuations need to be taken into account when valproate or carbamazepine are used. The optimal sampling time is then before the first dose, corresponding to trough level, if seizure control is not obtained, or at the time of probable maximum level if toxicity is suspected (Johannessen, 1981; Vajda & Aicardi, 1983). Repetitive tests are unnecessary when the epilepsy is under control, when compliance seems reasonably good, in the absence of intercurrent disorders and during periods of metabolic stability. In contrast, frequent determinations are mandatory in certain circumstances: when a loading dose is used, when dosages outside the usual range are given, or in infants immediately following the neonatal period.

Termination of drug therapy when indicated (see below) should be gradual, especially when phenobarbitone, clonazepam and, to a lesser extent, carbamazepine are being used. Reduction rates of the order of 0.01 g every month with phenobarbitone, 0.05 g per 2 weeks with carbamazepine, and 0.1 mg per week with clonazepam, are generally acceptable.

Non-drug treatments
These are used only in highly selected, intractable cases.

The ketogenic diet

It has long been suggested that ketosis and acidosis produced by a special diet may help to control seizures. Several variants of the ketogenic diet are now available.

The classical 4:1 diet provides about 75 cal/kg, 80% of which is fat, and 1 g/kg of protein. It should be strictly enforced and since it is un-palatable and rigid the parents need to be intelligent and well-motivated to ensure success. Ketosis should be controlled twice daily by urine testing and always be positive.

The medium chain triglycerides (MCT) diet is simpler and more flexible as it can be worked on an exchange system, similar to that used in diabetic patients (Berman, 1978). In the usual MCT diet 60% of the calories are provided as MCT oil, 11% as saturated fat contained in other foods, 10% are from protein and 19% from carbohydrates. A recent variant is the 'John Radcliffe diet' (Schwartz *et al.*, 1983) in which 30% of the calories, instead of 60%, are given as MCT oil, the remaining 30% as double cream.

The ketogenic diets are especially advocated in myoclonic epilepsies or the Lennox syndrome, as a last resort treatment due to the practical difficulties involved. Satisfactory results have been reported in 30–40% of the patients treated (Berman, 1978; Bower, 1980; O'Donohoe, 1985).

The relative merits of the diets are still uncertain although good results have been obtained with the MCT diet. Diarrhoea, vomiting, steatorrhoea and failure to thrive may complicate the use of the diet. The help of a skilled and dedicated dietitian is mandatory, and initial hospitalization and frequent controls are required.

Neurosurgical therapy

The aim of surgical treatment of the epilepsies is to suppress the area of origin of partial seizures or to interrupt the propagation of epileptic discharges. Removal of an epileptogenic area has been the most widely used technique (either by *en bloc* temporal lobectomy or by cortical resection after depth electrode location of the focus) (Purpura *et al.*, 1975; Talairach *et al.*, 1974; Ward, 1983). Amygdalotomy, division of the corpus callosum or other similar techniques are still in the experimental stage, as is electrical cerebellar stimulation (Wada, 1980; Ward, 1983).

Surgical treatment is reserved for partial epilepsies with a single or a clearly preponderant focus in patients refractory for 4–5 years to correct medical therapy and over 10 years of age. Surgery must be preceded by complete investigation and performed in a specialized centre.

General management

Patients with seizure disorders need not be treated entirely in hospital centres, even though their initial referral and subsequent visits to such centres are highly desirable. Whenever several physicians are in charge of the same patient, close co-operation is essential as unco-ordinated changes in therapy are extremely damaging psychologically and prevent any organization and control of therapy.

Management after a single seizure

Single seizures of grand mal or partial types may remain isolated in an unknown but significant proportion of patients. The decision to start on long-term treatment that will also 'confirm' the unproven diagnosis of epilepsy, is therefore better deferred until a second seizure supervenes. The decision, however, is a highly individual one and should take into account the desires (and fears) of the patient and his family, the possible risks of a seizure, the availability of prompt medical care, etc. Untreated patients should remain in close contact with their doctor or hospital.

Management of established epilepsy

In this case, drug treatment is advisable, except in cases in which avoidable triggers are regularly present (e.g. television epilepsy in which simple measures may be sufficient) (Jeavons & Harding, 1975). The need for uninterrupted and prolonged treatment should be clearly explained to the parents and child. Difficulties in obtaining control vary tremendously, from the benign cases in which minimal treatment is enough to the intractable ones that may defy any form of drug or other treatment. In these difficult patients, one must refrain from 'pushing' therapy up to unacceptable levels detrimental to the child's behaviour and learning.

Duration and discontinuation of therapy

Treatment is continued as long as seizures are occurring. How much time without seizures should elapse before withdrawal of drugs is contemplated is an unsolved question. If the epilepsy is part of a recognized syndrome with a fairly predictable outcome a decision can be made, knowing the usual course of the syndrome. Thus, in benign partial epilepsy, therapy can be stopped within 18 months of the last fit if the patient is over 7–8 years of age; in pure petit mal, 2 years without absences is probably sufficient. In contrast, severe epilepsies like the Lennox-Gastaut syndrome necessitate over 5 years of freedom from seizures.

If the epilepsy is not a part of a definable syndrome, the decision to discontinue therapy is more arbitrary, 2–5 years after the last fit being a 'safe' delay according to various authors (Annegers *et al.*, 1979; Gordon, 1982; Holowach *et al.*, 1972). There is some evidence (Emerson *et al.*, 1981; Rowan *et al.*, 1980) that features such as an onset after the age of 3 years, the absence of a cerebral lesion as a cause, normal mental and neurological functions and, possibly, the absence of EEG abnormalities, are associated with a low recurrence rate (less than 10−20%). In such cases, a 2-year duration is probably reasonable. The lack of these features, possibly the occurrence of a large number of major seizures, and certain types of seizures, would indicate a higher recurrence rate and more prolonged treatment (Emerson *et al.*, 1981; Holowach *et al.*, 1972).

The risk of stopping therapy should be explained and discussed, at times with some degree of persuasion. It seems highly desirable to stop treatment in adolescents before they leave school, as this removes the label of epilepsy, helps to restrict professional limitations and prevents interference with obtaining a driving licence. Stopping therapy is best done at a time when the patient is unlikely to be exposed to exceptional stresses, and should always be done gradually over a period of a few months. The possibility that one or two seizures occur as a result of drug withdrawal is hard to prove, but is accepted by experienced neurologists. If the epilepsy is not too severe and if the psychological effect of a late recurrence can be accepted, such seizures may not necessitate resuming treatment.

Management of social and educational aspects

Psychological aspects

The impact of a diagnosis of epilepsy on the family and the child is enormous so that appropriate information about the disease in general and the child in particular must be offered. Several interviews are necessary since the shock brought about by the diagnosis makes rational understanding difficult. From the first interview, however, it is essential that parents understand the necessity for regular and prolonged treatment but also that it is not a life-long one. Possible side-effects of therapy should be discussed to facilitate the difficult period of initiation of treatment. Thereafter, it will be necessary to explain the nature and cause of the disorder and its foreseeable course in an effort to repel the fears associated with seizures and the prejudices attached to the 'disease'. This should be done in an objective way but with emphasis on the positive aspects of each particular situation. Care should be taken to use terms appropriate not only to the socio-cultural background, but also to the emotionally disturbed state induced by the situation. It is important to avoid delivering messages that can be regarded as ambiguous by the family, like indicating a benign prognosis while requesting a large number of sophisticated and impressive examinations.

Personal restrictions should be limited to a reasonable minimum. Parents ought to be reassured that normal methods of discipline are in no way provocative. Common sense will indicate that some seizures, e.g. exclusively nocturnal or regularly provoked by specific stimuli, do not require any restriction, while completely unpredictable ones may be quite dangerous, even if rare and brief. Restrictions should also be adjusted to the personality of the patient as well as to practical ways of life, and some flexibility is imperative. Most sporting activities can be allowed, except in very severe cases, including swimming with proper supervision, or skiing. Rock climbing, wall bars and high diving are obviously contraindicated. Cycling with friends on quiet roads is permissible. Motor cycles are unsafe for anyone and should not be allowed before full seizure control is achieved. It should be recalled that apparently peaceful occupations may be dangerous to epileptic patients, e.g. practical cooking and, especially, unsupervised baths and showers if the risk of burns from hot water is not eliminated by a safe device. The slight increase of risk which results from a liberal policy is more than compensated for by the avoidance of segregation and over-protection, as well as by the increased responsibility of the patient. The latter should be encouraged also by favouring self-administration of drugs, under reasonable control. Special compartment boxes containing the tablets for a week are very useful in this regard. In the case of uncontrollable seizures, especially with falls, physical protection of the child is the first aim. Protective headgear is a necessity even though no model is ideal, especially as far as chin protection is concerned.

Education and schooling

The vast majority of children with uncomplicated epilepsy should and do attend ordinary schools. Special schools are useful only for a small minority of children with intractable epilepsies. Such patients can benefit from a multiprofessional approach to their care and education as available in these schools. School problems, however, are more common among children with convulsive disorders than in the general population (Holdsworth & Whitmore, 1974), even though intellectual normality is the rule (Rutter *et al.*, 1970). Learning problems and educational under-achievement are relatively common in epileptic children, and may be related to attentional deficits as well as to specific difficulties with language and abstract thinking (Stores & Hart, 1976). Behaviour problems are also common. However, both learning difficulties in children with epilepsy, and conduct disorders, are not essentially different from those in non-epileptics, so that the same remedial help within the normal school system as used for other children is adequate. Every effort should be made to avoid drugs that disturb behaviour, such as phenobarbitone, or the effects of which on the memory and learning processes may be detrimental, such as phenytoin.

The choice of a career should be discussed with the patients. It would be disastrous to prevent adolescents from choosing a specific career when they have benign, self-remitting epilepsies (with the exception of those requiring a public service or vehicle driving licence, which are specifically prohibited). In cases less certain to remit before adulthood, the patients should be advised to avoid careers involving the use of dangerous devices or depending on obtaining a driving licence.

General rules of life and other problems

Although a normal style of life is strongly advised, certain rules should be followed, with reasonable flexibility. Sleep deprivation and alcohol use in adolescents, long watching sessions at the television set in children are to be discouraged, as well as exposure to any other recognized precipitant. These problems are particularly difficult with adolescents who resent the differences manifested by prohibitions and the need for taking drugs, so that some allowance should be made for an occasional intemperance provided the main lines of treatment are accepted and followed. The question of a possible interference by anti-epileptic drugs with hormonal contraception, with resultant failure, is now a frequent problem. Anti-convulsants increase only very slightly the risk of failure of oral contra-ception even though the risks of accelerated metabolism through enzymic induction is theoretically well-established (Perucca & Richens, 1980; Schmidt, 1981). Mechanical devices are not generally advised in this age group, so that the use of normal dosage 'pills' and, whenever possible, of non-inducing anti-epileptic drugs (e.g. valproate, benzodiazepines) is probably preferable.

Management during intercurrent illnesses and vaccinations

Families should be instructed not to interrupt drug therapy during common illnesses or when surgical operations have to be carried out. If oral intake is not permitted for a relatively long period, oral treatment should be replaced by the same (or a similar) amount of parenteral drugs. For a brief period, a load of a long half-life drug may suffice. Physicians should be aware of the possible interference of some antibiotic drugs (macrolides, e.g. erythromycin, spiramycin; chloramphenicol) on the metabolism of anticonvulsants, and of the occasional diminution of efficacy of certain drugs as a result of anti-epileptic treatment (antibiotics, steroids, digoxin, etc.). Although these effects are usually insignificant, they need be considered when anomalous responses occur (Perucca & Richens, 1980).

Most vaccines can be given to infants with epilepsy with the exception of whooping cough immunization. When fever is expected (e.g. measles vaccine) anticonvulsant prophylaxis may be indicated if there seems to be a risk of precipitating fits.

Special problems

Status epilepticus

Any seizure that lasts, or repeats without recovery of consciousness, for more than 30 minutes is currently termed status epilepticus. Although there are as many types of status as of epileptic seizures (Gastaut, 1982), the most serious problem is posed by major convulsive status, with a mortality rate of 6–12% and the possibility of sequelae (Aicardi & Chevrie, 1982). Any convulsive status (i.e. tonic-clonic, partial or unilateral clonic, tonic) should be investigated in search of an acute treatable cause, since 26% of cases among children are symptomatic of an acute brain insult or of metabolic disorders (Aicardi & Chevrie, 1970). Lumbar puncture is mandatory with fever. Magnesium, calcium, glucose and electrolyte levels should be obtained, and other examinations (e.g. CT scan) are done according to clinical indications. Treatment requires hospitalization.

Aetiological treatment is clearly necessary when feasible, but does not obviate the need for anticonvulsant treatment in most cases.

Symptomatic treatment includes the immediate application of vital measures: adequate oxygenation of brain and adequate cardio-respiratory function (intubation is usually necessary); stabilization or correction of lactic acidosis, dehydration and other metabolic inbalances; detection and correction of any visceral complication. An intravenous (i.v.) line is required both to provide fluids and to obtain blood samples for vital constants and blood levels of anticonvulsants. Rapid termination of seizure activity should be obtained, using a drug whose blood level is readily built up and which crosses readily the blood–brain barrier.

Diazepam (occasionally clonazepam) by i.v. route enters the brain within 10 seconds and promptly stops seizures in nearly 90% of cases (Browne & Penry, 1973). Dosage is 0.2–0.5 mg/kg by slow (2 mg/minute) 'push' injection while monitoring respiration and with resuscitation material available (mainly if phenobarbitone has been previously administered). As an initial measure, intrarectal diazepam (0.3–0.5 up to 1.0 mg/kg of the injectable solution) can be administered, e.g. at home or pending the establishment of an i.v. line. Diazepam may be sufficient to stop an episode of status. Recurrence is, however, frequent after 15–20 minutes, due to rapid redistribution of the drug out of the intravascular space (Wilder & Bruni, 1981). A continuous i.v. drip of diazepam (Treiman & Delgado-Escueta, 1980) or the experimental diazepine lorazepam (Walker *et al.*, 1979) may prevent recurrence. However, most workers now favour the use of a long-lasting agent, following the immediate use of diazepam, or at least if two successive administrations fail.

Phenytoin is the drug of choice and is used as a loading dose of 15 mg/kg which produces blood and brain levels of over 16 µg/ml by the end of a 45–60 minute infusion, with a success rate of 80% (Wilder *et al.*, 1977). Some authors advocate loading doses of 18–25 mg/kg to obtain blood levels of 25 µg/ml (Treiman & Delgado-Escueta, 1980). With these large doses blood levels remain 'therapeutic' for 12–24 hours. The total loading dose may also be divided into two injections an hour apart or more widely spaced (Albani, 1977). Phenytoin should be given at a rate no greater than 80 mg/minute in saline, not glucose, solutions. Cardiovascular effects are usually slight in children.

Phenobarbitone is also very effective and some physicians prefer it to phenytoin in neonates, especially if diazepam has not been used. The depression of consciousness by the large doses employed is a drawback. In large doses phenobarbitone seems to rapidly penetrate the CNS. The initial dose is 10–15 mg/kg given at a rate of 100 mg/minute (Ramsay *et al.*, 1979). In patients refractory to phenytoin, it can be given immediately following a full loading dose of phenytoin without potentiating CNS depression.

Paraldehyde is still considered a very useful drug by some, especially outside hospital. It can be given intramuscularly at 0.15 mg/kg or intravenously as a 2% solution, 0.1–0.2 ml/kg. Additional doses of 0.1 mg/kg can be given as necessary at 2–4 hour intervals (Browne, 1983). Due to its local and general reactions diazepam is now preferred.

Lignocaine is used by some (Perucca & Richens, 1980; Wilder &

Bruni, 1981) in refractory status at a rate of 4 mg/kg/hour, continued for several days.

Chlormethiazole (heminevrin) in a 0.8% solution administered as a slow drip may be useful (Harvey *et al.*, 1975), but has a marked depressive action.

Whenever possible, EEG monitoring is advisable as subtle convulsive activity can easily go unrecognized. Further reference to the management of status will be made in Book II.

Neonatal seizures
Seizures occurring during the first 28 days of life may be difficult to recognize as they may present only with ocular phenomena, apnoea, and vasomotor disturbances (subtle seizures). They are most often the presenting manifestation of serious neurological disturbances since the common metabolic disturbances are now much rarer, except for hypoglycaemia in the first 48 hours of life among dysmature babies, and hypocalcaemia at 5−7 days of life. Uncommon metabolic conditions still exist and their diagnosis is important since some of them can be effectively treated. Therefore, blood glucose, calcium, magnesium and electrolytes should be routinely measured. In resistant cases of unknown cause, an intravenous injection of 50 mg of pyridoxine should be given. Lumbar puncture is essential since infection is the most common treatable cause. Neonatal seizures, though occurring in isolation, tend to be repeated over a few days (Volpe, 1981) so that an immediately effective treatment schedule, adapted to the special metabolism of anti-epileptic drugs at this age, is imperative. Once an adequate airway and an intravenous line have been established, 3−5 ml/kg of 25% glucose is given to treat any hypoglycaemia, after blood has been drawn for chemical determinations. Calcium gluconate (5 mg/kg in 5% solution) and magnesium sulphate (20−50 mg/kg in 2% solution) are given if necessary.

Anti-epileptic drugs are used when no obvious metabolic disturbance is present. *Diazepam* (0.08 mg/kg up to 2.7 mg/kg) is frequently used (Lombroso, 1978, 1983) but is a short-acting drug and may produce apnoea. If the clinical profile makes repeated seizures likely or if fits are persistent, the parenteral administration of long-lasting drugs is recommended. *Phenobarbitone* is generally the first choice, *phenytoin* being used when phenobarbitone is ineffective. Both drugs are best given as *loading doses* since conventional schedules produce low blood levels initially, followed, on days 4−5, by excessive levels with possible toxicity, as a result of the very long half-life of anti-epileptic drugs in neonates

(Lockman *et al.*, 1979; Painter *et al.*, 1981) Loading doses of 15–20 mg/kg (with either drug) will give effective blood levels that can be maintained by giving 2.5–4.0 mg/kg day over the next few days (intravenously if phenytoin is used). Blood levels should be regularly monitored as toxicity is difficult to assess and since rapid changes in concentration may occur. Treatment need not usually be maintained for more than 1 month, although no agreement has been reached on this point (Volpe, 1981). Other drugs (valproate, carbamazepine, primidone) have been used only occasionally in this age range.

Febrile convulsions
Febrile convulsions are defined as epileptic seizures, which occur mainly between 5 months and 5 years of age, with fever not due to intracranial infection or disorder. Their course is usually benign: the risk of a febrile recurrence is 30–40% and that of chronic residual epilepsy about 5% (increased to up to 10% when the initial seizure is long, unilateral, repeated, or supervenes in a previously neurologically abnormal infant) (Nelson & Ellenberg, 1978). The risk of brain damage, incurred as a result of a long-lasting febrile seizure, is small although somewhat controversial (Aicardi, 1980).

The single most important investigation in the acute stage is CSF examination, which is imperative in infants under 6 months and widely indicated below 18 months of age. Lumbar puncture is also compulsory in patients of whatever age with meningeal signs and in those who do not rapidly recover following the fit (Aicardi, 1980; Nealis, 1981). Other investigations, except those needed to establish the cause of the fever, are of little help, as is the EEG (Aicardi, 1980). Prolonged febrile convulsions must be terminated rapidly as they can produce brain damage, and this is best achieved with intravenous *diazepam* (see status).

Prophylactic treatment with anticonvulsants should certainly be discussed with parents after a prolonged focal fit or recurrence of febrile fits. It may be used to try and prevent recurrences of febrile convulsions. It has been shown that this objective is attainable in part by continuous prophylaxis with *phenobarbitone* (4 mg/kg to obtain a blood level of over 15 μg/ml) (Wolf *et al.*, 1977) or with *sodium valproate* (20–30 mg/kg/day) (Ngwane & Bower, 1980). Behavioural side-effects are common with phenobarbitone (up to 20–40% of the patients), although there is no evidence that cognitive development is impaired (Wolf *et al.*, 1981). Valproate is better tolerated but the risk of severe hepatic disease must be better evaluated before the drug is given to such a large population.

Other drugs (primidone, phenytoin, carbamazepine) are either ineffective or have not been properly tested. Intermittent prophylaxis is largely ineffective. Some studies (Knudsen & Vestermark, 1978) indicate that diazepam might protect against seizures if given early enough after onset of fever. At present, most workers favour continuous prophylaxis after the first fit only for selected patients: those under 13 months of age, those with focal and/or prolonged seizures, those with CNS abnormality prior to or at the time of the first seizure, and possibly those with a strong family history of epilepsy (Nelson & Ellenberg, 1981). Such a regime may not prevent acquired brain damage since (i) long-lasting seizures are the first ones in 75% of the cases, and (ii) it may supervene at any time and in any child with febrile convulsions. Brain damage, however, could probably be avoided by having an effective emergency treatment for prolonged seizures quickly available. Intrarectal diazepam using the intravenous preparation (0.5 mg/kg) seems suitable for that purpose as it can be easily administered without delay by a doctor, nurse or by the parents themselves if they are reliable enough. Intrarectal preparations are available in some countries in a convenient form (Knudsen, 1979) and respiratory depression has not been reported, so far, following rectal instillation. This method of management is becoming increasingly acceptable for selected families, as it does avoid the many problems of long-term prophylactic treatment.

There is no evidence that prophylactic treatment prevents the occurrence of later epilepsy.

Infantile spasms
Infantile spasms (West's syndrome) are a resistant form of seizures. ACTH and/or adrenal steroids are effective in controlling the spasms and suppressing EEG abnormalities in 40−70% of the patients (Jeavons et al., 1973). The recurrence rate is high, however, and the effects on the long-term mental and neurological development of affected infants are still controversial (Lacy & Penry, 1976). There is no agreement as to the relative potency of ACTH and steroids. The difference, if any, is certainly small (Hrachovy et al., 1983). Suggested dosages commonly range from 20 to 40 IU of ACTH (or 0.25−10 mg of tetracosactide) and from 3 to 20 mg/kg of hydrocortisone (2.0 mg/kg of prednisone, 0.3 mg/kg of dexamethasone). Recommended lengths of treatment vary from 3 weeks to several months (Aicardi, 1980; Lacy & Penry, 1976). Due to the marked side-effects, we prefer brief treatment durations (4 weeks) and use hydrocortisone 15 mg/kg/day, thus avoiding injections and facilitating

treatment outside the hospital, which helps to limit infections.

The prognosis depends heavily on the cause of the syndrome (a normal mental development can be expected in up to 40% of the crypto-genic cases whilst it is essentially nil in symptomatic ones), on the age of onset, association of other seizure types, etc. It may also be related in part to the delay of therapy in the cryptogenic cases (Chevrie & Aicardi, 1971; Lombroso, 1983).

Non-hormonal treatment with the benzodiazepine drugs (nitrazepam, 0.6—1.0 mg/kg/day; clonazepam, 0.1—0.3 mg/kg/day; and more recently, clobazam, 0.5—1.5 mg/kg/day) may be effective against the seizures, but the effects on mental development have not been assessed. Sodium valproate (30—60 mg/kg/day) also seems to be effective on the seizures in some of the children (Pavone *et al.*, 1981), but further evaluation is needed. The ketogenic diet has also been recommended (Huttenlocher *et al.*, 1971). At this moment we prefer to use hormonal treatment in all cryptogenic or dubious cases, and we reserve other drugs for symptomatic cases and for failures of hormonal therapy. ACTH or steroids are also occasionally used in other epileptic syndromes, mainly the Lennox-Gastaut syndrome (Aicardi, 1980). We believe that they should be employed only for brief periods, to tide the patient over a particularly difficult episode, and not on a long-term basis.

Intractable epilepsy
Even with the best drug therapy, a significant proportion of the epilepsies of childhood remain uncontrolled, especially those cases associated with mental retardation and/or neurological abnormalities. Before the refrac-tory character of an epilepsy is accepted, a complete reassessment of the patient is mandatory. Particular attention should be directed to the possibility of a progressive neurological disorder, especially a brain tumour or metabolic disease, to the possible inadequacy of drug therapy (e.g. non-compliance, improper drug or combination of drugs for the particular seizure disorder, drug interactions that influence not only total, but at times only free plasma levels) and to the role played in some patients by physical or emotional stresses, excessive fatigue, etc. In rare patients, the difficulties with control may stem, paradoxically, from excess drug therapy (Johannessen, 1981). In such difficult cases, hospitalization may be indicated for intensive EEG and drug monitoring, and/or for withdrawal of excess drugs in selected patients, as this may improve not only alertness but also certain types of seizures (Viani *et al.*, 1977).

In any intractable case it should be remembered that dosage escalation and drug multiplication are seldom, if ever, the solution to the patient's problem. Sleepiness, drooling, ataxia are the usual results, whilst seizure frequency is rarely decreased significantly. Many patients are better off when excessive treatments are diminished or even discontinued, especially if their seizures are of relatively limited consequence (i.e. without falls and injury).

Conclusion

In spite of recent advances, anti-epileptic therapy remains far from satisfactory, as it is still largely based on empiricism. Most therapeutic rules are more the reflection of habits or personal prejudices than a result of scientific evidence. For example, we still do not know with any certainty whether two (or more) drugs are better than one, when therapy should be started or discontinued or which patients will benefit from surgery. Our criteria for evaluating anti-epileptic drugs were quite inadequate in the past and are still imperfect. Most trials performed have suffered many drawbacks: insufficient number of patients, too short duration of the trials, imprecise classification of the patients, polytherapy, use of inadequate controls or complete lack of them. The same criticism can apply to recent techniques, such as blood level monitoring, whose global impact upon anti-epileptic therapy has not been assessed, even though it has contributed enormously to a better understanding of drug treatment and is undoubtedly useful in selected cases (Vajda & Aicardi, 1983).

Standardized methods of evaluation are indeed very difficult to apply in a collection of heterogeneous disorders such as epilepsy. Therefore, clinical judgement and common sense remain essential tools in the treatment of epileptic patients and cannot be replaced by sophisticated laboratory techniques, however useful these may be when intelligently used.

References

Aicardi, J. (1980) Seizures and epilepsy in children under two years of age. In *The Treatment of Epilepsy* (ed. J.H. Tyrer), pp. 203–250. MTP Press, Lancaster.

Aicardi, J. (1982) Childhood epilepsies with brief myoclonic atonic or tonic seizures. In *A Textbook of Epilepsy* (eds J. Laidlaw and A. Richens), 2nd edn. pp. 88–96. Churchill Livingstone, Edinburgh.

Aicardi, J. (1985) Myodonic epilepsies of infancy and childhood. In *Myoclonus* (eds S. Fahn, C.D. Marsden & M. Van Woert). Raven Press, New York.

Aicardi, J. & Chevrie, J.J. (1970) Status epilepticus in infants and children. A study of 239 cases. *Epilepsia*, **11**, 187–197.

Aicardi, J. & Chevrie, J.J. (1983) Consequences of status epilepticus in infants and children. In *Status Epilepticus: Mechanisms of Brain Damage and Treatment* (eds A.V. Delgado-Escueta, C.G. Wasterlain, D.M. Treiman and R.J. Porter) pp. 115–125. Raven Press, New York.

Albani, M. (1977) An effective dose schedule for phenytoin treatment of status epilepticus in infancy and childhood. *Neuropädiatrie*, **8**, 286–292.

Annegers, J.F., Hauser, W.A. & Elveback, L.R. (1979) Remission of seizures and relapse in patient with epilepsy. *Epilepsia*, **20**, 729–737.

Berman, W. (1978) Medium-chain tryglyceride diet in the treatment of intractable childhood epilepsy. *Developmental Medicine and Child Neurology*, **20**, 249–250.

Bower, B.D. (1980) Epilepsy in childhood and adolescence. In *The Treatment of Epilepsy* (ed. J.H. Tyrer) pp. 251–273. MTP Press, Lancaster.

Brodie, B.B. & Hogben, C.A.M. (1957) Some physicochemical factors in drug action. *Journal of Pharmacy and Pharmacology*, **9**, 345–380.

Browne, T.R. (1983) Paraldehyde, chlormethiazole, and lignocaine for treatment of status epilepticus. In *Status Epilepticus: Mechanisms of Brain Damage and Treatment* (eds A.V. Delgado-Escueta, C.G. Wasterlain, D.M. Treiman and R.J. Porter), pp. 509–517. Raven Press, New York.

Browne, T.R. & Penry, J.K. (1973) Benzodiazepines in the treatment of epilepsy: a review. *Epilepsia*, **14**, 277–310.

Bruni, J. & Wilder, B.J. (1979) The toxicology of antiepileptic drugs. In *Handbook of Clinical Neurology* (eds P.J. Vinken and G.W. Bruyn), Vol. 37, Part 2, pp. 199–222. North-Holland, Amsterdam.

Cavazzuti, G.B., Cappela, L. & Nalin, A. (1980) Longitudinal study of epileptiform EEG patterns in normal children. *Epilepsia*, **21**, 43–55.

Chevrie, J.J. & Aicardi, J. (1971) Le pronostic psychique des spasmes infantiles traités par l'ACTH ou les corticoïdes. Analyse statistique de 78 cas suivis plus d'un an. *Journal of Neurological Sciences*, **12**, 351–357.

Commission on Classification and Terminology of the International League Against Epilepsy (1981) Proposal for revised clinical and electroencephalographic classification of epileptic seizures. *Epilepsia*, **22**, 489–501.

Eadie, M.J. (1980) Unwanted effects of anticonvulsant drugs. In *The Treatment of Epilepsy* (ed. J.H. Tyrer), pp. 129–160. MTP Press, Lancaster.

Emerson, R., D'Souza, B.J., Holden, K.R., Mellits, E.D. & Freeman, J.M. (1981) Stopping medication in children with epilepsy. Predictors of outcome. *New England Journal of Medicine*, **304**, 1125–1129.

Gastaut, H. (1970) Clinical and electroencephalographic classification of epileptic seizures. *Epilepsia*, **11**, 102–113.

Gastaut, H. (1982) Classification of status epilepticus. In *Status Epilepticus: Mechanisms of Brain Damage and Treatment* (eds A.V. Delgado-Escueta, C.G. Wasterlain, D.M. Treiman and R.J. Porter) pp. 15–35. Raven Press, New York.

Gordon, N. (1982) Duration of treatment for childhood epilepsy. *Developmental Medicine and Child Neurology*, **24**, 84–88.

Harvey, P.K.P., Higgenbottam, T.W. & Loh, L. (1975) Chlormethiazole in treatment of status epilepticus. *British Medical Journal*, **ii**, 603–605.

Holdsworth, L. & Whitmore, K. (1974) A study of children with epilepsy attending normal schools. I. Their seizure patterns, progress and behaviour in school. *Developmental Medicine and Child Neurology*, **16**, 746–758.

Holowach, J., Thurston, D.L. & O'Leary, J. (1972) Prognosis in childhood epilepsy. *New England Journal of Medicine*, **286**, 169–174.

Huttenlocher, P.R., Wilbourn, A.J. & Sigmore, J.M. (1971) Medium chain triglycerides as a therapy for childhood epilepsy. *Neurology*, **21**, 1097–1103.

Hrachovy, R.A., Frost, J.D.. Kellaway, P. & Zion, T.E. (1983) Double-blind study of ACTH vs prednisone therapy in infantile spasms. *Journal of Pediatrics*, **103**, 641–645.

Jeavons, P.M. & Harding, G.F.A. (1975) *Photosensitive Epilepsy*. Clinics in Developmental Medicine, **56**, S.I.M.P., Heinemann, London.

Jeavons, P.M., Bower, B.D. & Dimitrakoudi, M. (1973) Long-term prognosis of 150 cases of 'West syndrome'. *Epilepsia*, **14**, 153–164.

Johannessen, S.I. (1981) Antiepileptic drugs: pharmacokinetic and clinical aspects. *Therapeutic Drug Monitoring*, **3**, 17–37.

Knudsen, F.U. (1979) Rectal administration of diazepam in solution in the acute treatment of convulsions in infants and children. *Archives of Disease in Childhood*, **54**, 855–857.

Knudsen, F.U. & Vestermark, S. (1978) Prophylactic diazepam or phenobarbitone in febrile convulsions: a prospective controlled study. *Archives of Disease in Childhood*, **53**, 660–663.

Lacy, J.R. & Penry, J.K. (1976) *Infantile Spasms*. Raven Press, New York.

Lockman, L.A., Kriel, R., Saske, D., Thompson, T. & Virnig, R. (1979) Phenobarbital dosage for control of neonatal seizures. *Neurology*, **29**, 1445–1449.

Lombroso, C.T. (1983) Differentiation of seizures in newborns and early infancy. In *Antiepileptic Drug Therapy in Childhood* (eds P.L. Morselli, C.E. Pippenger and J.K. Penry), 85–102. Raven Press, New York.

Morselli, P.L. (1977) Antiepileptic drugs. In *Drug Disposition during Development* (ed. P.L. Morselli), pp. 311–360. Spectrum, New York.

Nealis, J.G.T. (1981) Management of febrile seizures by pediatricians in the United States. In *Febrile Seizures* (eds K.B. Nelson and J.H. Ellenberg), pp. 81–86. Raven Press, New York.

Nelson, K.B. & Ellenberg, J.H. (1978) Prognosis in children with febrile seizures. *Pediatrics*, **61**, 720–727.

Nelson, K.B. & Ellenberg, J.H. (eds) (1981) *Febrile Seizures*. Raven Press, New York.

Ngwane, E. & Bower B. (1980) Continuous sodium valproate or phenobarbitone in the prevention of 'simple' febrile convulsions. Comparison by a double-blind trial. *Archives of Disease in Childhood*, **55**, 171–174.

O'Donohoe, N.V. (1985) *Epilepsies of Childhood*. 2nd edn., Butterworths, London.

Oxley, J., Janz, D. & Meinardi, H. (eds) (1983) *Chronic toxicity of anti-epileptic drugs*. Raven Press, New York.

Painter, M.J., Pippenger, C., Wasterlain, C., Barmada, M., Pitlick, W., Carter, G. & Abern, S. (1981) Phenobarbital and phenytoin in neonatal seizures. Metabolism and tissue distribution. *Neurology*, **31**, 1107–1112.

Pavone, L., Incorpora, G., La Rosa, M., Li Volti, S. & Mollica, F. (1981) Treatment of infantile spasms with sodium dipropylacetic acid. *Developmental Medicine and Child Neurology*, **23**, 454–461.

Perucca, E. & Richens, A. (1980) Anticonvulsant drug interactions. In *The Treatment of Epilepsy* (ed. J.H. Tyrer), pp. 95–128. MTP Press, Lancaster.

Petersén, I., Selldén, U. & Eeg-Olofsson, O. (1975) The evolution of the EEG in normal children and adolescents from 1 to 21 years. In *Handbook of Electro-encephalography and Clinical Neurophysiology* (ed. A. Redmond), Vol. 6, Part B, pp. 31–68. Elsevier, Amsterdam.

Pippenger, C.E. (1980) Rationale and clinical application of therapeutic drug monitoring. *Pediatric Clinics of North America*, **27**, 891–925.

Purpura, D.P., Penry, J.K. & Walter, R.D. (1975) *Neurosurgical Management of the Epilepsies*. Raven Press, New York.

Ramsay, R.E., Hammond, E.J., Perchalski, R.J. & Wilder B.J. (1979) Brain uptake of phenytoin, phenobarbital and diazepam. *Archives of Neurology*, **36**, 535–539.

Reynolds, E.H. (1975) Chronic antiepileptic toxicity: a review. *Epilepsia*, **16**, 319–352.

Reynolds, E.H. & Shorvon, S.D. (1981) Monotherapy or polytherapy for epilepsy? *Epilepsia*, **22**, 1–10.

Richens, A. (1976) Clinical pharmacology and medical treatment. In *A Textbook of Epilepsy* (eds J. Laidlaw and A. Richens), pp. 185–247. Churchill Livingstone, Edinburgh.

Rowan, A.J. Overweg, J., Sadikoglu, S., Binnie, C.D., Nagelkerke, N.J.D. & Hünteler, E. (1980) Seizure prognosis in long-stay mentally subnormal epileptic patients: interrater EEG and clinical studies. *Epilepsia*, **21**, 219–226.

Rutter, M., Graham, P. & Yule, W. (1970) *A Neuropsychiatric Study in Childhood. Clinics in Developmental Medicine*, 35–36, S.I.M.P., Heinemann, London.

Rylance, C.N. & Morland, T.A. (1981) Saliva carbamazepine and phenytoin level monitoring. **56**, 637–639.

Schmidt, D. (1981) Effect of antiepileptic drugs on estrogen and progesterone metabolism and on oral contraception. In *Advances in Epileptology: XIIth Epilepsy International Symposium* (eds M. Dam, L. Gram and J.K. Penry), pp. 423–431. Raven Press, New York.

Schmidt, D. (1982) *Adverse Effects of Antiepileptic Drugs*. Raven Press, New York.

Schwartz, R.H., Eaton, J., Aynsley-Green, A. & Bower, B.D. (1983) Ketogenic diets in the management of childhood epilepsy. In *Research Progress in Epilepsy* (ed F.C. Rose), pp. 326–332. Pitman, Bath.

Stephenson, J.B.P. (1980) Reflex anoxic seizures and ocular compression. *Developmental Medicine and Child Neurology*, **22**, 380–386.

Stores, G. (1971) Cognitive function in children with epilepsy. *Developmental Medicine and Child Neurology*, **13**, 390–393.

Stores, G. (1973) Studies of attention and seizure disorders. *Developmental Medicine and Child Neurology*, **15**, 376–382.

Stores, G. (1978) School children with epilepsy at risk for learning and behaviour problems. *Developmental Medicine and Child Neurology*, **20**, 502–508.

Stores, G. (1983) Behavioural aspects of childhood epilepsy. In *Research Progress in Epilepsy* (ed F.C. Rose), pp. 221–223. Pitman, Bath.

Stores, G. & Hart, J. (1976) Reading skills of children with generalised or focal epilepsy attending ordinary school. *Developmental Medicine and Child Neurology*, **18**, 705–716.

Talairach, J., Bancaud, J., Szikla, G., Bonis, A., Geier, S. & Vedrenne, C. (1974) Approche nouvelle de la neurochirurgie de l'épilepsie. Méthodologie stéréotaxique et résultats thérapeutiques. *Neurochirurgie (Paris)*, **20**, Suppl. 1, 3–240.

Treiman, D.M. & Delgado-Escueta, A.V. (1980) Status epilepticus. In *Critical Care of Neurologic and Neurosurgical Emergencies* (eds A.A. Thompson and J.R. Green), pp. 53–99. Raven Press, New York.

Trimble, M.R., Thompson, P.J. & Huppert, F. (1980) Anticonvulsant drugs and cognitive abilities. In *Advances in Epileptology: XIth Epilepsy International Symposium* (eds R. Canger, F. Angeleri and J.K. Penry), pp. 199–204. Raven Press, New York.

Vajda, F.J.E. & Aicardi, J. (1983) Reassessment of the concept of a therapeutic range of anticonvulsant plasma levels. *Developmental Medicine and Child Neurology*, **25**, 660–671.

Viani, F., Avanzini, G., Baruzzi, A., Bordo, B., Bossi, L., Canger, R., Porro, G., Riboldi, A., Soffientini, M.E., Zagnoni, P. & Morselli, P.L. (1977) Long-term monitoring of antiepileptic drugs in patients with the Lennox-Gastaut syndrome. In *Epilepsy, the 8th International Symposium* (ed. J.K. Penry), pp. 131–138. Raven Press, New York.

Volpe, J.J. (1981) *Neurology of the Newborn*. W.B. Saunders, Philadelphia.

Wada, J. (1980) New surgical treatment through experimental models. In *Advances in Epileptology: Xth Epilepsy International Symposium* (eds J.A. Wada and J.K. Penry), pp. 195–204. Raven Press, New York.

Walker, J.E., Homan, R.W., Vasko, M.R., Crawford, I.L., Bell, R.D. & Tasker, W.G. (1979) Lorazepam in status epilepticus. *Annals of Neurology*, **6**, 207–213.

Ward, A.A. (1983) Surgical management of epilepsy. In *Epilepsy, Diagnosis and Management*, (eds. T.R. Browne and R.G. Feldman), pp. 281–296. Little, Brown and Co., Boston.

Wilder, B.J. & Bruni, J. (1981) *Seizure Disorders. A Pharmacological Approach to Treatment*. Raven Press, New York.

Wilder, B.J., Ramsay, R.E., Willmore, L.J., Feussner, G.G., Perchalski, R.J. & Shumate, J.B. (1977) Efficacy of intravenous phenytoin in the treatment of status epilepticus. *Annals of Neurology*, **1**, 511–518.

Wolf, S.M., Carr, A., Davis, D.C., Davidson, S., Dale, E.P., Forsythe, A., Goldenberg, E., Hanson, R., Lulejian, G.A., Nelson, M.A., Treitman, P. & Weinstein, A. (1977) The value of phenobarbital in the child who has had a single febrile seizure: a controlled study. *Pediatrics*, **59**, 378–385.

Wolf, S.M., Forsythe, A., Stunden, A.A., Friedman, R. & Diamond, H. (1981) Long-term effect of phenobarbital on cognitive function in children with febrile convulsions. *Pediatrics*, **68**, 820–823.

Chapter 12
The Falling Sickness: a Reorientation to Hysterical Epilepsy

David Taylor

What other essential wisdom have
I based on misinformation
And, unaware of deformation
Leaned on a world that isn't there

Jenny Joseph: *False Postulate*

Epilepsy and hysteria are two of medicine's most prejudice-laden concepts. The terms are ancient too and they carry with them into the late 20th century the dross of their former usage. Behind the word *epilepsy* lurks fear of dyscontrol, deterioration and death; behind *hysteria* lies morbid sexuality, mystery and deceit. The double danger of drawing them into diagnostic conjunction is evident in the confused literature.

A paper, read by Worster-Drought (1934) to the British Psychological Society only 50 years ago, stands at the watershed between ancient and modern practice. Written just after the invention of the EEG, it is the most modern paper on hystero-epilepsy to reveal the dilemma of the physician trying to help a patient with fits but faced only by their behaviour, or worse by an account of their behaviour. 'It is extremely difficult', he said, 'in fact almost impracticable to draw a hard and fast line between hysteria and epilepsy.' On what basis could he have made the distinction? Before 1857, when Locock introduced bromides (originally it might be remembered for the treatment of hysteria), it was of academic interest only, because there was no treatment for either hysteria or epilepsy (Locock *in* Temkin, 1971). In the absence of electro-encephalography, Worster-Drought was forced to draw his conclusions on his best understanding of his patients' whole situation. Fifty years later, for the most part, even with our split screens and portable EEG apparatus, so are we. Despite being able to say with more confidence that our patient is not at the moment suffering from an epileptic fit as we now understand it, we are not much wiser than Worster-Drought, or Aretaeus (Trimble, 1983) come to that, about what they are suffering from. Whereas the late 19th-century concept of epilepsy as an electrical discharge from neurones, spreading by progressive recruitment, has been vindicated and developed down to neurochemical levels by biomedical research, with hysteria we are still encumbered with ideas based on psychic energy or flux which can be blocked, diverted, repressed or converted, which have led nowhere. This contrast could be regarded as a poignant reminder of the relative failure of psychiatry. But it is actually more suggestive that hysteria is not a biomedical sort of thing. For Worster-Drought and his predecessors, epilepsy and hysteria might not only be confused, they were phenomena of equivalent conceptual status. Since then epilepsy has been recognized as an electrophysiological process. Because hysteria has not proved to be a thing of that sort, it has been suggested that it does not exist at all. Yet, as Aubrey Lewis wrote (1982), hysteria outlives its obituarists. This is because there are sicknesses that are not things or processes. These sicknesses are demanding of medical time, they are common, troublesome, even lethal. Some psychiatrists are aware of all this and their concept of hysteria has moved from being an outcome of personal psychopathology to being an aspect of social process. Non-psychiatrists, medical and lay alike, tend still to be more influenced by the more ancient formulations.

In this paper I shall use personal experience of a relatively large number of people with hysterical epilepsy to promote this alternative view of hysteria as an aspect of social process. I promote this view in the context of a general theory about sickness (Taylor, 1982) where I divide *sickness* into *diseases* (which are essentially things) and *illnesses* (which are processes and roles) and *predicaments* (which are personal situations). My triad owes something to Popper's three worlds (Popper & Eccles, 1977). Hysteria turns out to be, in Karl Popper's language, not in World I, the world of things; nor even in World II, a psychological world; but in World III, a human artefact, like a story. Hysteria will be one possible outcome of a predicament; it will have been scripted and is being enacted. Yet it is not a fiction—partly because the acting out of a play is not itself a fiction, and partly because all the other participants function at World I or II levels, providing it with apparent integrity. Much ink has been spilled to defend the hysteric from the accusation of 'putting it on'. But the validity of a sickness is not measured on a continuum between the unconscious and the conscious, but between innocence and malice. Given a proper understanding of the predicaments concerned, the excuse afforded by the concept of an unconscious process can be dispensed with. What is true for hysterical epilepsy will be seen to be true for pains, paralyses, sensory losses, and the modern refinements such as sneezing and total allergy. Essentially, we are involved with the building of a sickness.

Case histories

The danger is that the method of case by case analysis, which is traditional in medicine, is a major factor in perpetuating just exactly the disease concept which is so inappropriate to hysteria. In 1895, Breuer for example regarded hysteria 'as a clinical picture which has been empirically discovered and is based on clinical observation in just the same way as tubercular pulmonary phthsis' (Breuer & Freud, 1955 edition).

This of course is just what it is not. A clinical picture is not in the same universe of discourse as pulmonary tubercules. Indeed, the very act of drawing together people who aspire to have fits as opposed to people who have aspirations of other sicknesses already threatens to impose a spurious categorization. Of course, it is possible to proceed in that manner, noting the age, the sex composition of the sample, the social class of parents, age of onset, IQ, previous illness record and so on. The result would be a pastiche of the average hysteric but a representation of none. A better style is analogous to the group photograph in which each individual is discernible, something of their characteristics as a group is revealed as well as the sort of place and time in which they were identified as coming together.

CASE   Alice. One story is that she presented to a neurology clinic aged 15 with recent attacks of unconsciousness. No eyewitness account was available, but there was no history of convulsive movements, tongue biting or urinary incontinence. Her headteacher said that they were not typical fainting attacks and she might pass out three times in 10 minutes and then sleep for an hour. Because of bi-temporal abnormalities in her EEG she was given 50 mg of phenytoin bd; and because of a high level of parental anxiety they were given reassurance. The phenytoin produced a rash so it was changed to phenobarbitone. Neither drug affected her attacks. Phenobarbitone was stopped and the parents asked for a second opinion. She reached a psychiatrist 1 year after the first attack.

Another story is that she is the second of three children born to a meticulous couple of artisans with high standards and aspirations. Her clever older brother has broken away and is therefore regarded as 'selfish', but there are no secrets between the rest of them and they do everything together all the time. The school nurse came to know Alice around her menarche. She was said to be asthmatic.

'When she had an attack we would give her one of her own tablets which she carried with her. She would become extremely tense and rigid ... She would huddle up and cling to me and not let go until the tablets finally made her go to sleep. The physical contact seemed to reassure her. Her last asthma attack was on 23.3.1981. About that time it was said that she did not suffer from asthma and she was then taken off medication.'

For five months she did not attend the nurse. Then 'blackouts' began and recurred every few days. Friends said that some hours before an attack, she became quiet, pale and quick-tempered. Then headache, dizziness, and rapid breathing supervened, her eyes glazed and she placed her head on her arms on her desk.

'More often than not she will 'black out' and fall to the ground. On recovery she is coherent but not co-operative; she will not move even from a corridor or busy staircase. No matter how long she is left to rest where she falls she always 'blacks out' when I move her.'

A perceptive teacher who had taken her on holiday abroad in a small group noticed that the child's life was regimented, 'not so much pressurized as guided all the way along the line. Home life plays a big role, she goes home for dinner and was unable to stay for an extra class with her peers because she had to go home.' Her appearance was outmoded, similar to that of her younger sister whom she closely resembled in every way. 'It is as if she was struggling subconsciously with her own personality crisis.'

Pressures from expectation of success at school were evident in seven of the 15 girls in the series. Often the expectation was beyond the level of performance that might be predicted from their IQ. These aspirations were not different in quality from those of many striving families. But they were associated with family groupings of grossly anomalous construction with considerable interpersonal deceit. Or else they were normally constructed families but had precluded ordinary communication about situational distress, the possibility of failure, personal isolation, or the sexual pangs of adolescence.

CASE Bernice. This girl had been placed at an expensive private school at great personal sacrifice by her parents because of her impossible behaviour at her local school. Her specific learning difficulties were overlooked by both schools. A problematic knee joint kept her away from school for a year until she was finally operated upon. Standing in front of her GP waiting to be discharged back to school she developed her first right-sided focal epileptic attack. These soon became very frequent and were investigated in the finest detail and treated with carbamazepine without effect. More, and more bizarre, attacks occurred during several months of psychiatric therapy. She was transferred to the Park Hospital for Children where anti-epilepsy therapy was withdrawn and her attacks were ignored until they ceased. On her return, after many weeks of no attacks, she entered into a grossly bizarre fit as she crossed the threshold. This was interpreted to her as being just her way of telling the psychiatrist that he was useless. Subsequently, her occasional small lapses at home have been ignored and she is making good progress in an appropriate college.

Eight girls experienced problems at the prospect of changing from school to a job of work or further education. Four were in families of unusual constitution.

CASE Claudia. This illegitimate child was reared by her elderly grandmother as if she was her daughter, though everyone knew that she was her daughter's daughter. Her real mother absolutely denies her any maternal attention but treats her as a sister. She suffered a febrile convulsion at 13 months. Aged 11 years she was seen again having been noted to be 'glassy-eyed, chomping and inaccessible'. On carbamazepine 200 mg bd fits were no problem, and 2 years later, following normal EEGs, medication was withdrawn just before her menarche. Grandmother now began sporadic interference in her treatment and a variety of people became involved such that, at the time of her referral to the adolescent service, a consultant paediatrician, paediatric neurologist, psychiatrist, psychologist, psychiatric social worker, general practitioner and various casualty officers were regularly involved in her case.

Real epilepsy might have occurred at some time in the biography of seven of the girls. For none of them, however, was difficulty with the management of their genuine seizures their core problem.

CASE Doreen was suspended from professional training because the frequency of her psychomotor seizures was disrupting the work of her entire class. Fifty seizures a day were reported. A focal discharge over the left temporal lobe was eventually recorded. She coyly confessed to her psychiatrist that her seizures were genuine though she had told her neurologist who referred her, equally coyly, that she feigned them. Being older and more independent of her parents, she was able to move from one therapist to another, persuasively derogating her former therapists in the sort of way which her current therapist transiently enjoyed.

Competing with an academically successful sister, she had had her first seizure during examinations. She had had a spontaneous abortion while still a school girl. Both her mother and her boyfriend's mother had professional experience with epileptic patients.

There was a member of the 'caring professions' among six of the parental couples. They played a significant part in orchestrating their child's sicknesses.

CASE Elaine. The mother of this girl was secretary to their GP and she was present when Elaine fainted whilst receiving an injection designed to reduce the frequency of her infectious diseases. She twitched in her syncope. As she came round her doctor asked if there was a 'family history of epilepsy'.

Actually the family history was rather a painful mystery, since both the child and her mother were illegitimate and fatherless. Mother had been raised by the sister of her real mother. All these facts were concealed but became known to Elaine when she glimpsed the family history in a bible at the age of 11, around the time of her menarche. Previously, she had never been sick; subsequently, she entered upon 7 years of infections, allergies, joint disorders and surgery, culminating in 'epilepsy' which rapidly became incapacitating and threatened her employment. The 'epilepsy' ceased immediately after a 'postictal' EEG, which had been insisted on, showed no abnormality. This was followed by a year of supportive psychotherapy. She, like others, made no use of the opportunity afforded to discuss the self-apparent painful issues and situations in her life, and gained only from a reassuring friendship which was based on a mutual, but unspoken understanding, about the nature of the seizures. A year later she answered the psychiatrist's follow-up enquiry letter by appearing dressed in her full motor cycle outfit.

The question of driving motor vehicles posed problems to at least three of the girls.

CASE Freda possibly experienced a grand mal convulsion at the age of 14 which had pitched her down the stairs while her mother was out. Mother had vomited copiously in her pregnancy and lost weight. At birth, Freda weighed 4 lb 8 oz (2000 g) and was cold. She was in an incubator for 2 weeks. When she was sent from a consultant neurologist aged 16, I gave great attention at the first consultation to the possibility of genuine epilepsy. Immediately following the second psychiatric consultation, her mother telephoned to say that over the weekend Freda had experienced 54 fits the following day and 72 the next; she had already had 42 that morning. An EEG done immediately showed no abnormality despite the persistence of her fit-like behaviour.

The 'seizure disorder' had for 2 years provided a reason for such irregular school attendance as to allow her to fail the family aspirations. Mother was a 'quality controller' by profession too. The girl's IQ was just below the normal range and the parents' aspirations had been well beyond her. Subsequently, the epilepsy persisted sporadically but Freda was suddenly very keen to be without it when she saw that it would preclude her from driving.

CASE Geraldine was school-phobic and her 'epilepsy' played a part in keeping her out of school. Her biography revealed a number of the features found in the other patients. The family consisted of four women: grandmother and mother who were each divorced, and her younger sister who was moderately severely physically handicapped by spina bifida. Each had a chronic illness. Mother was also house-bound and preoccupied with the care of the handicapped sister. Although only 16, Geraldine had the demeanour of a 40-year-old management consultant. The household was in some awe of her, but each member was very dominating in her own way. It is likely too that Geraldine had originally a grand mal induced by television. But the management of her sporadic grand mals was as nothing compared with the situational chaos she could create. When, as a group, they were offered treatment via an adolescent unit, grandmother said that Geraldine would refuse, a sentiment with which mother agreed. Geraldine obligingly refused.

In the course of being sick with an hysterical disorder, some people use a tremendous amount of health care resources.

CASE   Helen was known at seven hospitals at least in the course of 3 years between her first and last known seizures. Epilepsy was diagnosed when she was 13 on the basis of described seizures. Taken in evidence was the fact that her sister was a 'known epileptic'. (In fact her sister was just being placed in a long-stay mental hospital for persistently overdosing herself with anticonvulsants which she was taking for a seizure disorder of rather uncertain basis.) Within 5 months Helen was overdosing too but her father refused permission for psychiatric intervention. Recurrently she was assessed on an emergency basis following a seizure and was usually regarded as a 'known epileptic' despite the very atypical nature of her seizures. Two paediatric neurologists who saw her in a fit thought them 'put on'. Her seizures and her overdosing became even more problematic after her sister had entered a persistent vegetative state following a cardiac arrest of unknown cause but probably related to pharmacological abuse. She said that they had agreed a death pact. Reluctantly, her parents now let Helen go to an adolescent unit. Although she was difficult and her discharge within 3 months was unplanned, she appears to have relinquished her 'seizures' at that time. Professionals visiting the house became aware of the grossly abnormal family, functioning with a powerful, large, very dominating father, a psychiatrically sick mother, and an older brother who had already been turned out of the house. It was never possible to know precisely what factors influenced the girls' sickness behaviour. Helen remains a rather over-enthusiastic hospital attender at a variety of clinics.

Discussion

Some people behave in a way that makes others wonder whether they might be having fits. Fits are socially stigmatizing to the sufferer and frightening to witnesses. They claim attention, and doctors will be consulted about them.

Mostly, what people say to doctors about how they are is true as they understand it, and doctors quite properly work on that basis. But the language of human distress is coextensive with the language of sickness and, throughout childhood, most parents recognize that a child's somatic complaints sometimes have only token value. Should parents become alarmed, they turn to the doctors who give back-up reassurance about most of these distresses. Seizures, however, being ephemeral but regarded as of serious potential significance, are liable to evoke standard responses from doctors. These responses reveal that physicians are not primarily oriented towards people who suffer sickness but to the sicknesses people suffer. Their fail-safe strategy is to exclude disease rather than to explore the predicament. This tactic commits them to entertain possible physical illnesses which might provoke such behaviours. This inevitably re-enforces such possibilities in the mind of the patient and others who are involved. Besides, the predicament may be unrecognized by the presenter of the sickness. Or else discussion of the predicament is so unacceptable to the family that a disease, however hideous, is their preferred explanation. Doctors can hardly believe this and they have preferred to believe that a dissociative state is needed to explain how a person can maintain their disorder, and endure the subsequent tedious investigations. Further, they tend to believe that psychiatric illness is a complex process which is fashioned deep in the unconscious, rather than an understandable response within a limited repertoire of human responses to distress, as is readily apparent given even a minimum of enquiry.

Fingarette (1969) on the subject of self-deception writes, 'As the individual grows from infancy to adulthood he identifies himself as a person of certain traits of character, having certain virtues and views, a certain bodily shape, having allegiances, enemies, obligations, rights, a history.' These are qualities that Fingarette sees as being 'avowed' and that can be 'disavowed'. They are not mere descriptions. I think that sickness can be such an avowal, and this means that the resultant conversion hysteria shares something of the quality of sudden religious conversion. The conditions under which mass hysterias occur are similar to those under which other people have made their solemn avowals. In both circumstances the states of mind are mostly transient, but some are very enduring. The facility with which these states can be induced is proof against serious psychopathology being their basis. Recently, for example, a girls' band was ravaged in this way; crop spraying nearby was blamed, but in fact little girls who had gone to play in the band, banded up in a play; and in a play an avowal must be made, a conjecture entertained.

In the building of an hysterical sickness the raw materials and the plan are fairly standard. First, a life situation that ranges from difficult to excruciating. Any means by which this might be discussed or altered should be blocked. Sexual abuse by a father provides an extreme but historic example, but Bernice, above, was actually finding punitive the school for which her parents were making such sacrifices. Second, an ally is needed to help in the promotion of the sickness. A person in some way involved in the caring professions, especially someone with their own problem to promote, or a family tradition of sickness, or an absolute priority to cover over the real issues, will each serve. Third, to complete the predicament, a model should be available, either in previous experience, or opportunistically, or else contrived within a situation. The question 'Is there a family history of epilepsy?', innocently asked, will do. Fourth, someone with sufficient social skill and status to manage the presentation of the sickness is needed. Perhaps that is why young children rarely provide adequately for an hysteria, unless accompanied by an angry adult with an axe to grind. Doctors, of course, can excellently fulfil most of the above roles and can do so quite unwittingly. They can do this by not being interested in or listening to the life situation, by being over-inclined to settle on a physical diagnosis, by having a problem with non-organic phenomena, or by not wanting to know unpleasant things about people.

Sickness is always a social event which has meaning, but it is particularly important in an hysteria to monitor what that meaning seems to be. For example, most sick people are only too willing to be reassured. The relatives of these people are unhappy about being reassured because in the creation of an hysteria they will have been required to participate and the illness will have been meaningful to them too. They may not readily give up the idea simply because the 'sufferer' proves not to conform to the required specification for a real disease. Another feature of hysterical illness is self-justification. Instead of responding to simple measures there is often marked deterioration at the beginning of treatment. If one fit is unconvincing, then another and another will claim the necessary attention. The illness is repeated in an effort to justify what has occurred previously.

However, as Slater (1982) and others have pointed out, disease does have a part to play. Feeling unwell for no apparent reason, feeling depressed without knowing it, suffering a disease, or having a treatment that tends to reduce the ordinary modes of coping, are all known to provide the opportunity for an hysterical elaboration which may not necessarily even be in the same bodily system as the disease. For these reasons, as well as just being misunderstood, there is likely to be a high morbidity of disease among these patients.

Recent studies of hysterical conversion in childhood such as those of Dubowitz & Hersov (1976) and Maloney (1980) and Goodyer (1981) do not support a psychopathological basis for the disorder. They tend more to support the views of Slater (1982) and Kendell (1982) and Rabkin (1964) that hysterical conversion is a social construction set up in the doctor–patient relationship. While I concede that it is validated there, in ways that are socially very powerful, I believe that the conversion hysterias are vehicles of human communication. They are tokens offered and accepted, at times mistakenly, and at times gladly, in service of the needs of the group. In childhood they seem often to start as innocent misunderstandings of token sicknesses. By the time they are offered to doctors they may have become quite elaborate. Usually, by the time they reach the psychiatrist, attitudes have become entrenched.

Viewed in the way, I have suggested that the conversion hysterias are more obviously related to the 'mass hysterias' which, in their turn, support the irrelevance of personal psychopathology. This view of hysteria also suggests that, at times, communication through somatic complaints, well rehearsed in childhood or adolescence, can become a way of being, such as is now called Briquet's syndrome by the St Louis group (Woodruff *et al.*, 1982).

The difference between hysteria and malingering is perhaps not a difference between two cerebral states but between two sets of motives. People vary in what sensations or feelings of sickness they choose to express. There is thus a moral component in the evaluation of every sickness, and hysteria is only an extreme case. Throughout the history of medicine there have always been devices that deflect responsibility for sickness away from the sufferer: in the animistic phase, people were the playthings of the Gods and anything might happen; in the naturalistic phase, people participated, transiently, in His order; in the empirical phase, doctors constructed entities out of observable phenomena in Nature and looked towards neurophysiology; most recently, the notion of unconscious process and society have been placed between persons and their ultimate responsibility for their well-being. This responsibility is now beginning to be assumed in a variety of ways, but most of the initiative comes from outside medicine.

The outcome of these disorders is not always good. Very persistent illness behaviour and loss of function can occur and life-threatening situations arise. Disease may supervene.

Nevertheless, there is an urgent need to stop all kinds of physical interference with drugs, regimes or investigations. This clarifies the doctor's and the patient's mind. It allows any physical process to declare itself and it stops re-enforcing illness behaviour.

An 'exit ploy' must be devised whereby the patient can be provided with a means of recovery. At the same time, alterations can be made in the situation that was productive of distress. In the absence of psychopathology, the psychiatrist plays the part of an expert negotiator in human affairs. Toleration of uncertainty, and the capacity to accept that doctors need not necessarily always be 'right' in the structural sense to serve the greater good, are also useful prophylactics against hysteria.

References

Breuer, J. & Freud, S. (1955) *Studies on Hysteria*, Standard Edition, Vol. 2, pp. 259–292. Hogarth Press, London.

Dubowitz, V. & Hersov L. (1976) Management of children with non-organic (hysterical) disorders of motor function. *Developmental Medicine and Child Neurology*, **18**, 358–368.

Fingarette, H. (1982) Self-deception and the 'splitting of the ego'. In *Philososphical Essays on Freud* (eds R. Walham and J. Hopkins), pp. 212–226. Cambridge University Press.

Goodyer, I. (1981) Hysterical conversion reactions in childhood. *Journal of Child Psychology and Psychiatry*, **22**, 179–188.

Kendell, R.E. (1982) A new look at hysteria. In *Hysteria* (ed. A. Roy), pp. 27–36. John Wiley, Chichester.

Lewis, A. (1982) The survival of hysteria. In *Hysteria* (ed. A. Roy), pp. 21–26. John Wiley, Chichester.

Maloney, M.J. (1980) Diagnosing hysterical conversion reactions in children. *Journal of Pediatrics*, **97**(6), 1016–1020.

Popper, K.R. & Eccles, J.C. (1977) *The Self and Its Brain*. Springer, Berlin.

Rabkin, R. (1964) Conversion hysteria as social maladaptation. *Psychiatry*, **27**, 349–363.

Slater, E. (1982) What is hysteria? In *Hysteria* (ed. A. Roy), pp. 37–40. John Wiley, Chichester.

Taylor, D.C. (1982) The components of sickness: diseases, illnesses and predicaments. In *One Child* (eds J. Apley and C. Ounsted), pp. 1–13. Spastics International Medical Publications.

Temkin, O. (1971) *The Falling Sickness*, 2nd edn, p. 298. John Hopkins Press, London.

Trimble, M. (1983) Pseudoseizures. *British Journal of Hospital Medicine*, **29**, 326–333.

Woodruff, R.A., Goodwin, D.W. & Guze, S.B. (1982) Hysteria (Briquet's syndrome). In *Hysteria* (ed. A. Roy), pp. 117–129. John Wiley, Chichester.

Worster-Drought, C. (1934) Hystero-epilepsy. *British Journal of Medical Psychology*, **14**(1), 50–82.

Chapter 13
Children with Paroxysmal Disorders which are not Epilepsy

John Stephenson

The episodic and reversible alterations of cerebral function described in this chapter may cause much distress to the families involved but are only rarely of danger in themselves. *Primum non nocere* is thus the first principle.

Careful diagnosis is coupled with reassurance based on full explanation. Therapy often involves more an adjustment of attitude and lifestyle than pharmacological manipulations. The use of drugs is restricted and conservative: the treatment must not be worse than the predicament.

Breath-holding attacks

In my opinion, the term breath-holding attack should be confined to the situation in which holding the breath in forced expiration appears to be responsible for the disturbance of cerebral function which follows. In this well-known phenomenon, the child when annoyed or hurt stops crying, goes dark blue, and becomes limp or opisthotonic after 30–40 seconds, and recovers when gasping respirations resume.

It seems to me unhelpful to include under this heading the 'white' attacks or reflex anoxic seizures in which cardiac asystole is responsible (see reflex anoxic seizures), even though some children have both kinds of attack. It may be that there is often respiratory arrest in such asystolic syncope or seizures, but this is as it were a by-product, an epiphenomenon, as is the respiratory arrest in most epileptic seizures. No one would describe a tonic epileptic seizure with apnoea as a breath-holding attack: the same discrimination should, I think, be applied to asystolic seizures.

The diagnosis of breath-holding attacks depends entirely on the history. Unlike asystolic (reflex anoxic) seizures, they seem to occur exclusively in close proximity to caring adults who therefore witness both the provocation and the evolution of the attack. From this it follows that the diagnosis should present no difficulty. I cannot see the justification for ordering an EEG in this situation, unless the physician wishes to use the recording as a magical instrument of reassurance, and is prepared to employ deceipt should the child be one of the 2% or so who happens to show EEG spikes at that particular age.

In many families an explanation and reassurance that these horrifying attacks are harmless and will be outgrown is enough. In others one needs to go further. It is helpful to regard the attacks from the point of view of the child, and from the point of view of the adult witness. The child only breath-holds in the presence of, or very near to the caretaker whose behaviour he hopes to influence. The breath-holding is a type of non-verbal communication of great emotional content. It is a directional signal, with the possibility of reinforcement or inhibition depending on the response. Any active response may be reinforcing, whether it be waking up in his mother's arms, or receiving panic-stricken resuscitation. To the caring adult, who is always on hand to respond, there is powerful motivation both to terminate the attack to prevent death or brain damage, and then to show immense relief that the child is safe, sensible and alive. Stopping this two-way reinforcement is the objective of management in the more difficult cases.

Although time-consuming, counselling on the scope and methods of disciplining may be necessary to reduce the other behaviour disorders which often accompany breath-holding attacks, the crux of the problem of the attacks themselves is to convince the parents that the best response from them is no response. They must come to believe that the attacks are harmless with no risk of death or immediate disaster, no risk of secondary epilepsy in the medium term, and no risk of consequent mental handicap in the long term. Then there is a chance that the advice that the child should be left untouched and ignored may be accepted.

If, however, the breath-holding attacks are very frequent, 'severe', and easily induced, and the parents indicate that they are not convinced of the need to do nothing, then the next step is the induction of an attack in their presence. One has to warn the parents what one is about to do (or one may be assaulted oneself!) without in any way warning the child. Then, if one is lucky, a sudden pinch to the achilles tendon will induce breath-holding, and the examiner must watch impassively till the attack is concluded. (If only crying occurs, one tells the parents that if an attack had occurred one would still have done nothing—it is not possible to try this kind of provocation twice). This demonstration of inactivity through-out and after an attack is an application of the technique of modelling and is more effective than verbal advice alone. It is better in the case of (cyanotic) breath-holding attacks *not* to connect the child up to an EEG/ECG recorder in advance, for in this type of child the constraints necessary for the application of the electrodes may both induce crying without full breath-holding and remove the element of surprise from the deliberate noxious stimulus. Admittedly, it is nice to see the anoxic EEG response characteristic of a breath-holding attack, with EEG flattening despite uninterrupted tachycardia, but it is so rarely possible to induce an attack under such circumstances that the effort is not worthwhile. Further, with an EEG recorder attached, one runs the risk of finding irrelevant spikes which are better not disclosed.

Reflex anoxic seizures

Although vasovagal syncope is probably uncommon in young children, cardiovagal syncope is by no means rare. Arrest of the heart for about 10 seconds induces a convulsive seizure, and it is thus no surprise that most syncope in the young is convulsive syncope. I have defined (Stephenson, 1980) anoxic seizures as 'a particular type of fit which is neither epileptic nor due to breath-holding, but rather results from brief stoppage of the heart through excess activity in the vagus nerve.' It must be admitted that the statement that cardiac asystole is responsible for these non-epileptic seizures was in the main a prediction, only recently confirmed by continuous ECG/EEG monitoring. However, the confirmation of the prediction allows more confident reaffirmation of the principles of management.

As in the case of breath-holding attacks, the diagnosis may often be made by obtaining a precise and lucid history. Commonly, a minor blow to the head, particularly to the occiput, or other painful surprise is followed within seconds by the seizure. There is collapse, upward deviation of the eyes, flexion of the upper limbs with fisting, extension, mild cyanosis, eyes staring, brief jerks, snorting, eyes closed, limpness, awakening, drowsiness and pallor, in that order. In some cases there may be only pure syncope with pallor and limpness, in others extensions may be more violent and repeated two or three times. In either case, incontinence, usually urinary, may occur, and rarely tongue-biting during the tonic extension. Vomiting at the conclusion is a rare but potentially hazardous complication, especially if a panic-stricken parent attempts mouth-to-mouth respiration and blows the vomit down the airway (Paulson, 1963). The range of provoking stimuli elicited by history-taking include all varieties of bumps and surprising pain, including internal pain (such as in passing a constipated stool), together with fright, fear, sudden excitement and tickling. In infants and toddlers the stimuli traditionally associated with breath-holding attacks may also induce reflex anoxic seizures—a conflict of wills, annoyance, frustration. Other stimuli to the face and its orifices may be powerful provocations, for example bathing the eyes, cleaning the nose, examining the ears, eating ice cream or a chunk of ice lolly. In young infants laryngo-tracheal stimulation from oesophageal reflux may be responsible. Hair cutting, hair brushing and blow-drying are common precipitants in older children. In the adolescent, horror, fear and trepidation relating to things medical (dentists, blood, injections, allergy testing) have similar effect and thus induce convulsive syncope.

Diagnostic difficulty may arise because, unlike breath-holding attacks, reflex anoxic seizures have no predilection for occurring in the presence of parents or other caring persons. They may occur at home in a distant part of the house so that a mother hears only a bump with no succeeding cry. The infant may topple backwards onto the carpet so quietly that no one notices till he is in the fit. The child may fall over in the street or the playground. The school child may drop without warning and stiffen on the floor of the classroom. Even more difficult is the situation with young infants in whom it may be very hard to elicit a story of any significant provocation at all.

If the history is adequate for diagnosis, then, as with breath-holding attacks, a detailed explanation and reassurance may be all that is required. However, in the case of reflex anoxic seizures, both diagnosis and the provision of reassurance may be more difficult, and one often has to go further. I favour the use of ocular compression as a diagnostic and therapeutic aid. The method has been described in detail elsewhere (Stephenson, 1978, 1980). I continue to use it daily, unmodified, except that I no longer have any concern about the need for special emergency resuscitation facilities. Indeed, I rather think they are contra-indicated. In brief, the procedure is as follows. The supine child is connected for combined EEG and ECG. The parent present is told that brief pressure on the closed eyes may reproduce an attack, and if so, that this will be valuable. The operator then exerts firm pressure over the closed eyelids for up to 10 seconds, and allows the parent to witness the anoxic seizure if one is induced—which it is in more than 50% of cases. Meanwhile the operator does not touch the child further, watching impassively till recovery occurs. At this stage one is able to reinforce two observations which the parent will have made, inwardly at any rate. First, it is a relief to the parent that an attack has been reproduced (even though less severe than the natural attack) and seen by a professional. Second, it is apparent that (even allowing for the induced attack being somewhat mild) the child recovers with no need for help from onlookers. Then the parent is shown the record of the ECG and EEG, and focused on the stoppage of the heart at the time of touching the eyes, and the reappearance of the ECG signal at a time when the child was in the seizure or looking 'dead'. This is a suitable moment to explain the fail-safe organization of the child's physiology, in that cessation of blood flow to the head end of the vagus nerve means that the heart must restart automatically. It is also the time to point out the *possible* value of being flat at the time of failure of the circulation to the brain, and the possible hazards of picking the child up. I always mention the action of atropine in preventing the reflex heart stopping, but in most cases the 'modelling' therapy with the natural visual aids which I have described is sufficiently reassuring, and drug treatment is not required.

It is worth adding a word about the diagnostic power of ocular compression. As I have indicated, its main value is in the *reproduction* of attacks, identical in detail to those previously witnessed. This is helpful even when provocations have not been obvious. There are difficulties when there have not been reliable witnesses, and it must be remembered that anoxic seizures can be induced in a small percentage of the general population with the same order of frequency as spikes can be found in the EEG. Proof of cardiac arrest as the mechanism of what appears to be a reflex anoxic seizure demands ECG/EEG ambulatory monitoring (e.g. Medilog), but is only practicable when attacks are more frequent than once daily—even then, the child may be inhibited by the apparatus from normal robust activities for the first couple of days.

I reserve atropine for use when there remains much anxiety after ocular compression based reassurance, if attacks are sufficiently frequent to disrupt family life (in effect, this means more than once daily, with post-ictal sleep), if attacks appear to have been life-threatening (Stephenson, 1979), or if diagnostic uncertainty remains—as a therapeutic trial. Those who do not employ ocular compression will use atropine more often for this last reason.

Atropine sulphate can be used orally with effect. The starting dose is 0.01 mg/kg daily in three divided daytime doses, but this may be increased to at least 0.01 mg/kg/dose, titrating against dry mouth (and dry nose). A solution may be made up, but needs replacing every 2 weeks. Alternatively, one may use powders, or tablets (600 μg) in older children. Theoretically, one might expect atropine sulphate to impair cognitive processes (especially memory), since it enters the brain to some extent and blocks acetylcholine at muscarinic sites. This dementing effect is well known in the case of hyoscine which enters the brain much more readily, but to date we have not detected cognitive impairments with atropine sulphate. However, concern about this has led to the use of atropine methonitrate whose quaternary structure keeps its distribution extracerebral. Atropine methonitrate comes as drops (Eumydrin 0.2 mg/drop) and is started at a dose of 0.4 mg/kg/day in three day time doses. As with atropine sulphate, the dose may be raised till oral and nasal dryness limit further increase. How long an atropine compound is given depends on the reason for its use, but commonly would be no more than a matter of months. I only use prophylactic atropine compounds alone in young children. In adolescents and adults, reflex anoxic seizures may be replaced by attacks which more resemble vasovagal syncope. In such circumstances, atropine only blocks the vagal component, and if full prophylaxis is absolutely necessary an ergotamine-containing preparation such as Bellergal (belladonna alkalids, ergotamine and phenobarbitone) used to be employed. One would not recommend this today. Animal experiments suggests that GABA is important in central automatic regulations (Di Micco *et al.*, 1979; Williford *et al.*, 1980), and future work may clarify the role of GABA agonists in syncope (Quest *et al.*, 1977). Following this, the chlordiazepoxide and anticholinergic (clidinium) combination Libraxin might be considered in the older individual with syncope.

Migraine

It is evident that the earlier in life the child with migraine presents, the less clear-cut will be the symptomatology, but in practice the diagnosis should not usually present difficulties. Children tend not to be sent to the paediatric neurologist until they are old enough for a good history to be obtained. The referral is often because it comes as a surprise that migraine should present in childhood, whereas in fact it commonly does so.

In the evolution of the condition there may at first be episodes of being 'off-colour' called either 'acidosis' with vomiting or recurrent bellyache. Such attacks of abdominal pain and vomiting may be very severe: a family history of migraine is reassuring if malrotation of the gut has been excluded. Later, the picture of common migraine develops, with headache, vomiting, dislike of bright light, pallor, and a desire to lie down. Classical migraine, with visual phenomena, and less often other focal neurological symptoms, tends to become manifest in older childhood, but a young child may reveal much detail of scintillating sootomata and fortification spectra if given encouragement and a supply of crayons. I do not propose to discuss in any detail the less common manifestations of migraine when the headaches may be associated with opthalmoplegia, hemiplegia, hemianopia, and dysphasia. The very fact that these complications are rare may indicate that there are additional factors at play, such as defects of coagulation. Investigation of such possibilities is justifiable in the hope of finding treatable causes, although in general the therapeutic approach is not different from that in the more common variety.

The initial consultation is an important part of the management of the child with migraine. The history needs to be probed for possible triggers, psychological or dietary. I undertake a concise neurological examination and blood pressure measurement, but the only physical sign elicited at all frequently is optic nerve Drusen appearing as pseudo-papilloedema (Santavuori & Enkkila, 1976). Reassurance by the opthalmologist may be necessary to support one's own reassurance to the patient and parents in such cases. Further investigations in childhood migraine are seldom needed on medical grounds, though it is possible to use an EEG, for example, as a demonstration of the 'normality' of the brain—provided that the actual record is available, and that trivial and irrelevant observations are ignored.

In childhood, migraine management may require no more than a confident pronouncement and explanation of the diagnosis. Parents on the whole will steer the right course between completely ignoring or rejecting the attacks and over-protection. Altering life-style in a radical way is commonly not practicable, but the use of food diaries and elimination diets has at the least some placebo potential. (The use of oral disodium cromoglycate against intractable food allergy is too rare a possibility for discussion in this chapter.)

Some parents may be frightened of giving the simple analgesics aspirin or paracetamol in adequate doses for headache. Normal dosage and the limits of safety need explanation. Possibly more effective against the pain are compound tablets containing codeine in addition, such as Paracodol or yellow Migraleve. If straight analgesics given at the onset of an attack, or in anticipation, are ineffective, then the most rational addition is metaclopramide (Maxolon) which increases gastric motility and should propel the analgesics into absorptive gut if given soon enough. Soon enough is 15 minutes beforehand. The metaclopramide is of course also a powerful anti-emetic, but from time to time causes acute dystonic reactions in children. It can be given as the combination Migravess. Another anti-emetic, which seems less troublesome but which does not increase gastric motility, is contained in pink Migraleve tablets. Ergotamine preparations are best avoided as treatment of individual attacks in children, in my opinion.

The need for regular drug prophylaxis of childhood migraine arises when attacks continue to interfere with life and lead to frequent absences from school despite initial counselling. What is 'frequent' is an individual judgement, and will depend on the stage in school career, examinations etc. The choice of drug may depend on for how long the prophylaxis is required.

For short periods, regular daily *aspirin* may have fewer side-effects and be of more benefit than the alternatives.

Clonidine originally seemed effective without side-effects, but I am not now clear that it is better than placebo.

Propranolol is safe enough for use in the over-anxious.

Pizotifen (Sanomigran) is now available as a paediatric syrup as well as in tablet form, and has been used in very young children. Drowsiness and possible appetite increase are the only notable side-effects.

Amitryptiline is now a sufficiently well-known drug to make its use safe, provided that the very dangerous prospect of accidental overdose is stringently guarded against.

I do not have any great experience of the use of *clonazepam* in childhood migraine, but there may be situations where a very small nightly dose may be effective and without the side-effects of drowsiness or bad temper. The main potential danger of the use of this drug, or carbamazepine, or low dose phenytoin, is that the migraine may be misconstrued as epilepsy.

If, despite good counselling and careful drug therapy, migraine attacks remain frequent and severe, formal psychological therapy deserves consideration. Of the various psychological treatments, relaxation exercises or hypnosis can certainly be effective, with perseverance.

For those parents who wish a reasonable discussion of the subject at greater length than can be provided in ordinary consultantion, I recommend the short monograph by Rose & Gawel (1979).

Rarer forms of paroxysmal disorders in childhood will not be considered but good reviews have been published recently on benign paroxysmal vertigo (*British Medical Journal*, 1979) and the Gilles de la Tourette syndrome (Corbett & Turpin, 1985).

References

British Medical Journal (1979) Benign recurrent vertigo. **ii**, 756.

Corbett, J.A. & Turpin, G.C.H. (1985) Tics and Tourette's syndrome. In *Child and Adolescent Psychiatry: Modern Approaches* (eds M. Rutter and L. Hersov), p. 516. Blackwell Scientific, Oxford.

Di Micco, J.A., Gale, K Hamilton, B. & Gillis, R.A. (1979) GABA receptor control of parasympathetic outflow to heart: characterization and brainstem localisation. *Science*, **204**, 1106–1109.

Paulson, G. (1963) Breath-holding spells: a fatal case. *Developmental Medicine and Child Neurology*, **5**, 246–251.

Quest, J.A., Freer, L.S., Kunec, J.R. & Gillis, R.A. (1977) Chlordiazepoxide inhibition of reflex vagal bradycardia in the cat. *Life Science*, 659–666.

Rose, F.C. & Gawel, M. (1979) *Migraine*. Oxford University Press, Oxford.

Santavuori, P. & Erkkila, H. (1976) Neurological and developmental findings in children with optic nerve drusen. *Neuropadiatrie*, **7**, 283–301.

Stephenson, J.B.P. (1978) Reflex anoxic seizures ('white breath-holding'): non-epileptic vagal attacks. *Archives of Disease in Childhood*, **53**, 193–200.

Stephenson, J.B.P. (1979) Atropine methonitrate in management of near-fatal reflex anoxic seizures. *Lancet*, **ii**, 955.

Stephenson, J.B.P. (1980) Reflex anoxic seizures and ocular compression. *Developmental Medicine and Child Neurology*, **22**, 380–386.

Williford, D.J., Hamilton, B.L. & Gillis, R.A. (1980) Evidence that a GABA-ergic mechanism at nucleus ambiguus influences reflex-induced vagal activity. *Brain Research*, **193**, 584–588.

Chapter 14
Emotional and Behavioural Disorders in Children with Neurological Disorders

David Thursfield

Introduction

Clinical interest in the psychosocial predicament of neurologically impaired children has been gathering momentum within the last decade, guided by experiences gained from the poliomyelitis epidemics in the United States in the 1940s and encouraged by Benders' classic studies of the deficit states of the victims of encephalitis lethargica (Bender, 1956). In the UK, the Reid report (DHSS, 1969) was responsible for the setting up of one special centre for children with epilepsy at the Park Hospital, Oxford, and more recently the special and residential educational needs of children with neurological and learning disabilities have been supported by the Warnock Report (Committee of enquiry into the education of handicapped children and young people, 1978). The Court Committee (Committee on Child Health Services, 1976) stressed the need for a better organized psychiatric and psychological support service for the handicapped child, following on the Isle of Wight study research findings (Rutter *et al.*, 1970a). Neuropsychiatric research has been beset by methodological inconsistencies which made it difficult to draw firm conclusions from past research.

In the fields of epilepsy and cerebral trauma, Stores and his colleagues in Oxford, and Rutter in London have made significant contributions to the literature in recent years. A comparative study of the emotional adjustment of 70 epileptic children (Stores & Piran, 1978) demonstrated striking sex differences between them: anxiety, inattentiveness, social isolation and dependency were characteristically more frequent in epileptic boys. A subgroup of boys with left temporal lobe dysfunction were significantly more disturbed in their behaviour, irrespective of seizure frequency or type of anticonvulsant therapy. Brown's prospective study of 31 children with severe head injury (Brown *et al.*, 1981) found rates of new psychiatric disorder to be twice as high as those of matched controls, although the relationship between brain injury and emotional disorder was less strong than that found in a parallel study of children with post-traumatic learning deficits (Chadwick *et al.*, 1981).

Rates of disorder were found to be greatly increased within the first follow-up period of 4 months and remained at a high level for the duration of the study. The authors found no specificity to the pattern of psychiatric disturbance, with the exception of one socially disinhibited child diagnosed as suffering from a frontal lobe syndrome. It is somewhat surprising in the light of our knowledge that children who are traumatized are more likely to have shown abnormal behaviour before their accident and to have experienced more family adversity (Craft *et al.*, 1972; Brown and Davidson, 1978). The latter found no association between over-activity and head injury.

Seidel *et al.*, (1975), investigated the impact of cerebral palsy and hydrocephalus on a group of 33 school children of normal intelligence. Compared with a group of 42 children with conditions involving either the spinal cord, peripheral nervous system and muscles only or a range of orthopaedic conditions, 24% of the brain-lesioned group showed psychiatric disorder with substantial social impairment, a rate twice that of the 'peripheral' group; a figure that compares with similar studies in the United Kingdom (Rutter *et al.*, 1970a) and the United States (Freeman, 1970; Minde, 1978). Within the handicapped group, overcrowding, anomalous family situations, marital discord and psychiatric disorder in the mother were all significantly associated with child psychiatric disorder, suggesting that behavioural disturbance stems from a combination of psychosocial adversity and biological vulnerability. The authors discuss the relevance of this concept and its contribution to current clinical neuropsychiatric practice. The success of a planned psychological support/treatment programme rests ultimately on the development of a working hypothesis for the individual child and his family. Adjustment problems of the disabled adolescent and children with learning disabilities are dealt with elsewhere (Chapters 8 & 15). There is probably a reservoir of undiagnosed and untreated psychiatric morbidity amongst neurological patients. (Bridges & Goldberg, 1984; Nabarro, 1984).

Only the more persistent signs of emotional disturbance will be considered: irritability, aggressive and antisocial behaviour, impulsivity and hyper-activity, fear states and some of the difficulties underlying long-term personal adjustment to neurological handicap.

Taking the psychiatric history

As an integral part of the neurological examination, symptoms of emotional disturbance should routinely be enquired into. The four most common areas of conflict are: immaturity, negativism, relationship difficulties and insecurity. Parents with a disturbed child may not recognize their own child's difficulties in the early stages, feeling that the child is wilful, stubborn or lazy and that if left their child 'will grow out of it'. Psychiatric disorders differ quantitatively from normality, therefore repeated questions may be necessary over several clinic visits to elicit a significant change of behaviour or the intensification of one specific symptom. Vigilance will avoid the situation of the profoundly distressed wheelchair child who attempts to 'run' away from home or the deeply depressed epileptic child who poisons himself with his own anticonvulsants. Frequency and severity of symptoms are indications of emotional disturbance, the greater the number of symptoms the more likely a child is to have a clinically significant disorder. Allow parents to talk freely about their difficulties, pose supplementary questions as necessary, aiming to quantify the severity, frequency and duration of symptoms. The following outline scheme indicates areas of possible enquiry.

1   Behaviour
Is the child co-operative or oppositional, constructive or destructive, irritable or placid, moody, prone to temper tantrums, telling lies, stealing, wandering from home, a delinquent gang member, fearful, sensitive, tearful, happy, easygoing? Friendships at school and home, any serious antisocial behaviour, previous court appearances for delinquent acts, under supervision or subject of a Care Order, probation, and placements away from home should be recorded.

2   Mood
Is the child depressed, excitable, angry, defensive, fearful? Do the child's moods fluctuate in a predictable or unpredictable manner? Are moods related to neurological status or hospitalization?

3   Temperamental characteristics
How adaptable is the child to new situations? Enquire about intensity of emotional reactions, quality of mood, persistence at tasks, attention span, distractability. Is he active, a creature of habit, does he like routine, hate uncertainty, is he easy to train in basic selfcare skills?

4 Thought processes and imagination

Is the child imaginative; what games does he play? Does he dream, day-dream, have any special ambitions, heroes and anti-heroes, any bizarre or eccentric ideas, any unusual religious experiences, inner-voices or hallucinatory experiences or imaginary companions?

5 School

Does he like or dislike school? Enquiry should be directed towards relationships with teachers and pupils, academic progress, fighting in school, truancy, school attendance, excessive amounts of time lost from lessons with specified 'illness', school refused, bullying or stigmatization by handicap.

6 Self-image

How does the child value himself? Is he confident, assertive, timid or anxious? Does he have an optimistic view of the world? How does the disabled teenager see his future, social relationships, marriage pro-spects? Are there any doubts about his effectiveness as a parent or wage earner, or doubts about sexual competence? How stable is his neurological state? Is it likely to interfere with future independence?

CASE Andrew a boisterous and roguish 4-year-old was referred to the psychiatric out-patient clinic by his family doctor after complaints from his mother of his aggressive behaviour, persistent headbanging and use of foul language. On interview, Mrs. S presented a catalogue of complaints from clinging and demanding attention at home, premeditated destruction of his elder brothers toys, kicking, hitting and throwing heavy objects at friends when provoked, spitting and urinating on neighbour's children, and pouring drinks over himself and his siblings. Reports of him being a bad mixer at school, with no special friends and unable to participate in group activities were not confirmed subsequently by Andrew's teacher. Mrs. S's management of her son's oppositional behaviour was to shout, smack him and send him to bed often in an unpredictable or inconsistent way. Her husband, however, disagreed frequently with his wife's approach and would punish Andrew with threats that invariably were not carried out. The developmental history was significant; Andrew had been different from his 9-year-old brother in a number of respects. From birth Andrew had been a restless, active baby, demanding of mother's time. Brother Gary had always resented the new baby's arrival and would constantly provoke his brother to fight. Gary was an outward-going and carefree individual, his brother shy and sensitive; Andrew fearful and lacking in self confidence, his brother fearless and egocentric.

Twelve months prior to Andrew's psychiatric referral, Mr. S had left the navy to be nearer home and support his wife but had been made redundant soon after successfully applying for a machine operator post. Mr. S had accepted the reversed role of house-husband whilst his wife became the family bread-winner, as a secretary. She found her job satisfying and it provided her with a social life. Mr. S, normally a placid but moody individual, found the boys to be demanding, despite his efforts to give them a great deal of his time and attention. His expectations of his children's behaviour were high. There were frequent open arguments between the parents. Whilst at the peak of the domestic crisis and coincidental with Andrew's entry into primary school, Mrs. S began to notice that the boy was having absences, initially weekly attacks, later becoming regular daily occurrences, characterized by cessation of movement, eyes rolling upwards, tremors of both arms and transient masticatory movements of one to two minutes duration, after which he would appear perplexed and clinging to a familiar adult. Neurological examination proved negative. A combination of anticonvulsant therapy initially, and later a simple behavioural modification programme using 'time-out' procedures were successful in re-establishing a positive atmosphere in the home. Despite improvement in Andrew's adjustment, little change was seen within the marriage and parent counselling has continued.

Poor peer relationships have been shown to be not only a strong indication of current emotional disorder (Rutter *et al.*, 1970b) but a good predictor of persisting disorder (Sunby & Kreyburg, 1968; Cowen *et al.*, 1973). Aggressive behaviour in combination with school failure is strongly predictive of future delinquency in boys (Robins, 1972). Age and sex appropriateness of behaviour have to be considered. Because behaviour disorders are situation-specific, information should be sought from several different sources: the child, parents, school and interested professional third parties. Child psychiatric disorders must be regarded in interreactional terms and not viewed simply as a disease state or as intrapsychic conflict. When enquiring about the developmental history, special note should be made of significant milestones of development (Erikson, 1965), temperamental characteristics, (Thomas *et al.*, 1968), toilet training methods and the child's responses to them, and overall adaptability to new situations, e.g. entry into playgroup, admission to hospital, reactions to significant family losses or parental illness, birth of siblings and finally, entry into formal primary education. The preparation of a life-event chart will often highlight significant associations between family crises, emotional disturbance and changes in the child's neurological status. Caution is necessary in respect of the accuracy of parental reporting, particularly in relation to retrospective and developmental information. Threatening events, frightening experiences or situations that evoke a great deal of anxiety tend to be underreported; major crises are more likely to be remembered than minor ones, mothers of pre-school children being especially prone to underestimating the child's true difficulties (Yarrow *et al.*, 1964). The use of symptom checklists and behavioural questionnaires may encourage parents to be more objective (Richman & Graham, 1971; Rutter *et al.*, 1970a, Connors, 1973, Connors, 1981). As standardized information systems for Child Psychiatric Services are developed, behavioural data on all registered neurologically handicapped children will become available, a trend that can only be of benefit (Synderman *et al.*, 1980).

Interviewing the child

There are two main functions of the interview with the child: first, to grasp the quality of that child, his individuality, his self worth; and second, to determine his ability to share and relate to his family and friends around him. Early in the interview, the child should be given the opportunity to give an account of his own difficulties or worries, depending on his age and capacity and willingness to talk. Pre-school children will require play materials to communicate through, whilst older children and teenagers can be interviewed rather as one would a parent. A flexible approach to examination is necessary. By interviewing parents first, the sensitive or guilt-prone child may feel he is being discredited or censured.

The first step towards assessing a child's mental state is to establish a trusting relationship with him. A child needs to feel respected and that his point of view is valued; indeed, the child's perception of his disability or disorder will be a guiding factor in future management. Low self-esteem and a poor self-image are precursors of poor personality adjustment in adult life (Pless & Satterwhite, 1975). The examination room setting should be friendly and informal, possibly replacing the time-honoured examination couch with a comfortable reclining armchair. A selection of toys should be made available appropriate to the age and ability of the child, but perhaps not immediately open to view. A not unfamiliar experience will be the total disruption of an assessment by the over-stimulated hyperactive child who in his agitation and frustration makes marauding assaults on parents or the examiner, the interview invariably ending in tears. For the younger child, a selection of modelling and drawing materials, dolls, puppets and constructive toys is appropriate (Beiser, 1955). The older and literate child may be content to complete one of the wide range of pencil and paper projection tests available

(Winnicott, 1971; Raven, 1951). Problem checklists with anxious and defensive teenagers can produce a high yield of otherwise unsolicitated information about family and school life, friendships, attitudes to health and self perception (Mooney, 1950). Once a child's confidence has been gained, it is best to talk on topics unrelated to symptom areas; their interests or hobbies, heroes and heroines on film and television, comics and magazines they read, games they play, their neighbourhood, family outings, holidays, home life, friendships and ambitions. Enquire about nice and nasty dreams, secret wishes, fears and worries. In the course of a thirty minute interview the following areas may be assessed:

1.   Mode of dress and general appearance

Does the child look happy, tearful, anxious? Does the child easily relate to the interviewer? Is the child overactive, can he write, draw a human figure? It is worth noting whether he is talkative or mute and the content of his conversation. Does the child's stream of thought flow in a logical manner? Does the child exhibit bizarre or eccentric thoughts or delusional ideas? Is the child hallucinated?

2.   Mood

Is he bright, cheerful, sad, tense and anxious, resentful and hostile, suspicious, tearful? Has he ever thought of running away from home, going to sleep and never wanting to wake up, wishing he were dead, had thoughts of harming himself or contemplated taking his own life? Enquire about specific fears and worries and any rituals or compulsive habits.

3.   Fantasy Life

Enquire about dreams and ambitions, three magic wishes. Useful questions, though not to be rigidly used, include: what is the best or worst thing that could happen to a child? Who would he choose to be in his team on a journey to the moon or a jungle exploration? If he could change into an animal or a bird which one? Make up a short story about a dragon, a giant and a baby.

4.   Social Life

Ask how many friends he has or if he has one special friend. Are they also handicapped? What are his interests and hobbies and affiliations to young people's organizations? How confident is he with the opposite sex? Does he feel lonely or isolated from peers? Is he bullied or teased? Is he popular in school? Does he make enemies easily? Is he envious of more able children? Does he avoid social contact? Is he encouraged to mix by his family?

5. *Play*

What games does he play and with whom? How imaginative is he, can he concentrate? How constructive is play?

Free play activity is potentially a rich source of information and a much neglected clinical tool. It can indicate a child's developmental level (Newson & Newson 1980), his capacity to organize behaviour (Kalverboer, 1980) and emotional status (Kamp & Kessler, 1970). The observation of play behaviour in the clinic or ward setting allows the clinician to focus on problems that do not easily lend themselves to conventional forms of psychological testing such as attentional deficits, hyperactivity, disorder of language and socialization. Kalverboer's work with pre-school children with brain dysfunctions warrents further study. Using a specially designed playroom, video recordings of the child's behaviour are made through a one way screen. Aspects of motor, visual and verbal activity are scored by two trained observers. Data derived from observations of the child in a variety of structured settings are correlated with the child's neurological status (Touwen, 1979). Two levels of play activity were identified; boys with neurological deficits were shown to be less constructive at the lower play levels than those with better neurological scores.

Conclusion

In conclusion the first step towards remediation for emotional disorder is the accurate and detailed account of the child and his disability. An extensive range of screening questionnaires and standardized interview schedules are available to the clinician, but recommended only to complement the clinical formulation (Comrey *et al.*, 1973).

Family assessment

Interviewing all the family members together may give a vivid impression of family interactions but may make it more difficult to obtain factual historical details; whole family assessments may need to be reserved for domiciliary visits. Whilst the history is being taken, the background of each parent can be explored and a brief outline obtained of their origins and early experiences. Enquiry should always be made of any psychiatric illness in the family, and an assessment made of each parent's personality and an estimate of their relationship. How caring or rejecting are they of their handicapped child? Are they tense, anxious and overprotective, tolerant or intolerant? Are they consistant in their approach to discipline? Are they in accord with each other in matters of medical care, schooling, or meeting the day to day needs of the family? An extensive literature exists on interviewing and examining handicapped and non-handicapped children and their families (Rich, 1968; Rutter *et al.*, 1970a; Richman & Graham, 1971; Simmons, 1974; Cox & Rutter, 1975; Quinton *et al.*, 1976; Berg 1974; Stores & Piran, 1978).

The formulation

The formulation is a concise summary of the case in the light of all information available. It is not just a listing of factors, but a description of their interplay and relative importance. It should be a clearly written, logical and dynamic explanation, leading to a plan of treatment, management or further assessment. It should also give an indication of the expected outcome. It is important that strengths are mentioned as well as weaknesses. In multidisciplinary clinics, the formulation should be given at a conference attended by all team members.

1 *Predisposing factors.* Including constitutional factors; perinatal, temperamental, environmental and genetic.

2 *Precipitating factors.* Is emotional disturbance related to relapse of a condition, hospitalization or family crisis?

3 *Perpetuating factors.* Are there factors in the home or the child's environment reinforcing maladaptive behaviour?

4 *Protective factors.* What are child's and family strengths? What personal or intellectual skills will be of use to the child in adjusting to a long-term illness?

Child psychotherapy and counselling

Supportive psychotherapy is aimed at helping the child to cope more easily with a current anxiety, for example to stress relating to readmission to hospital or the emergence of new symptoms in a progressive neurological disease. For children with continuing stresses and family disturbance, psychoanalysis and psychotherapy aim to achieve a radical change in a child's personality structure. Between the two forms of therapy a range of psychological interventions exist, their techniques and application only being learned by regular contact with disturbed children, and necessitating a degree of supervision. Many paediatricians may feel they lack the conceptual background to be therapists. Supportive psychotherapy is seen to be unduly time-consuming and yet there are strong arguments for the clinician to remain the key figure in the administration of support services. Battle (1972) sees him as a professional ombudsman interpreting, integrating and implementing the total care of the handicapped child. Psychoanalysis is a highly specialized treatment requiring supervised training and is not routinely available in British clinics. There are wide variations in psychotherapy practice depending on the therapist's personality, the patient's age and the nature of his handicap. A therapist may take an active and more directive role in counselling, others prefer a passive, more interpretative stance. Common to all psychotherapies is the development of a working relationship with the child and using that relationship as the basis for encouraging self determination, and especially looking at new ways of adapting to and compensation for illness or disability.

CASE John, a highly intelligent 12-year-old, severely incapacitated with spinal muscular atrophy had been confined to a wheelchair for some years. A tendon transplant performed just before his twelfth birthday had proved unsuccessful in improving his mobility and John had become suicidally depressed at the final realization of his helplessness. Diagnosed hypotonic at birth, John had received unfailing parental support, the family negotiating all the natural crises of childhood, even the grief of suddenly losing father with a coronary thrombosis when John was 7 years old. When interviewed in the children's psychiatric clinic, John proved to be a friendly boy beneath his depression. He appreciated the opportunity of sharing his own concern for his handicap, his diminitive stature and his anxieties over chest infections that repeatedly hospitalized him and drew him away from home and friends. Since the death of his father, John had felt unable to share his feelings with his mother for fear of overburdening her. Mrs. T was a kindly, if forceful individual, helping to ensure her son led an independent life. She had failed to recognize her son's emotional needs only because of her own prolonged mourning over the death of her husband.

John received psychotherapy for 6 months, initially on a weekly basis, enabling him to take stock of his disability, allowing him to develop a positive view of his personal strengths and attributes, and to anticipate some of the difficulties of adolescence. A local youth group welcomed him to their membership and immediately took him off on holiday where he was able to compare notes with other wheelchair teenagers, and enter into friendly competition with his peers through a Wheelchair Olympics. Subsequently, he felt able to discuss his embarrassment over the need for supervision for his toileting and bathing, and discovered that showing his anger and frustration would not result in total abandonment by his mother. Some 4 years on, John has been accepted for residential sixth form college and plans an academic career.

Counselling parents

Pless and Satterwhite (1975) have made a major contribution to the literature on chronic childhood disorders by emphasizing the educative role of supportive counselling. Counselling is a means both of supporting parents to meet the needs of their handicapped child, and coping with their own personal vulnerabilities (Taylor, 1982). To quote Allen and Pearson's (1928) observation 'The child seems to adopt the same attitude to the disability that his parents do. If they worry so does he. If they are ashamed of it he will be sensitive too. If they regard it in an objective manner, he will accept it as a fact and not allow it to interfere with his adjustment'. The emotional reactions of parents to the handicapped child have been extensively reviewed by Steinhauer *et al.*, (1974) and MacKeith (1973) and include conflicting emotions of protection for the helpless and revulsion for the abnormality. The child is a reminder of their reproductive failure. Parents are often reluctant executors of treatment demands laid upon them by professionals. By actively encouraging contact with families, the counsellor may anticipate crisis periods: of hospitalization, adverse changes in health status, school placement, those long-term needs of preserving family self-esteem and buttressing a deteriorating marriage. Parents need time to unburden themselves of guilt, and acceptance of the diagnosis requires repeated explanation. Entrenched attitudes of denial and rejection of the handicapped child put him severely at risk. Equally damaging is the reaction of overprotectiveness towards the child and overdependence on professional resources. Some recent innovations in group counselling and the development of self-help groups deserves mention. A number of excellent publications are available for parents, as well as educational texts dealing with the theory and management of behaviour disorder and minimal brain dysfunction (Russell, 1978; Gardner, 1974). A counsellor may wish to seek the advice of a psychiatric colleague over new avenues to explore with a child, or refer the child or family to the psychiatric clinic for more intensive help. The referring paediatrician may then wish to retain interest and actively plan for continuing the care of a child on termination of psychiatric treatment.

Explaining handicap to the family

Whether a particular family whose child has a neurodevelopmental disability is referred to a psychiatrist, a developmental paediatrician or a neurologist is affected by the preferences of the referral source, the range of local specialist services and the attitudes of the family to the child and to the medical services. There will be a substantial overlap between the case-mix seen by each type of specialist. For each child the family needs help to understand the nature of the child's problem, the cause, the prognosis and the ways in which the child may be enabled to improve. The psychiatrist is especially equipped to assess the mental health of parents and children and to treat these in ways which facilitate coping. Although this can be a time-consuming process, so also is oncology or neurosurgery for instance. The effects of such treatment on the mental health of the family as a whole may be neglected by health service planners who only measure outcome by neglected by health service planners who only measure outcome by quantifying improvement in the patient. Nonetheless, improved mental health of the family usually leads to improvement in the patient's health.

Behaviour modification

Behavioural psychotherapy seeks to apply learning theory to the alteration of a child's behaviour, and notably to the training of parents and teachers in the use of behavioural techniques in the management of antisocial behaviour which has proved resistant to more traditional forms of psychotherapy (Berkowitz & Graziano, 1972; Levin *et al.*, 1976; O'Leary & O'Leary, 1977; Philipp, 1979). Parents may unwittingly reinforce undesirable behaviour in a child by ignoring 'good' behaviour and only attending to the misbehaviour. Because parent affection is a powerful reinforcer for children, they will repeat their misbehaviour even for negative attention. By selectively weakening misbehaviour and strengthening appropriate behaviour, undesirable behaviours may be phased out. The three common areas of application of behavioural psychotherapy are: those children who are deficient in certain age appropriate skills (self-care, delayed speech development, attentional deficits, social skills); the avoidance behaviours (school refusal, anorexia nervosa, animal phobias, social avoidance by the disabled) and finally, undesirable behaviours, non-compliance and temper tantrums. A number of simple approaches may be offered to parents initially. Ignoring behaviour and withdrawing attention from a child will gradually weaken behaviour. Once withdrawal of attention from certain target behaviour has been decided upon, other family members, friends and teachers may be called upon to consistently ignore it. Reinforcing good behaviour or 'catching them being good' is important. Children should be praised for playing quietly and amusing themselves, and not receive parental attention only when they misbehave. Emphasizing or reminding the child of his misdemeanors may reinforce undesirable behaviour. When a child is misbehaving, a request (i.e. a question) is inappropriate, but a firm friendly command specifies a desired behaviour. Anxious, unassertive parents will shrink from giving clear instructions to their handicapped children, lest they in some mysterious way 'damage' the child. Children need to know when a parent means business. Unless children learn to comply with the first command, parents lose credibility and the child continues to ignore subsequent commands. Used consistently and given immediately after the misbehaviour, mild punishments remind the child of the reason he is being punished. If ignoring a child proves ineffective, a time-out system (T.O.) should be considered; this means removing the child from the situation in which he is receiving reinforcement for misbehaving.

Because T.O. is a punishment, it needs to be consistently applied when used; the guidance of a psychologist may be necessary in initiating a T.O. system. Parents can remove themselves from the child when he is misbehaving or place the child in a designated T.O. area. A baseline measure of the frequency of the misbehaviour is useful before instituting a T.O. system, and aids the monitoring of the effectiveness of treatment. A simple explanation to the child of T.O. and its consequences will help secure his co-operation. A T.O. area should not be so isolated as to scare or harm the child but somewhere where a child can spend a short period of time without further reinforcement; a bathroom, bedroom, hallway or simply turning a chair to face a corner of the room.

When a child no longer responds to adult praise, desirable social behaviour can be reinforced using tokens, contingent on the completion of specified activities. Tokens need not be money; a combination of star chart and coloured counters, plastic money etc. may be sufficient as a form of self-monitoring and will generate further praise. Alternatively, tokens earned for achieving the desired goals can be exchanged at the end of each day or week for a predetermined more material reward, a trip to the cinema, staying up later with parents to watch a favourite television programme, buying a book or record. Excessive rewards should be avoided. Guilt-prone parents will offer lavish rewards for little effort, believing that large rewards bring instant cure. The process of negotiating an operant programme often proves to be a therapeutic bonus, clarifying parent and child expectations and leading to an overall improvement in family relationships.

A number of specialized techniques deserve mention, for example accelerator programmes to augment the acquisition of new skills; imaginal and *in vivo* desensitization by exposing phobic youngsters to an anxiety-producing stimulus in a structured mode. Flooding may succeed where desensitization has failed, although maximal exposure to a fear may be distressing for the younger child. Desensitization and flooding techniques are equally applicable to the anxious parents of the anxious child; indeed, unless parents are taught positive coping skills, the child will continue to model himself on his fearful adult counterpart. Token economy systems are being widely used within institutional settings, although some therapists are adopting a more cognitive stance with emphasis on self-control (Thoresen & Mahoney, 1974; Meichenbaum, 1977; Beck, 1976) and biofeedback techniques. Sterman's work with epileptic patients (Sterman *et al*, 1974) holds some promise for the future, making it possible for children to modulate their own brain waves and reduce the frequency of their seizures through voluntary control.

Residential psychiatric units for the treatment of neurologically impaired children

A number of units specializing in the assessment and habilitation of neurologically impaired children have now been established in Britain following the recommendations of the Reid report (D.H.S.S., 1969). In these units, child psychiatric services are closely integrated with paediatric neurological services within multidisciplinary-run residential units. Nevertheless, any well staffed child psychiatric unit should be able to cope with most disturbed, epileptic and neurologically handicapped children, assuming close links with paediatricians, neurologists and neurosurgeons. The psychiatrist in charge should have both an interest in neuropsychiatry and a willingness to train staff in the observation and treatment of such children.

When the Child Psychiatric Unit is unable to meet all the therapeutic needs of a disturbed and neurologically disordered child in the short term, residential special schools and community homes with education on the premises may appropriately meet their long-term requirements, as will a number of small specialist 'communities' run by voluntary organizations, and some independent boarding schools. Regrettably a few of the more aggressive, anti-social but often multiply handicapped adolescents continue to be accommodated on adult wards in psychiatric hospitals, a situation which can only be remedied by the creation of more specialist Child Psychiatric Units.

Drug therapy

Psychotropic drugs have a distinct but circumscribed role in the treatment of neurologically impaired children with emotional disorders. Careful surveillance for adverse effects is mandatory, dosages being minimized whenever possible. If long-term drug usage is envisaged, regular 'drug holidays' should be considered, thereby avoiding possible retardant effects on growth and cognitive function. Four major categories of drugs are currently prescribed for behaviour-disorder children in Britain: stimulants, neuroleptics, antidepressants and anticonvulsants.

Stimulants

The use of synthetic amphetamines has attracted considerable adverse publicity in recent years, opinions ranging from one of dismissal as a drug of dependency to that of outright condemnation as a psychotropic drug that suppresses any natural exuberance of a child and merely silences aggressive children without alleviating the cause. In his exhaustive review of 110 studies of the effects of stimulant drugs on more than 4200 hyperactive children, Barkley (1977) concludes that 75% of hyperactive children improve whilst on drugs, whilst 25% are unchanged or made worse by them. Psychophysiological research on stimulant drugs indicates that they do not act paradoxically or sedatively on the CNS of hyperactive children, but typically energize CNS responses. The main impact of stimulant medication in these children appears to be one of increased concentration or attention span and decreased impulsivity. Therapeutic doses of methylphenidate can be as low as 0.3 mg/kg/day, the total daily dose not exceeding 20 mg. Methylphenidate is active for 4–6 hours and is administered in a single morning dose or in divided doses, morning and midday. Treatment can be monitored using a combination of behaviour rating scales, completed by parents, teachers, clinicians or nursing staff (Connors, 1973). Failure to observe significant changes in behaviour within 2 weeks of commencing treatment would be a strong indication for discontinuing medication. Depressive reactions have been described in children with epilepsy or structural brain damage (Ounsted,

1955), and also transient dyskinetic states with fine hand tremors and orofacial tics (Bradley, 1950; Connors, 1973) not justifying cessation of therapy unless severe. When stimulants are prescribed, the clinicians must monitor the child's behaviour closely and ensure parental co-operation with the administration of the drug. The unexpected appearance of distressing side-effects, of irritability, tics, euphoria or nightmare (Werry & Sprague, 1974) will not only affect parental compliance with the treatment programme but may compromise any future psycho-pharmacological endeavours. Height and weight changes should be monitored on a percentile-related growth chart in view of Safer's findings of retarded growth over a 3-year period of treatment (Safer *et al.*, 1972). Regrettably, whilst stimulant drug therapy does facilitate short-term management of learning-disordered hyperactive children, research would suggest that it has little impact on the child's long-term social, emotional and academic adjustment (Minde, 1978; Huessy, 1974; Weiss *et al.*, 1975).

Tricyclic drugs

The biological mechanisms of antidepressant activity in the immature CNS remain a major research issue. Rapoport *et al.* (1974) have shown that imipramine has acute 'anti-hyperactive' effects, comparable with those of stimulants. The short-term efficiency of tricyclics, together with the observation from pharmacokinetic studies (Brown *et al.*, 1981), suggests that the main behavioural effects of stimulants are observed during the acute release of catecholamines, particularly noradrenaline. Winsberg *et al.*, (1972) in a double-blind trial found a significantly reduced rate of aggressive and overactive behaviour in two thirds of their group of 41 children, aged 5–13 years, treated with imipramine in a dose not exceeding 15 mg/day, 61% having an additional diagnosis of organic brain disease based on indices of high obstetrical adversity, the presence of developmental deviations and of accidents to the CNS.

Gittelman-Klein & Klein (1971) in a double blind trial, using dosages of imipramine in the order of 100–200 mg per day, after 6 six weeks' treatment reported that four-fifths of the treatment group were attending school, almost twice as many as the control group. There was a lessening of observed depressed mood, phobic avoidance behaviour and somatic symptoms in the imipramine group. Tricyclics can be prescribed to children with seizures who are already receiving anticonvulsant medication, but careful monitoring is required. In epileptic children presenting a recent mood change, a fall-off in academic achievement and a positive family history of depression, Weinberg *et al.* (1973) advocate a short-term trial of tricyclics. Imipramine's provocative action which may slightly increase the frequency of seizures means that dosages should be maintained at a low level. Young people do not show the delayed response effect recognized in their adult counterparts and if there is a failure to demonstrate results within 2 weeks, the drug should be abandoned.

Tricyclics are tolerated well by children. Used in therapeutic doses, side-effects are uncommon and may be relieved by a reduction in dosage. Children are less tolerant of sedative side-effects, of blurred vision and fine tremor, which not infrequently interfere with scholastic ability. Yepes *et al.* (1977) found ECG abnormalities among their population of children receiving imipramine pharmacotherapy. The United States Department of Health, Food and Drug Administration have recommended ECG monitoring of children as follows: when the total daily dose approaches 90 mg for an 18 kg child; 110 mg for 22.5 kg; 135 mg for 27 kg; 180 mg for 36 kg (Hayes *et al.*, 1975).

Major tranquillizers
A number of well controlled and carefully evaluated studies have shown that children with severe emotional behaviours may benefit from treatment with phenothiazines or butyrophenones (Garfield *et al.*, 1962; Anderton & Hoddinott, 1964; Werry *et al.*, 1976; Barker, 1975; Alexandris & Lundell, 1968). Response to medication is characterized by lessening of aggressive and oppositional behaviour; children become easier to manage, concentrate better and are less argumentative and aggressive with other children. Tranquillizers may reduce gross motor activity but have little effect on restless and fidgety activity. Le Vann (1971) in a double-blind trial comparing haloperidol with chlorpromazine in behaviourally disturbed mentally handicapped children, found a significant reduction in impulsiveness, hostility and aggressiveness, haloperidol being superior to chlorpromazine. McAndrew *et al.* (1972) noted rapid improvement in motor performance on the Stanford Achievement Battery tests in a small number of children after withdrawing them from long-term phenothiazine therapy. Clinically, benefits from improved concentration and a return to prosocial behaviour have to be weighed against simultaneous deficit of cognitive function.

Recommended dosage of haloperidol is 0.05−0.1 mg/kg body weight in 24 hours, in divided doses, increasing at fortnightly intervals until therapeutic response is obtained. Doses in excess of 0.07 mg/kg/day should warrant simultaneous administration of an antiparkinsonian agent (Barker, 1975). In the author's experience, older children and teenagers can be highly sensitive to haloperidol in high doses, with marked dystonic reactions and other extrapyramidal side-effects. Intravenous procyclidine produces a dramatic relief of dystonic symptoms. An increase in seizure frequency in epileptic children may be seen. Adverse effects from long term usage of major tranquillizers have been reported (Polizos *et al.*, 1973). A dyskinetic syndrome characterized by ataxia and choreiform movements, starting within 48–72 hours after discontinuation of medication is described by McAndrew *et al.* (1972). Symptoms abate with the reintroduction of phenothiazines but are unresponsive to antiparkinsonian agents, remitting spontaneously some months after drug withdrawal.

Anxiolytics

There is considerable doubt as to the effectiveness of benzodiazepines in young children (Zrull *et al*, 1964; Lucas & Pasley, 1969). Diazepam in daily doses of 5 to 20 mg failed to relieve anxiety and tension and in some cases seemed to increase anxiety and disturbed behaviour. Benzodiazepines continue to be widely prescribed by family doctors and paediatricians despite a significant lack of evidence in the literature of their long-term benefits.

Anticonvulsants

It has been claimed that anticonvulsants are effective in a variety of childhood disorders but they have not found a place in current child psychiatric practice. In one much quoted study (Dalby, 1971), 93 patients with psychomotor epilepsy were treated with carbamazepine for periods up to 6 years. More than 50% of the patients were psychiatrically disturbed at the outset and a substantial number of them improved during the treatment phase. These improvements were, however, significantly related to better control of seizures and to the withdrawal of previous anticonvulsant therapy with their socially handicapping side-effects. In five patients with known cerebral degeneration, the administration of carbamazepine was associated with the onset of severe mental disorder. Carbamazepine may therefore be contra-indicated in similarly brain-damaged individuals.

The large-scale controlled studies of Moffatt *et al.* (1970) and Al-
Kaishi & McGuire (1974) on sulthiame have reported significant reduction of excitement and aggression in severely mentally handicapped
patients suffering from epilepsy and showing gross behaviour disorder.
Phenytoin has been implicated in the development of a wide range of
psychiatric disorders, including conversion hysteria (Neidermeyer *et al.*,
1970) delusional states (Hoaken & Kane, 1963) and schizophrenia (Peters
1962), associated with long-term administration of the drug. The importance of recognizing a phenytoin encephalopathy cannot be too
strongly reiterated when there is a sudden change in a child's mood,
associated with an increase of fit frequency and the development of focal
neurological signs, choreoathetosis or dystonia (Glaser, 1972; McLellan
& Swash, 1974). Vallarta *et al.* (1974) and Logan & Freeman (1969) have
emphasized that toxicity may occur in children within previously well-
tolerated dosages and that cerebellar signs may be absent. Folic acid
deficiency in patients receiving long-term anticonvulsant therapy has been
associated with an increased incidence of pyramidal tract damage and
organic brain syndromes (Reynolds *et al.*, 1973). Depression and psychotic
states have been linked with high doses of sulthiame (Green & Kupferberg,
1972; Jeavons, 1975). These also occur as side-effects of ethosuximide
(Roger *et al.*, 1968). The debate on adverse effects of anticonvulsants on
cognitive processes in childhood continues. Barbiturates are known to
impair performance on vigilance tests; ethosuximide is capable of promoting a selective improvement in verbal skills in children with specific
learning disabilities (Smith *et al.*, 1968). The reading skills of epileptic
children taking phenytoin attending ordinary schools were found to be
significantly inferior to those taking other anticonvulsants over a 2-year
period (Stores & Hart, 1976). There is increasing evidence that long-term
use of anticonvulsants may be responsible for a variety of psychiatric
syndromes in childhood, those with structural brain damage being
particularly vulnerable.

On the basis of well-controlled drug studies, psychoactive medications
are effective in the management of the neuropsychiatrically disordered
child. However, the use of psychotropic medication in children will only
lead to the erroneous conclusion that the child's problems lie entirely
within himself and that the solution is medical rather than social or
political. Psychosocial factors should not be underestimated in planning
treatment programmes (Werry, 1979). Although psychiatric drug therapy
research is still in its infancy, positive trends are towards more target-
specific drugs, and for drugs to be used sparingly and with consideration

of a low incidence of long-term effects on cognitive function and behaviour.

Prognosis

There is a marked paucity of follow-up studies in the psychiatric literature on the neurologically impaired child population. Menkes *et al.* (1967) carried out a long-term study of 18 untreated brain-injured hyperactive children diagnosed retrospectively. Twenty-five years on less than one quarter (21%) were persistently hyperactive; one third were institutionalized with a psychotic illness; over one quarter were dependent on relatives. Of the 11 patients examined neurologically, eight had evidence of persisting neurological dysfunction, including intention tremor, poor co-ordination and impaired gait. One patient had a partial expressive and receptive aphasia and resting tremor. Six patients performed poorly on the Bender Gestalt test. From the Robins (1972) study, 17% of the epileptic and 33% of the post-traumatic group were diagnosed as sociopathic, these differences not achieving statistical significance. Ounsted (1981) offers an optimistic view of the adult adjustment of children diagnosed as having temporal lobe epilepsy and followed up for 30 years. Of the initial 74 patients diagnosed as suffering from TLE and concomittant psychiatric disorder, only 30% were disturbed as adults. Of the hyperkinetic subgroup, however, over half had developed psychiatric illness (two with a psychotic illness and five diagnosed antisocial). Of 29 children diagnosed as having pathological rage reactions in 1964, 16 (55%) were psychiatrically disturbed by 1977, indicating the significance of aggression as a prognostic indicator for poor social adjustment in adult-hood. One in 10 of the group had developed schizophreniform psychoses, eight males, one female. EEGs showed that seven of the psychotic group had left sided foci and two had bilateral discharges. All had continued on anticonvulsants and all had active seizures. Of the 10 males and two females exhibiting persisting antisocial behaviour, in six of the seven cases who were subsequently convicted it was for assault or criminal damage. Eleven of the 12 with antisocial behaviour had foci contralateral to the preferred hand, and 10 patients had had severe grand mal epilepsy in childhood.

The last decade has seen a revolution in the field of Child Psychiatry and Paediatric Neurology and the development of areas of common interest. New methods of treatment have been introduced, and clinical trials are currently being undertaken. Situational factors as contributors to illness have been more appreciated. No longer are specialists faced with their own feelings of helplessness and frustration when confronted by the severely handicapped child. Psychological techniques can be curative and offer a means of enhancing the handicapped child's self worth and of giving support to the family; in sum, effective preventive mental health.

Liaison psychiatry

Over the past two decades there has been an increasing involvement of the psychiatrist in general hospital practice to the benefit of many patients, particularly when there are problems of management. The psychiatric contribution includes the assessment of factors producing or maintaining symptoms, the treatment of psychiatric disorders arising in the setting of organic illness (Nabarro, 1984; Bridges & Goldberg, 1984) or when such disorders present with physical symptoms and help with the management of psychosomatic disorders such as asthma. Also, their advice can often be of benefit to the dying child and family, and to the staff of such units as intensive care and oncology (Gomez, 1981). Occasional joint ward rounds can play an important preventive role when problems likely to arise in the future can be discussed.

Many paediatric problems can be helped in this way. They may not be sufficiently complex to warrant a formal referral to a Child Psychiatric Department, which may be unacceptable to some parents, but the approach of the child psychiatrist is a necessary part of their assessment and investigation, with the emphasis on childhood and family illness experience and the chronology of life events (Gomez, 1981). A good example may be the diagnosis of unusual seizures. Are these of an epileptic nature, or are they of psychogenic origin, or does the child have attacks of both kinds? In the past, Departments of Child Psychiatry have tended to be isolated but this is no longer acceptable and they should be fully integrated into the work of a general hospital.

References

Alderton, H.R. & Hoddinott, B.A. (1964) A controlled study of the use of Thioridazine in the treatment of hyperactive and aggressive children in a children's psychiatric hospital. *Canadian Psychiatric Association Journal*, **9**, 239–247.

Alexandris, A. & Lundell, F.W. (1968) Effects of Thioridazine, Amphetamine and placebo on the hyperkinetic syndrome and cognitive area in mentally deficient children. *Canadian Medical Association Journal*, **98**, 92–96.

Al-Kaishi A.H. & McGuire, R.J. (1974) The effect of Sulthiame on disturbed behaviour in mentally subnormal patients. *British Journal of Psychiatry*, **124**, 45−49.

Allen, F.H. & Pearson, G.H.J. (1928) The Emotional Problems of the physically handicapped child. *British Journal of Medical Psychology*, **8**, 212−235.

Barker, P. (1975) Haloperidol. *Journal of Child Psychology and Psychiatry*, **16**, 169−172.

Barkley, R.A. (1977) A review of stimulant drug research with hyperactive children. *Journal of Child Psychology and Psychiatry*, **18**, 137−165.

Battle, C.V. (1972) The role of the paediatrician as ombudsman in the health care of the young handicapped child. *Pediatrics*, **50**, 191−196.

Beck, A.T. (1976) *Cognitive Therapy and the Emotional Disorders*. International Universities Press, New York.

Beiser, H.R. (1955) Play equipment for diagnosis and therapy in play techniques *American Journal of Orthopsychiatry*, **25**, 761−770.

Bender, L. (1956) Post-encephalitic behaviour disorders in childhood. In *Encephalitis, A Clinical Study* (ed. J.B. Neal). Grune and Stratton, New York.

Berg, I. (1974) A self-administered dependency questionnaire (SADQ) for use with mothers of schoolchildren. *British Journal of Psychiatry*, **124**, 1−9.

Berkowitz, B.P. & Graziano, A.M. (1972) Training parents as behaviour therapists: A review. *Behaviour Research and Therapy*, **10**, 297−317.

Bridges, K.W. & Goldberg, D.P. (1984) Psychiatric illness in inpatients with neurological disorders: patients' views on discussion of emotional problems with neurologists. *British Medical Journal*, **289**, 656−658.

Brown, G., Chadwick, D., Shaffer, D., Rutter, M. & Traub, M. (1981) A prospective study of children with head injuries. III Psychiatric sequelae. *Psychological Medicine*, **II**, 63−78.

Brown, G.W. & Davidson, S. (1978) Social class, psychiatric disorder of mother and accidents to children. *Lancet*, i, 378−381.

Chadwick, O., Rutter, M., Brown, G., Shaffer, D. & Traub, M. (1981) A prospective study of children with head injuries: II Cognitive sequelae. *Psychological Medicine*, **II**, 49−61.

Committee on Child Health Services (1976) 'Fit for the Future'. H.M.S.O., London.

Committee of enquiry into the education of handicapped children and young people. (1978) 'Special Educational Needs'. H.M.S.O., London.

Comrey, A.L., Backer, T.E. & Glaser, E.M. (1973) *A Sourcebook for Mental Health Measures*. National Institute for Mental Health, Maryland, U.S.A.

Conners, C.K. (1973) Rating scales for use in drug studies with children. *Psychopharmacology Bulletin Special Supplement to* **Vol. 9** Pharmocotherapy in Children, 24−84.

Conners, C.K. (1981) Rating scales. In *American Handbook of Psychiatry* (ed. S. Arieti *et al.*), pps. 675−685.

Cowen, G.L., Pederson, A., Babigian, H., Izzo, L.D. & Trost, M.A. (1973) Long term follow-up of early detected vulnerable children. *Journal of Consulting and Clinical Psychology*, **41**, 438−446.

Cox, A. & Rutter, M. (1975) Diagnostic appraisal and interviewing. In *Child Psychiatry: Modern Approaches* (eds M. Rutter and L. Hersov). Blackwell, Scientific, Oxford.

Craft, A.W., Shaw, D.A. & Cartlidge, N.E. (1972) Head injuries in children. *British Medical Journal*, iii, 200−203.

Dalby, M.A. (1971) Anti-epileptic and psychotropic effect of Carbamazepine (Tegretol) in the treatment of psychomotor epilepsy. *Epilepsia*, **12**, 325−334.

Department of Health and Social Security and the Welsh Office (1969) *People with epilepsy* (Report of a Joint Sub-committee of the Standing Medical Advisory

Committee on health and welfare of handicapped persons). H.M.S.O., London.

Erikson, E.H. (1965) The eight ages of man. Chap. 7 in *'Childhood and Society'*. Penguin Books, London.

Gardner, R. (1974) *Therapeutic Communications with Children: The Mutual Story-telling Technique*. Aronson, New York.

Garfield, S.L., Helper, M.M., Williott, R.C. & Muffly, R. (1962) Effects of chlorpromazine on behaviour in emotionally disturbed children. *Journal of Nervous and Mental Diseases,* **135**, 147–154.

Gittelman-Klein, R. & Klein, D.F. (1971) Controlled Imipramine treatment of school phobia. *Archives of General Psychiatry*, **25**, 204–207.

Glaser, G.H. (1972) Diphenylhydantoin toxicity. In *Anti-epileptic drugs* (eds D.M. Woodbury, J.K. Penry & R.R. Schmidt). Raven Press, New York.

Gomez, J. (1981) Liaison psychiatry. *British Journal of Hospital Medicine*, **22**, 242–246.

Green, J.R. & Kupferberg, H.J. (1972) Sulphonamides and derivatives; sulthiame In *Anti-epileptic drugs* (eds D. Woodbury, J.K. Penry & R.R. Schmidt). Raven Press, New York.

Hayes, T.A., Panitch, M.L. & Barker E (1975) Imipramine dosage in children: a comment on Imipramine and electrocardiographic abnormalities in hyperactive children. *American Journal of Psychiatry*, **132**, 546–547.

Hoaken P.C.S. & Kane F.J. (1963) Unusual brain syndrome with diphenylhydantoin and pentobarbital. *American Journal of Psychiatry* **120**, 282–283.

Huessy, H.R. (1974) The adult hyperkinetic. *American Journal of Psychiatry*, **131.6**, 724–25.

Jeavons, P.M. (1975) The practical management of epilepsy. *Hospital Update*, **1**, 11–22.

Kalverboer, A.F. (1975) Measurement of play: clinical applications, Chap. 8, in *A Neurobehavioural Study in Pre-School Children. Clinics in Developmental Medicine*, **54**, 100–22 Spastics International Medical Publications, William Heinemann, London.

Kamp, L.N.J. & Kessler, E.S. (1970) The world test: developmental aspects of a play technique. *Journal of Child Psychology and Psychiatry*, **II**, 81–108.

Le Vann, L.J. (1971) Clinical comparison of Haloperidol with Chlorpromazine in mentally retarded children. *American Journal of Mental Deficiency*, **75**, 719–723.

Levin, S., Rubenstein, J.S. & Streiner, D.C. (1976) The parent therapist programme: an innovative approach to treating emotionally disturbed children. *Hospital and Community Psychiatry*, **27**, 407–410.

Logan, W.J. & Freeman, J.M. (1969) Pseudodegenerative disease due to diphenyl hydantoin intoxication. *Archives of Neurology*, **21**, 631–637.

Lucas, A.R. & Pasley, F.C. (1969) Psychoactive drugs in the treatment of emotionally disturbed children: Haloperidol and Diazepam. *Comprehensive Psychiatry*, **10**, 376–386.

McAndrew, J.B., Case, Q. & Treffert, D.A. (1972) Effect of prolonged phenothiazine intake on psychotic and other hospitalised children. *Journal of Autism and Childhood Schizophrenia*, **2**, 75–91.

McLelland, D.L. & Swash, M. (1974) Choreo-athetosis and encephalopathy induced by phenytoin, *British Medical Journal*, **ii**, 204–205.

MacKeith, R. (1973) Feelings and behaviour of parents of handicapped children. *Developmental Medicine and Child Neurology*, **15**, 524–527.

Meichenbaum, D.H. (1977) *Cognitive Behaviour Modification*. Plenum Press, New York.

Menkes, M., Rowe, J. & Menkes, J. (1967) A twenty-five year follow-up study on the hyperkinetic child with minimal brain dysfunction. *Pediatrics*, **39**, 393–399.

Minde, K.K. (1978) Coping styles of 34 adolescents with cerebral palsy. *American Journal of Psychiatry*, **135**: (**11**), 1344–49.

Moffatt, W.R., Siddiqui, A.R. & MacKay, D.N. (1970) The Use of sulthiame with disturbed mentally subnormal patients. *British Journal of Psychiatry*, **117**, 673–678.

Mooney, R.L. (1950) *Mooney Problem Check List*. Psychological Compactim, New York.

Nabarro, J. (1984) Unrecognised psychiatric illness in medical patients. *British Medical Journal*, **289**, 635–636.

Neider-Myer, E., Blumer, D., Holscher, E. & Walker, B.A. (1970) Classical hysterical seizures facilitated by anticonvulsants toxicity. *Psychiatrica Clinica*, **3**, 71–75.

Newson, J. & Newson, E. (1980) Play and playthings N.I.M.H. (1973). *Psychopharmacology Bulletin*, Special Issue **9**, 196–239.

O'Leary, K.D. & O'Leary, S.G. (1977) *Classroom Management: The Successful Use of Behaviour Modification*. Pergamon, New York.

Ounsted, C. (1955) The hyperkinetic syndrome in epileptic children. *Lancet*, **ii**, **269**, 303–311.

Ounsted, C. (1981) In *Epilepsy and Psychiatry*. (eds E.H. Reynolds and M.R. Trimble). Churchill Livingstone, London.

Peters, H.A. (1962) Anticonvulsant drug intolerance. *Neurology*, **12**, 299.

Philipp, R. (1979) Conducting parent training groups: approaches and strategies. In *New Directions in Children's Mental Health* (ed S.I. Shamsie), Spectrum, New York.

Pless, I.B. & Satterwhite, B. (1975) *Chronic illness In Child Health and the Community* (eds R.J. Hoggarty, K.J. Roghmann, I.B. Pless). Wiley, New York.

Polizos, P., Engelhardt, D.M., Hoffman, S.P. & Waizer, J. (1973) Neurological consequences of psychotropic drug withdrawal in schizophrenic children. *Journal of Autism and Childhood Schizophrenia*, **3**, 247–253.

Quinton, D., Rutter, M. & Rowlands, O. (1976) An evaluation of an interview assessment of marriage. *Psychological Medicine*, **6**, 577–586.

Rapoport, J., Quinn, P.O., Bradbard, G., Riddle, K.D. & Brooks, E. (1974) Imipramine and Methylphenidate treatment of hyperactive boys. *Archives of General Psychiatry*, **30**, 789–793.

Raven, J.C. (1951) *Controlled Projection for Children*. H.K. Lewis, London.

Reynolds, E.H., Rothfield, P. & Pincus, J.H. (1973) Neurological disease associated with folate deficiency. *British Medical Journal*, **ii**, 398–400.

Rich, J. (1968) *Interviewing Children and Adolescents*. Macmillan, London.

Richman, N. & Graham, P.J. (1971) A behavioural screening questionnaire for use with 3 year old children. Preliminary findings. *Journal of Child Psychology and Psychiatry*, **12**, 5–33.

Robins, L.N. (1972) Follow-up studies of behaviour disorders in children. In *Psychopathological Disorders of Childhood* (eds. H.C. Quay and J.S. Werry). Wiley, New York.

Roger, J., Grangeon, H., Guey, J. & Lob, H. (1968) Psychiatric and psychological effects of ethosuximide treatment in epileptics. *Encephale*, **57**, 407–438.

Russell, P. (1978) *The Wheelchair Child*. Souvenir Press, London.

Rutter, M., Graham, P. & Yule, W. (1970a). *A Neuropsychiatric Study in Childhood Clinics in Developmental Medicine No. 35/36*. Spastics International Medical Publications, Heinemann, London.

Rutter, M., Tizard, J. & Whitmore, K (eds) (1970b) *Education, Health and Behaviour.* Longman, London.

Safer, D.J., Allen, R.P. & Barr, E. (1972) Depression of growth in hyperactive children on stimulant drugs. *New England Journal of Medicine*, **287**, 217–220.

Seidel, U.P., Chadwick, O.F.D. & Rutter, M. (1975) Psychological disorder in crippled children. A comparative study of children with and without brain damage. *Developmental Medicine and Child Neurology*, **17**, 563–573.

Simmons, J.E. (1974) *Psychiatric Examination of Children.* Lea and Febiger, Philadelphia.

Smith, W.L., Philippus, M.J. & Guard, H.L. (1968) Psychometric study of children with learning problems and 14–6 positive spike EEG patterns treated with ethosuximide (Zarontin) and placebo. *Archives of Disease in Childhood*, **43**, 616–619.

Snyderman, B., Magnussen, M.G. & Henderson, P.M. (1980) Standardised data collection. Chap 82, in *American Handbook of Psychiatry.* (eds Arieti, Silvano *et al.*), 657–673.

Steinhauer, P.D., Mushin, D.N. & Rae Grant, Q. (1974) Psychological aspects of Chronic Illness. *Pediatric Clinics of North America*, **21**, 825–840.

Sterman, M.B., MacDonald, L.R. & Stone, R.K. (1974) Biofeedback training of the sensorimotor electroencephalogram rhythm in man: effects on epilepsy. *Epilepsia*, **15**, 395–416.

Stores, G. & Hart, J. (1976) Reading skills of children with generalised or focal epilepsy attending ordinary school. *Developmental Medicine and Child Neurology*, **18**, 705–716.

Stores, G. & Piran, N. (1978) Dependency of different types in schoolchildren with epilepsy. *Psychological Medicine*, **8**, 441–445.

Sundby, H.S. & Kreyberg, P.C. (1968) *Prognosis in Child Psychiatry.* Williams and Wilkins, Baltimore.

Taylor, D.C. (1982) Counselling the parents of handicapped children. *British Medical Journal*, **284**, 1027–1028.

Thomas, A., Chess, S. & Birch, H.G. (1968) *Temperament and Behaviour Disorder in Children.* New York University Press, New York.

Thoresen, C.E. & Mahoney, M.J. (1974) *Behavioural Self-Control.* Holt, Rinehart and Winston, New York.

Touwen, B.C.L. & Prechtl, H.F.R. (1979) The Examination of the Child with Minor Neurological Dysfunction. *Clinics in Developmental Medicine No. 71.* Spastics International Medical Publications, Heinemann, London.

Vallarta, J.M., Bell, D.B. & Reichart, A. (1974) Progressive encephalopathy due to chronic hydantoin intoxication. *American Journal of Diseases of Children*, **128**, 27–34.

Weinberg, W.A., Rutman, J., Sullivan, L., Penick, E.C. & Dietz, S.G. (1973) Depression in children referred to an educational diagnostic centre: diagnosis and treatment. *Journal of Pediatrics*, **83**, 1065–1072.

Weiss, G., Kruger, E., Daniel Sen, U. & Elman, M. (1975) Effect of long-term treatment of hyperactive children with methylphenidate. *Canadian Medical Association Journal*, **112**, 159–165.

Werry, J.S., Aman, M.G. & Almpen, E. (1976) Haloperidol and methylphenidate in hyperactive children. *Acta Paedopsychiatrica*, **42**, 26–40.

Werry, J.S. & Sprague (1974) Methylphenidate in hyperactive children—effect of dosage. *Australian and New Zealand Journal of Psychiatry*, **8**, 9–19.

Werry, J.S. (1979) Principles of use of psychotropic drugs. *Drugs*, **18**, 392–397.

Winnicott, D.W. (1971) *Therapeutic Consultations in Psychiatry*. Hogarth Press, London.
Winsberg, B., Bialer, I., Kupietz, S. & Tobias, J. (1972) Effects of Imipramine and Dextroamphetamine on behaviour of neuro-psychiatrically impaired children. *American Journal of Psychiatry*, **128**, 1425–1431.
Yarrow, N.R., Campbell, J.D. & Burton, R.V. (1964) Recollections of childhood: a study of the retrospective method. *Society for Research in Child Development*, **35**.
Yepes, L.E., Balka, E.B., Winsberg, B.G., & Bialer, I.R.V. (1977) Amitriptyline and methylphenidate treatment of behaviourally disordered children. *Journal of Child Psychology and Psychiatry*, **18**, 39–52.
Zrull, J.P., Westman, J.C., Arthur, B. & Rice, D.L. (1964) A comparison of diazepam, d-amphetamine and placebo in the treatment of the hyperkinetic syndrome in children. *American Journal of Psychiatry*, **120**, 590–591.

Chapter 15
Adolescents with Chronic Neurological Disease

Lewis Rosenbloom

Chronic neurological disorder in adolescence

It is difficult to define either when childhood ends or to be specific on what constitutes adolescence. This is especially true when there are abnormalities or immaturities of neurological function producing physical or mental retardation in young people. Normally those processes of social, psychological, physical and sexual maturation that are termed adolescence will occur at some period between 12 and 20 years of age. Boys and girls at this time are concerned with their developing sense of personal identity, the need to conform with their peers, educational and vocational aspirations, their appearance, relationships with the opposite sex and not least, the need to break away from dependence on their parents. Their families likewise have to come to terms with all of these and effectively promote the adolescent's independence. Stress at this period is common and the additional stress of a chronic neurological disorder can not only produce specific management problems but can also jeopardise many of the aspirations of adolescence.

The commonest chronic neurological disorders of adolescence are mental handicap and epilepsy. Physical handicaps, especially cerebral palsy and spina bifida also have an appreciable incidence. In addition, there are a number of specific conditions, including Duchenne muscular dystrophy and other myopathies, the longer term effects of specific learning and language disorders and neurological problems arising *de novo* such as cerebral tumours, multiple sclerosis, psychoses and degenerative disorders.

The treatment of neurological disease during the adolescent period needs to be based upon a number of general considerations. Firstly, the natural history of the disorder needs to be known and it is significant that for many of the conditions enumerated, knowledge is far from complete. Secondly, the relevance of intervention and therapy programmes during infancy and childhood to the pattern of disability that will be seen later in adolescence needs to be considered in respect to both the children and their families. Thirdly, the effect and relevance of intervention and therapy programmes during the adolescent period itself merits consideration. Fourthly, there is a need for appropriate provision of health, social, educational and employment services for neurologically handicapped individuals both at adolescence and beyond.

In practice, it is well recognized that the interface between paediatric and adult neurological practice is not distinguished by well developed service models. To this must be added a lack of statutory educational or social provision for handicapped adolescents and this has produced the bizarre position in the United Kingdom in which often excellent services for the young handicapped children come to a halt as school leaving age is reached. In this chapter consideration will firstly be given to some aspects of specific neurological disabilities in adolescence. Thereafter, the wider issues that are common throughout the age group, notably the need to promote independence, will be discussed. Finally, a comment will be made on the provision of medical services for handicapped adolescents.

Mental handicap

Those adolescents whose primary disability is cognitive will normally have attended a special school for either moderately retarded (ESN(M)) or severely retarded (ESN(S)) children. A proportion will, however, have attended a normal school or some other type of special school such as one for delicate or physically handicapped children, whilst at the other end of the spectrum some profoundly handicapped individuals will have spent long periods of their childhood in institutions. The key issue for mentally handicapped adolescents relates to the degree of social independence which they can eventually attain and the evaluation and promotion of this should be paramount throughout childhood. Academic and social skills that are taught to individual mentally handicapped children should, as far as possible, be geared to this end. However, there are pitfalls to prediction. Whilst on the one hand it is usually possible to predict future competence within very broad limits as a result of assessment in the first 5 years, it is true also that there is ignorance of the natural history of certain aspects of development in the mentally handicapped. For example, the normal pattern and evolution of language development in this group of children is incompletely defined. It is known that children (no matter how severely retarded) can continue to learn and acquire social skills throughout adolescence and early adult life. Thus, formal education opportunities beginning from 2 years of age could extend for 20 years or more.

These points have implications for both educational methods and curricula and it is necessary to define and monitor teaching objectives and educational programmes. Appropriate teacher training should have a high priority and parental involvement in teaching children, especially beyond 16 years of age, is relatively untapped. Another resource that could be made available is the optional extension of the school leaving age for some mentally handicapped individuals to 19 or 20 years of age. In theory, therefore, there are opportunities for promoting learning in the mentally handicapped adolescent as a result of appropriate input both during adolescence and in earlier childhood.

Other learning disorders
Examples of these include developmental language disorders, specific disabilities (for example of reading) and poor motor learning, manifested clinically as clumsiness and often secondary to spatial or perceptual disorders. The natural history into adolescence of all of these is largely unknown but there is evidence that they do not always resolve. Thus, 50% of 5-year-olds who are placed in classes for those with language disabilities still have subtle linguistic difficulties of semantic and syntatic type when they leave school (Ludlow, 1980). Some individuals with specific reading disabilities retain these throughout life and may transmit them to their own offspring. The same would appear to apply to some children with perceptual problems and with other causes of poor motor learning producing clumsiness.

Whilst management of these problems before adolescence is aimed both at minimizing the primary disorder and reducing secondary emotional problems, treatment in adolescence itself can usually be geared towards by-passing the difficulty. For example, a clumsy adolescent no longer has to do physical education in school and one with poor handwriting can use a typewriter. In such children the emotional maturation that accompanies adolescence is important in enabling them to come to terms with their disability. Much the same can be said about the management of stammering; whatever the origins of this disorder of speech production, its treatment during childhood is often disappointing. On the other hand, group therapy of adolescents and young adults seems to offer a more appropriate setting and motivation for improvement. The key to the management of this loose grouping of not so severe learning disabilities therefore lies essentially in an appreciation of their chronicity.

Physical disabilities in the mentally handicapped

Many severely retarded individuals also have motor or sensory disabilities. In childhood it is usually pointed out that such problems can summate and that each needs to be tackled so that the individual may reach his or her full potential. Whilst this principle continues to hold during adolescence, it is equally true that realism with regard to both potential and achievement is essential. Thus, as a child becomes older the acquisition of new physical skills becomes less likely and decisions, for example, on how much independent walking should be promoted and on the management of such problems as hip dislocation and scoliosis, need to be made. The key in such circumstances is whether independence or overall care is going to be helped by treatment of physical disabilities in the multiply handicapped individual. Where progress is unlikely, then physical therapy regimes and orthopaedic procedures are inappropriate. Whilst it is sometimes hard not to offer help that is technically possible to such individuals, the decision is made easier if it is taken jointly with the parents as part of a long-term and multidisciplinary programme of advice and treatment for their child.

Behavioural difficulties in the mentally handicapped

A somewhat artificial but nevertheless helpful distinction can be made between those behavioural abnormalities that are co-incidental and those which can be considered to be an integral part of the primary disability of mental handicap. So far as the former are concerned there is an increased incidence in a mentally handicapped population of the same behavioural and psychiatric disorders that occur in the normal population. Their identification and management can be far from easy, largely as a result of the accompanying communication problems. This should be one of the roles of the medical specialist in mental handicap, although the availability of relevant resources varies. It is encouraging that this medical speciality is changing from a supervisory, custodial and administrative role to a psychiatric one, but problems of recruitment, expertise and relationships with other services remain.

Those behavioural abnormalities which are integral to mental retardation tend to be present from early in childhood and can occur initially as an exaggerated persistence of some of the characteristics of normal infancy. Behaviours such as hyperkinesis and poor attention, however, interfere with learning, making the mental handicap that much more severe. It is usually said that overactive behaviour gradually lessens throughout childhood and into adolescence. Clinical experience would appear to indicate that whilst this is true for less severely mentally handicapped individuals, it does not always hold for those who are severely handicapped. These individuals are not helped to learn by being over-active and disinhibited and the use of either stimulant or sedative drugs may well be worth a trial during adolescence. Their use needs to be closely monitored and to be part of an overall management programme in which therapeutic aims are clearly defined.

Autistic behaviour

The combination of social withdrawal, obsessional behaviour and linguistic abnormality usually carries an adverse developmental prognosis but this is particularly so when, as it usually is, there is associated mental retardation. Management both in childhood and adolescence of autistic individuals must not only concentrate upon the provision of some linguistic skills. Social skills must also, if possible, be taught with the appreciation that autistic individuals cannot generalize from the particular so that a lot of very specific behaviours need to be learned. Even given appropriate teaching, there needs to be an appreciation that autistic individuals will always be more socially inadequate and naive than can be expected from their mental level. Hence, in adolescence and beyond, autistic people will need a relatively greater degree of protection, and sheltered communities and similar provisions need to be made available.

Physical disabilities

Cerebral palsy

The evolving disorder of motor function that is the primary feature of cerebral palsy continues to change throughout adolescence and after-wards. In a probable association with the withdrawal of physiotherapy and educational and social support at school-leaving age, many young people with cerebral palsy lose a precariously acquired mobility, and there is also a significant increase in the development of contractures and deformities over the next decade. Given the importance of mobility in promoting any sort of independence, together with the discomfort and inconvenience of deformities, it is advisable that multi-disciplinary services, including physiotherapy, should continue to be available for individuals with cerebral palsy after they leave school.

Spina bifida

In addition to the general problems of withdrawal of school-based supporting facilities, many boys and girls with spina bifida face increasing
problems in their own right. Valve disorders continue to occur or present
afresh, renal failure can develop and scoliosis with its accompanying
danger of respiratory failure can become more obvious. Systems for the
integration of care for spina bifida children vary. They are usually co-
ordinated by either paediatricians or paediatric surgeons and there is
frequently a high degree of dependence of the child and the family on
either school or hospital based services. To lose both services, at a time
when the spina bifida sufferer's problems are not being reduced in any
way, commonly leads to deficits of care, and measures for alleviating these
are discussed subsequently in this chapter.

Muscular dystrophy

Those with a special interest in the care of neuromuscular disorders in
childhood are frequently strong advocates of an aggressive approach
towards maintaining independence and mobility in boys suffering from
Duchenne muscular dystrophy. There can be little doubt that the wise use
of appliances, surgery and other aids to mobility prolongs independent
walking. This approach is greatly devalued, however, if the relevant
support is withdrawn at about school-leaving age. Most boys with muscular dystrophy have the additional appreciation of their likely deterioration and short life span, and relevant support for them and their families
in the second decade is essential.

Epilepsy in adolescence

The majority of children with epilepsy become adolescents with epilepsy
and the disease can also arise *de novo* in this age group. The subject has
recently been reviewed by O'Donohoe (1985). When convulsions
commence for the first time in adolescence it is important that a diagnosis
be made. Primary generalized epilepsy of the grand mal type and temporal lobe epilepsy may present for the first time in the teens, as also may
the much less common myoclonic epilepsies of adolescence.

The other side of the coin is that the differential diagnosis of epilepsy
in adolescence also includes syncopal attacks and hysteria. The principles

of successful management must be based on obtaining the co-operation of the patient, and both boys and girls need constant support and encouragement, together with family counselling and vocational planning. Drug treatment presents not only difficulties of compliance but also of side-effects, both cosmetic and depressant. Activities should be limited as little as is legal and possible, but a history of convulsions should always be declared on a driving licence application. It may be advisable for the young person with epilepsy to wear an identification bracelet. The question of withdrawal of anticonvulsant medication often arises during adolescence and there is much to be said for the attempt being made in order to avoid the employment and social disadvantages of the epilepsy label. A seizure-free period of up to 2−4 years in individuals of normal intelligence and without underlying neurological disease or serious psychological disorder, and slow and cautious drug withdrawal, are all factors in favour of successful cessation of therapy.

Puberty

For all practical purposes sexual maturation will occur in all adolescents with chronic neurological handicaps. Mental and physical disability, however, adds a number of practical problems to those that face all adolescents. Thus, there are major differences between the handicapped and normal populations in how children learn about puberty, sexual maturation, relationships and specific topics such as conception, contraception, birth, abortion and sexually transmitted disease. The normal population not only has the availability of a partially informed peer group but also, more often than not, a specific sex education curriculum. Normal children are also more likely to obtain relevant information from their own families.

The handicapped population loses out on all of these counts. The peer group with its wide age range and limited social opportunities has virtually no knowledge, inaccurate or otherwise, to pass on. In special schools, sex education curricula are often token or non-existent. Where the subject is taught, much time is often given to imparting biological information and little to discussing relationships or offering practical advice. The position in schools for the moderately severely mentally handicapped (ESN(M)) has been fully discussed by Watson and Rogers (1980). They point out that ESN(M) children are usually found to be lacking in knowledge, but can be helped by appropriately structured teaching programmes. Families too are more likely to fight shy of discussion of sexual matters with their handicapped offspring, in part because of communication difficulties and in part because it is not traditional to accept their developing sexuality.

For those individuals who, because they are severely mentally handicapped or have multiple disabilities cannot reasonably be expected to function independently within society, a number of practical problems need to be faced. For girls the first of these is the problem of menstruation. Here it is most reasonable to await events and it is surprising how few individuals cannot cope with normal menstrual hygiene. In exceptional circumstances, control of menstrual flow by use of progesterone derivatives may be helpful and rarely hysterectomy is indicated, although the problem of obtaining informed consent does not make this a popular option (Kreutner, 1981). Masturbation in both boys and girls can usually be managed, as can other inappropriate self-stimulating behaviours by a suitable behaviour modification programme, and other specific measures are not normally indicated. The severely handicapped population has not hitherto needed a large input of advice on such matters as contraception, abortion and sexually transmitted disease. However, increasing moves towards integration into the community and mixing of the sexes within institutions imply that consideration will have to be given on how best to provide both protection and appropriate information. In situations where abortion and sterilization are involved, there is again the difficult problem of what constitutes informed consent.

For more moderately mentally or for physically handicapped individuals who might reasonably be expected to function independently within society, the problems are somewhat different. Historically, sexuality, marriage and reproduction have been discouraged for this group, with eugenic reasons being cited. Whilst these are no longer prominent, the children's own education and experiences, together with current social attitudes and economic constraints, continue to act as deterring factors. It has to be said also, that for the offspring of some handicapped individuals there is an increased chance of their having genetically transmitted disorders, whilst for many there is likely to be a poverty of cultural and social experience as a result of their parents' limitations. Where possible, therefore, informed genetic counselling to handicapped adolescents intending to have children must be offered.

In practice, a balance has to be drawn between giving moderately handicapped adolescents freedom to run their own lives on the one hand, and constraining them and protecting them for their own safety and for the sake of their offspring on the other. Our uncertainty is hardly ever satisfactory for either the individuals concerned or for helping agencies, and says much for our ignorance of how to promote independence and to provide relevant help.

Independence, employment and leisure

The fundamental question facing the handicapped adolescent relates to his potential capacity for independence. The likelihood that youngsters will be capable of coping alone depends on their inherent intelligence, drive and mobility. Beyond these, however, the willingness of the family to withdraw its total care, the problems of finding suitable accommodation and the major task of finding a job in a world where work even for the able bodied school leaver is difficult are all significant obstacles.

In practice, the majority of families continue to care for their handicapped children into and beyond adolescence and accept that they should do so. Even when this is particularly likely, however, because of the profundity of the child's handicap it is imperative that families are helped to make their own reasoned decisions at an early stage on how much independence they want both for their handicapped child and themselves. There is nothing more tragic than the mother of a totally dependent adolescent with multiple handicaps who has never spent a day or night apart from her child. The seeds for separation need to be sown very much earlier, and consistent and practical counselling is needed on this point.

Other provisions for handicapped school leavers have been detailed by Chamberlain (1981). The alternatives include entry to youth opportunity programmes, where they must compete with the able bodied, or entering further, or higher education or vocational training. Within the group of provisions, facilities for the physically handicapped are somewhat better than for the mentally handicapped, largely because of the contribution made by voluntary organizations such as the Spastics Society. There is, however, an appalling lack of local provision in many areas in the United Kingdom.

The handicapped school leaver can enter open or sheltered employment, but any sort of employment is available only to the smallest minority of children. In the former case adequate mobility, especially for the physically handicapped, is crucial. A further minority have day or residential care provided for them by local authorities or by the health service, but such care may be part time and the number of places and range of provision is very limited. These difficulties are exemplified in a recent study by Castree and Walker (1981) on young adults with cerebral palsy and spina bifida. They showed that less than one third of these individuals are in open employment while two thirds either attended day centres or were unoccupied. This study again emphasized that mobility is of over-riding importance in obtaining and maintaining employment.

Only a minority of handicapped adolescents aspire to live away from home. Whilst the majority have a theoretical interest in acquiring boy or girl friends and being married, in practice very many lose the social contacts they had at school and become increasingly socially isolated. The use of leisure by mentally handicapped adolescents has been investigated by Cheseldine and Jeffree (1981). An investigation into the national provision for leisure time activities by organized bodies showed in theory that this was reasonably comprehensive. Nevertheless, a subsequent survey of more than 200 individual families demonstrated that these leisure facilities were largely unused. Instead, the young people mainly participated in solitary passive activities which were family orientated (with the exception of attendance at special clubs). It is likely that this situation derives from the attitudes of parents who fully accept a role as sole providers of care and recreation. This contributes to a lack of awareness of social provisions and needs, as also does a lack of local friendships for handicapped adolescents outside their school environment.

The promotion of more independence would entail more realistic counselling of parents at a very early stage, the provision of more employment facilities including the availability of transport and the education of the young people themselves at an earlier age towards a more realistic appreciation of their disabilities and how to circumvent them. Special schemes such as those for sheltered housing, as well as employment, need to be developed.

Service development and provision

An account of chronic neurological disorder in adolescence is more illustrative of the gaps in available therapy than of successful management schemes. The gaps are medical, educational and social. The withdrawal of paediatric support and co-ordination of medical care at this period is not balanced by the introduction of other patterns of medical help. Given that educational continuity is also usually lost at this time, the argument could be put forward that where health care is needed for the handicapped adolescent this should continue to be provided by a paediatric service. This has implications for the training of paediatricians and how they should use the resources available to them. It could mean, for example, rather less investment in the early identification and care of young handicapped children and correspondingly more provision of facilities at the other end of the paediatric age range. This could be specifically relevant for the organization of community child health services. A degree of development of both in-patient and out-patient paediatric care would be needed. For in-patients it could be envisaged that those few handicapped adolescents who require hospital admission would be in an adolescent ward in which a paediatrician had overall medical administrative charge but which was attended by other relevant adult and paediatric specialists as needed. For out-patients there is much to be said for having specific facilities for adolescents. Again, it could be envisaged that their medical care would normally be undertaken by an appropriately trained paediatrician working in consultation with other specialists when necessary. Fuller involvement in the medical care of adolescents, therefore, could well be considered to be part of the natural evolution of paediatrics, especially if it is appreciated that the speciality is likely to change in any case as a result of changing patterns of childhood disease and its treatment.

Running parallel with the need for co-ordination of medical care is a need for more research and investment in the educational, employment and social needs of adolescents with chronic neurological disorders. The school leaving age of 16 is often voluntarily extended by some individuals and institutions. As the school population falls this could become more common, but does need to be combined with more knowledge on the best ways to teach mentally handicapped teenagers and on how to promote more independence for the physically handicapped. Resources need to be made available both for these developments and for more integration of the handicapped with the able bodied in further and higher education. Financial constraints normally limit initiatives that could provide handicapped young people with work and it might be appropriate if voluntary organizations could establish individual initiatives. For some organizations this might well involve a switch in their use of resources from concentration upon the needs of young handicapped children.

A similar argument can be developed with regard to housing. At a time when mental subnormality hospitals are no longer either encouraged or considered to be appropriate residential placements for handicapped people who are not in need of medical or nursing treatment, there is a poverty of alternative provision. It might be appropriate if local authorities, working in conjunction with voluntary organizations, could contribute towards sheltered housing, and this also might involve a redeployment of financial resources.

For the present, the care of the individual adolescent with a chronic handicap provides a multidisciplinary challenge. Much can be provided even given the present limited resources if there is early, appropriate and realistic counselling of the family, and if the adolescent is involved as fully as possible in making any decisions. These at least are better alternatives than the more common one of a virtual total lack of help for handicapped adolescents after they have left school.

References

Castree, B.J. & Walker, J.H. (1981) The young adult with spina bifida. *British Medical Journal*, **2**, 1040–1042.

Chamberlain, M.A. (1981) The handicapped school leaver. *Archives of Disease in Childhood*, **56**, 737–738.

Cheseldine, S.E. & Jeffree, D.M. (1981) Mentally handicapped adolescents: their use of leisure. *Journal of Mental Deficiency Research*, **25**, 49–59.

Kreutner, A.K. (1981) Sexuality, fertility and the problems of menstruation in mentally retarded adolescents. *Paediatric Clinics of North America*, **28** (2), 475–480.

Ludlow, C.L. (1980) Children's language disorder; recent research advances. *Annals of Neurology*, **7**, 497–507.

O'Donohue, N.V. (1985) *Epilepsies of Childhood*, p. 131–137. 2nd edition, Butterworths, London.

Watson, G. & Rogers, R.S. (1980) Sexual instruction for the mildly retarded and normal adolescent. *Health Education Journal*, **39**, 88–95.

Chapter 16
Children with Impaired Hearing

Ian Taylor, Jean Huntington &
Alan Huntington

The treatment of the child with impaired hearing

This chapter considers some of the problems of hearing-impaired children, a term used to cover all degrees of hearing loss. Deafness may be of conductive or sensori-neural type. The former includes all those conditions which impede the transmission of sound from the outside to the cochlea, and the latter arises from maldevelopment or degeneration of the cochlea or to damage to the auditory nerves and tracts.

The commonest cause of conductive deafness is exudative otitis media, characterized by negative pressure in the middle ear, with a variable pure tone audiometric threshold and an abnormal pressure and compliance curve determined by an electro-acoustic impedence bridge. Most causes of conductive deafness are amenable to medial or surgical treatment. Sensori-neural deafness is often of genetic origin (Taylor *et al.*, 1973, 1975), and among the exogenous causes, virus infections are of particular significance. The morbidity of congenital rubella seems to have altered, with fewer hearing-impaired babies showing other manifestations of the condition. This may be the result of the widespread practice of therapeutic abortion (Taylor, 1980). The incidence of congenital rubella will fall if the immunization programme is more vigorously implemented. Cytomegalovirus infection is also a cause of deafness and so far there are no effective means of controlling this disease. The relationship between perinatal factors and sensori-neural deafness is uncertain. In a prospective study of asphyxiated neonates by D'Souza and his colleagues (1981), only one child had such a disability. In the follow-up of children who have suffered from bacterial and viral meningitis the possibility of deafness must always be considered, though it is not common.

In practice, it is of particular importance to differentiate between the baby who is deaf from an autosomal recessive syndrome and the one whose deafness follows maternal rubella when there are no other disabilities. If incorrect genetic advice is not to be given, a careful check must be made for other manifestations of rubella such as the typical

344

rubella retinitis, and serological tests must be done on the mother and baby. Sensori-neural deafness is often associated with conductive deafness in childhood. The parents may be the first to suspect that their baby is deaf and their worries must be taken seriously. The parents should always be asked about this in the first few months of the baby's life and suitable tests carried out if doubts are expressed. One technique is the use of a microprocessor to identify and process the information given by respiration and other movements evoked from sounds fed into the baby's ear (Simmonds & Russ, 1974; Bennett & Wade 1980). The results of such studies are encouraging but validation is still awaited. Other methods include Auditory Evoked Responses in the newborn, and the Brain Stem Electrical Response (Sohmer & Feinmesser, 1967). The latter test evaluates auditory thresholds. This is of particular value in assessing the baby's disability, but the interpretation of the data is much more difficult than assessing the baby's responses to sounds fed into the ear.

If such tests are to be done, the necessary expertise on how to proceed and how to give parental guidance must be available. There is much still to be learnt about the importance of early diagnosis, although the sooner a disability is recognized the sooner future management can be planned. Until more is known about the effects of impaired hearing, or of fluctuating hearing loss, in early infancy on development, particularly of language, it must surely be reasonable to make such a diagnosis, and to control carefully the effects of various forms of intervention. Also, if conductive deafness is diagnosed, this is often amenable to treatment. If a child of any age does not pass the appropriate screening test for hearing, the ears, nose and throat are examined to identify any abnormality. If there is the possibility of a temporary disorder, a second screening is done four weeks later. If there seems to be hearing impairment, the child is referred to the appropriate centre where there are personnel with the necessary skill and experience in paediatric audiology.

Audiological procedures

Audiological procedures for diagnostic purposes have two parts:

1 The medical examination and investigation of the infant, including serological and other special tests such as an electrocardiograph and thyroid function tests, and particularly an examination of the eyes. The investigation should include the routine examination of the hearing of all the immediate family and relations when available.

2 Testing children's hearing requires experience. Tests used depend on the child's developmental level, and range from the application of distracting techniques to the point when the child is able to undertake puretone audiometry. The value of the latter procedure is the securing, as early as possible, of a definition of the air and bone thresholds to determine whether or not the hearing is sensori-neural or conductive.

One of the important technical advances has been the introduction of the electro-acoustic impedance bridge which allows an evaluation of the state of the middle ear and the stapedial and tensor tympanic reflexes, without the individual under test having to play any active role. The basis of this procedure is the notion that sound passes maximally from the exterior to the inner ear through the middle ear if the pressures on either side of the tympanic membrane are the same. If, in the event, the middle ear offers an increased resistance to the passage of sound because of disease in the middle ear (such as exists where an exudate is present), then more sound will be reflected from the tympanic membrane than would be the case in the physiological state. The electro-acoustic impedance bridge is designed to evaluate the conductive or resistant state of the middle ear and any changes in the pressure relative to the atmospheric pressure. By the use of the electro-acoustic bridge easy corroboration of the state of the middle ear is possible.

The value of such an investigation can be understood in the clinical situation often posed when an infant of a few weeks old is found to have a raised auditory acuity. The demonstration of normal middle ear function would indicate that the likely nature of the hearing loss is sensori-neural, rather than conductive. The electro-acoustic impedance bridge is a refined instrument which helps in the identification of abnormality of the tympanic membrane, and is sensitive to gradations of abnormality of the middle ear from a mild negative pressure to a severe problem of middle ear function due to the ear being full of fluid or glue from advanced exudative otitis media. Several readings during the course of treatment will help to evaluate the effectiveness or otherwise of the medical or surgical treatment undertaken.

The brain stem evoked response is essential in the determining of auditory thresholds in many infants impossible to test using standard procedures. The evaluation of the responses is a specialist procedure but in skilled hands differentiation can be made between a sensori-neural and conductive deafness by attention to the latencies of the response obtained.

The assessment of the handicap which results from sensory disability of the auditory system is undertaken by an evaluation of medical, audiological and psychological factors. The help which can be offered to the families of hearing-impaired children is now understood to be vital to the future development of the child. Although there are those who agree that some form of manual communication is desirable or even essential for the development of the hearing-impaired child and the family, the philosophy and practice in the United Kingdom is generally based on the view that the majority of, if not all, deaf children will have the best opportunities to develop their potential by the acquisition of linguistic skills, using an aural-oral method. The potential for reaching this goal is made even more likely now that there is a greater number of skilled workers who are able to give professional guidance to the families, and to the significant advances made in the technical aspects of hearing aids and their use.

The philosophy and practice of aural-oral management is based on the fact that the great majority of parents of deaf children communicate by the spoken word and not by a contrived system of signs and finger spelling which requires much practice to acquire fluency and competence. It is self-evident that hearing and speaking parents are immediately faced with the problem of having a deaf baby with no time, even if it were desirable, to acquire any esoteric system of communication; nor is there any evidence that such systems aid the problems facing parents unfamiliar with the communication practices of a minority of deaf adults. For most families the opportunity is open to continue with the usual methods of communicating with their children.

Hearing aids are now available to all hearing-impaired children of whatever degree of disability which will ensure the best possible opportunity to hear the spoken word. Important technical advances have been made, both with the design of hearing aids and in the manufacture and fitting of ear-moulds for children. The work of Nolan and Tucker (1977) has shown that good fitting moulds should be availabe for the deafest children, and since the National Health call-off contract in 1974 made available the best commercial aids to all, there is now no reason why hearing-impaired children in the UK should not receive the benefit of continuous and consistent listening experience. It is not enough to be satisfied with technical proficiency unless the child is exposed to the usual environment of speaking as a normal human experience.

The present trends in research suggests that where normal spoken language is used, then the spoken language of the children will follow a usual pattern. It would appear that abnormal spoken patterns for deaf children can be traced to the use of unusual and abnormal speech from those around them. In the management of deaf children the emphasis is on the necessity and desirability of normality, not in the sense that deaf children do not have a disability, but rather than their needs to acquire language competence will more likely be attained if their experience of the spoken word is as normal as possible.

The Warnock Report has reflected the philosophy and practice of encouraging, and indeed expecting, as many handicapped children as possible to be taught in normal school, although the need for continuation of special schools is readily recognized.

There are several interesting trends in the development of educational provision for hearing impaired children in the UK:

1   Firstly, there does seem to be a real reduction in the number of deaf children being born. Taylor (1980) found a significant reduction in the numbers of severely deaf children. There is also a change in morbidity mainly due to the reduction in the number of babies born with multiple disabilities with the disappearance of deafness from rhesus incompatibility and tuberculous meningitis, and a reduction in the incidence of deafness from perinatal disorders. There are fewer babies deafened from the rubella virus who have additional handicaps.

2   Secondly, there has been a considerable growth in the numbers of special classes and units in ordinary schools, and in the number of hearing-impaired children now educated in ordinary classes.

3   There has been a reduction in the numbers of hearing-impaired children attending special schools.

The most up-to-date figures available from the Department of Education and Science in the UK show that in 1979 there were 3524 children in maintained and non-maintained schools for the deaf and 2092 children in schools for the partially hearing. Now that the Special Education Act 1981 is in effect abolishing all categories, it is reasonable to consider that there were 5616 children in special schools in England and Wales in 1979.

So far as units are concerned, these are usually divided into full-time and part-time pupils. The official figures available for 1979 were:

	Deaf	*Partially Hearing*
Full-time	248	2497
Part-time	44	977
Total	292	3474

A more recent survey by the British Association of Teachers of the Deaf report the following statistics for 1981:

In schools for the deaf or partially hearing	3722
In units for hearing-impaired	3782
In local schools seen by peripatetic teachers	23,072

There is thus a tendency away from placement of hearing impaired children in schools for the deaf and partially hearing.

Language development and deafness in childhood

The essence of first language acquisition is learning to relate a particular system of sounds and visual systems to meaning in an organized and consistent way. In other words, the baby has to 'crack the code' and in order to do so he must have sufficient opportunity to observe the code in operation. If his exposure to the particular system of sounds which constitute his native language is reduced or debased to any appreciable degree, the child will be slow to acquire language.

The auditory basis of language learning

Hearing impairment which reduces or even suppresses completely the essential auditory input to the brain makes the deaf infant reliant for language acquisition on acoustic cues which, if perceived, are distorted, and on visual cues which are often unreliable indicators of linguistic differences. No English speaker with normal hearing confuses 'penny' and 'many', 'sell' and 'tell', 'biscuit' and 'biscuits', 'wash' and 'washed', 'probable' and 'improbable', '*re*fuse' and 're*fuse*', 'Is *Jack* coming with us?' and 'Is Jack coming with *us*?', or 'I do like that' and 'I don't like that'. Yet each pair of words or sentences would be exceedingly difficult, if not impossible, to distinguish by lipreading alone even if the receiver of the messages had perfect vision and knew the English language well. This is because some phonemes, such as /p/ and /m/, are identical in appearance and others, such as /s/, /t/ and /n/ are barely visible, as are some unstressed affixes in English like '-nt', 'im', '-ed' and '-s', which carry information about the important concepts of negation, tense and plurality. Similarly, stress pattern and intonation may dramatically alter the meaning of spoken sentences but these prosodic features have no visual correlates; they are only accessible through hearing.

The fact that auditory transmission is the basis of all natural languages means that, in their comprehension, vision is only a very second-rate substitute for hearing, as many deafened adults ruefully lament. The child who suffers an impairment of hearing during the normal period of language learning is not, like the deafened adult, trying to decipher faint differences in sounds of which he knows the linguistic significance. He has a more difficult task. He is attempting to deduce from the behaviour of those around him which of the dimly perceived differences in the speech signal have significance and which do not. He has to try to discover which sequences of sound recur in his environment and what their referents are in the external world. He must try to organize the data he abstracts into a system which coincides with the system adopted by the community in which he finds himself. It is, therefore, of supreme importance that hearing-impaired children are given the best experience of interesting and relevant spoken language which efficient amplification can make available to them, and this at the earliest possible opportunity.

Is sign language an acceptable alternative to verbal language?
The difficulty of the task of acquiring language leads some educators and some deaf adults to recommend that severely hearing-impaired children should experience an alternative or supplementary first language to their native English tongue. They advocate exposure to a language of manual signs in which linguistic differences are visually cued. It is rarely suggested that a sign language should be the only language to which deaf children are exposed for the obvious reason that to live successfully in the world and to earn one's living one must know the verbal language of the wider community. So non-verbal language systems, such as British Sign Language and the Paget-Gorman Sign System, are, if employed by parents or teachers, usually used in conjunction with spoken and written English. The claim of those who use a sign language is that it will accelerate the child's acquisition of a first (manual) language and so quickly satisfy the child's emotional and cognitive needs for a means of communication. The intention is then to replace the sign language gradually with English which is inevitably learned as a second language.

Finger spelling and Cued Speech are in quite a different category from sign language in that they are visual systems of signalling information about verbal language. They represent by hand configurations either the letters of the alphabet or selected features of speech sounds and are intended to reduce perceptual difficulties. The term 'Total Communication' is used to describe a composite medium in which signs, gestures, finger spelling and spoken English may be used concurrently. Interpretations of the term 'Total Communication' vary and its practice is unstable (Clare, 1981). For instance, users may adopt the one-handed or two-handed finger alphabet, they may use some signs which are standardized and others which are regional or peculiar to particular schools. Users may sign only the key concepts in a sentence or attempt to sign complete sentences including syntactic features. They may use finger spelling when no sign for a concept exists or sign the equivalent of a word root and finger spell word affixes. It is acknowledged that users find synchronization of manual and oral systems difficult so they may labour their speech, omit part of the spoken message, abbreviate the manual signs or finger spell only initial letters of words. The child may thus be expected to attend to multiple media, none of which is presented in its complete and regular form.

Manual communication is a solution by no means free from difficulty. There are the problems of simultaneous attention to a variety of sensory inputs and the problem of children being required to co-ordinate two diverse cognitive processes. Verbal languages are essentially abstract in that words in no sense represent or resemble the objects or concepts they stand for. The words 'seat' and 'eat' sound alike but have no connection in meaning; the words 'seat' and 'armchair' are totally dissimilar in form but their meanings are closely related. Traditional sign languages on the other hand, contain many representational or pictorial signs for objects and the more recently developed sign systems consciously exploit the connection between the visual appearance of the sign and the reality it stands for. For instance, in the Paget-Gorman System there is a basic sign for 'animal' and each species of animal is shown by this basic sign with additional features describing the recognizable characteristics of the animal. Thus, a horse is an animal with a bit in its mouth; a dog is an animal which barks; a giraffe is an animal with a long neck, and so on. (Notley, 1981). Children required to learn both sign and verbal languages at the same time, or in sequence, are being asked to symbolize external reality in two very disparate ways. Furthermore, deafness is a handicap which reduces experience of all kinds and in particular limits experience of language which the deaf person can never overhear or attend to casually. It is difficult enough to arrange for a hearing-impaired child to receive sufficient exposure to one language, expecting him to become bilingual seems unrealistically demanding.

Most of us show little facility in learning languages except when we are very young and when we are daily surrounded by fluent speakers of the new language. In order to learn a sign language in the same way and at the same rate as normally hearing children learn English, a hearing-impaired child would need to be brought up in a home where the parents always signed correctly and fluently. When these unusual conditions operate, the child may acquire a first language as rapidly as normally hearing children do, as a study by Klima and Bellingi (1972) illustrates. They describe a child in a manually communicating family whose level of language development in American Sign Language at the age of 2 years 7 months was comparable to that of hearing children of the same age in spoken English. However, most deaf children are born to hearing parents who do not have the opportunity to achieve competence in signing in time for their children's critical language learning years.

Sign language may be an appropriate first language for two special groups of deaf children. The first group are deaf children of deaf parents who themselves communicate almost exclusively through signs. Such children will need to learn English as a second language if they are to make successful social contacts in a wider circle than the family, and to gain the knowledge and information which is accessible through communication by verbal language. The second group comprises a very small proportion of hearing-impaired children, those who are severely mentally handicapped or have specific handicaps in addition to profound deafness. Some of these children may achieve only the bare essentials of communication, sufficient for the protected environments of their homes and schools.

[Having stressed the important differences, it may be an overstatement to imply that signing and spoken English are two languages in that non-verbal communication and signing are part of normal communication supplementing speech. The majority of signs used in the Makaton or Amerind signing systems can be identified by untrained observers. Some children, other than those mentioned, having become more relaxed about communication by using signs, seem to utter speech more readily. However, if signing is introduced, this has to be planned in discussion with the school and parents to avoid a half-hearted or unsustained programme. This will have to be an individual decision, and obviously for the majority it is best to teach the child to listen, which is becoming increasingly possible with improved hearing aids, even for the most severely deaf.— EDITORS]

Deafness and the acquisition of verbal language

For the majority of hearing-impaired children the language to be acquired is spoken English learned through social interaction with family and friends and later in the social environment of the school. There is no exact relationship between degree of hearing impairment and linguistic achievement, but in general deafer children learn to understand language more slowly, have smaller vocabularies, more deviant grammar, less intelligible speech and are more seriously retarded in the secondary linguistic skills of reading and writing. Even children with very slight hearing impairment who are able to follow the curriculum of ordinary primary and secondary schools are, as a group, linguistically and educationally retarded, although the effects of the retardation are not necessarily apparent in casual social exchanges. Individual children may not exhibit any retardation at all. By the time hearing-impaired children leave school, linguistic achievement by individuals ranges from parity with normally hearing pupils of the same age, to similarity with normally hearing pre-schoolers in size of vocabulary but with deviant grammar and pronunciation.

The effects of hearing loss on linguistic achievement are well illustrated in a study carried out by Gemmill and colleagues (1977) in the Department of Audiology, University of Manchester. Samples of spoken language were obtained from 215 hearing-impaired children aged 9–11 years and drawn from schools for the deaf and partially hearing in different parts of the country. The children's speech was recorded as they described a sequence of pictures which told a story and their efforts were graded into five categories, A to E, reflecting different degrees of skill and fluency in handling oral language. Whilst this is not a measure of children's linguistic knowledge, their expressive powers are a reflection of their underlying linguistic competence. The mean hearing loss of the 215 children was 81 dB (average of 0.5kHz; 1kHz and 2kHz in the better ear) and the standard deviation was 21.88. Samples allocated to category A were of this kind:

> One day the little boy saw some eggs in a nest in the tree. He went to climb up the tree and get the egg. And he nearly fall over. And he fall over and he broken all the eggs. And starts to cry.

Such a sample was judged by the researchers to be comparable with samples of spoken language obtained in the same recording situation from normally hearing children age 9–10 years. Samples allocated to category B were similar to samples from hearing children aged 7–8 years. For example,

> The, the boy was looking for a nest. The boy was climbing. He had the egg in his hand. He fell and the egg smash. That's all.

An example from Category C was as follows,

> A boy want egg. The boy climb a tree. The boy get egg. Boy fall down tree. A boy cry.

The following are examples from categories D and E.

Boy egg for tree. Tree climb. Egg tree climb egg fetch. Egg fall the tree. Tree boy cry. Egg.

Saw eggs. Climb. Catch—(unintelligible). Fall. Cry. Broken. Finish.

It will be seen that even the children with the poorest spoken language have sufficient vocabulary to tell the rudiments of the story; it is the deterioration in the structure of sentences from category A to category E which is so marked. A table showing the mean hearing losses of children allocated to each category illustrates the *general* correspondence between language development and increased severity of hearing handicap.

Language Category	*Mean Loss*	*S.D.*
A (n = 17)	61 dB	18.60
B (n = 43)	66 dB	16.04
C (n = 74)	83 dB	21.73
D (n = 49)	85 dB	17.39
E (n = 32)	98 dB	18.01

Number of children in each of five language categories, mean hearing loss and standard deviation for each category.

However, when a group of 72 children who had losses in the range 70−90 dB were extracted from the main sample and their results examined, there was found to be no significant relationship between language category and level of hearing loss. Linguistic achievement in this middle range of hearing loss appeared to be more dependent on factors in the children's language environments at home and at school than on the degree of handicap. Furthermore, 4 children from the main sample with losses greater than 90 dB were placed in categories A and B; that is to say, some children with profound hearing impairment had developed language similar to that of normally hearing children. By the time they were about 10 years old, these few children had almost 'caught up' despite drastically reduced experience of language.

Facilitating language development in hearing impaired children
Normally hearing children have mastered the phonology and syntax of their native language by the time they are about 4 years old and by 5 they have a vocabulary of about 2000 words which they can use and a considerably larger vocabulary which they understand. The rapidity with which this grasp of the structure and meaning of their native language is

gained by children is thought to be the product of a species-specific innate capacity which requires for its activation an unknown amount of exposure to spoken language (Chomsky, 1965; Lenneberg, 1967). There is obviously a required minimum exposure below which learning does not take place. The major task in the treatment of hearing-impaired children is ensuring that the transmission of linguistic experience is efficient enough, begins early enough and is sufficient in quantity to release their innate language learning capabilities. The children with profound hearing impairment who develop language similar to normally hearing children's show that it is possible to provide the necessary experience even for the most handicapped. Those severely deaf children who have more modest linguistic achievements show that good practice can ameliorate a grave disability.

Studies of development during the earliest months of life provide evidence of the attention normally hearing babies pay to the human voice, their appreciation of and responsiveness to the one-sided 'conversations' their mothers hold with them and of the ability they show to make sound discriminations related to the speech sounds of their native language. There appears to be no pre-lingual stage in the child's experience (Byers Brown *et al.*, 1981). He is prepared for the development of language from the outset. If the hearing-impaired child's propensity to attend to language is to be capitalized upon and all the experience available to him used, then the earliest detection and treatment of deafness is of supreme importance. The authors (Nolan & Tucker, 1981) of a recent book directed mainly to the parents of deaf children suggest that 'the language of hearing impaired children suffers delay related to an absence of early stimulation.' They assert that the age of diagnosis of hearing impairment throughout the United Kingdom is at present too high, with the result that valuable experience at a crucial stage of development is lost.

It was emphasized at the beginning of this section that in normal circumstances languages are transmitted auditorily and that the perception of linguistic features depends on hearing. It sometimes seems a wilful disregard of the deaf child's disability to insist that every effort be made to give him auditory experience of the speech of others and of his own voice. But the child who uses his remaining hearing to sort out the phonological system, grammar and semantics of his native language learns more about the principles governing the operation of languages than one who relies exclusively on the visually salient features of speech. Deaf children who from their earliest days are enabled to hear some speech through amplification develop natural voice quality, rhythm and intonation which is difficult to match in children without such auditory experience. The fact that many children cannot discriminate between consonants in isolation or even hear them at all does not mean that in their perception of running speech these phonemes are not accessible to them. There is information in the low frequency components of the spoken message about the high frequency (and generally weaker) components which children who are experienced in listening can detect. Of course the child will supplement his incomplete auditory perception with lipreading and should be encouraged to do so.

To facilitate perception, the input of spoken language to hearing-impaired children will ideally have the greatest degree of clarity which good amplification of well articulated, natural speech can achieve. But children are interested in the content of language, not in its form, and it is the clarification of meaning which is important. In research involving nursery school children, Tizard and her colleagues (1972) found that it was the amount of informative talk by adults, their willingness to answer children's questions and the amount of active play they initiated which resulted in the achievement of better comprehension and expressive language scores by children. Parents and teachers have to make clear to children, whether normally-hearing or hearing-impaired, the correspondence between linguistic and non-linguistic events. This is accomplished through personal interaction in social contexts, in conversations where there are real exchanges of meaning between adult and child. The adult needs to be alert to the child's thinking and interests, anticipating and responding to his incomplete and often unintelligible parts of the conversation. From his longitudinal study of language development, Wells (1977) attempts to distinguish between the characteristics of 'enabling' and 'non-enabling' homes. Listening to recordings of spontaneous conversations between children and parents in their home surroundings, Wells does not find 'that it is in the differential frequency of logical reasoning or of the other complex functions (Tough, 1977) that stands out as the characteristic distinguishing between the 'enabling' and 'non-enabling' home . . . . But rather it is in the presence or absence of genuine reciprocity and collaboration . . . . And it seems to be the *sharing* that is so crucial. Certainly this quality characterises the speech at home of all the children who are making above average progress after one year at school.'

The achievement of this 'sharing' or 'genuine reciprocity' in conversation is obviously more difficult when the child partner in the conversation is very young and very deaf as the adult may, at first, receive so little feedback about the child's comprehension. The parent may lose confidence and doubt the appropriateness of the language input; teachers likewise may become despondent when a large input of spoken language produces few returns in expressive language from the child. They should be encouraged to persevere because it is the comprehension of language that is the necessary precursor of speech, reading and writing. There is evidence that parents and teachers may be reasonably confident that the form of their spoken language will be appropriate to the language level of the children they address since adjustments of sentence length, sentence complexity, repetitions, vocabulary and so on seem to be instinctive (Snow & Ferguson, 1977). What is important is concentration on understanding and being understood, on engaging the child's mind and not restricting oneself to language the child is thought to know already.

Choosing hearing aids for hearing-impaired children

In an excellent essay on this subject, Ross and Tomasetti (1980) affirm, 'For most hearing impaired children, the early and appropriate selection and use of amplification is the single most habilitative tool available to us.' Three key words appear in this single sentence; 'early', 'appropriate' and 'use'.

There is evidence that the basis of normal language development lies in sounds heard *early* by infants, long before their first spoken words are recognized (Fry, 1977; Benedict, 1978; Crystal, 1979; Stark, 1979). It is thus of paramount importance that, once deafness is diagnosed, sound be made available as early as possible to the hearing-impaired infant so that linguistic milestones, in his case too, may coincide as nearly as possible with chronological ones. In pursuit of this aim, top priority must be accorded to the fitting of an appropriate hearing aid. The urgency of this cannot be overstressed, though there are, as yet, no published data on the follow-up of children supplied early with hearing aids.

What, then, are the considerations that will determine which aid is selected as appropriate for the hearing-impaired infant? At this stage so much desirable information is simply not available; perhaps all that one has is the clear result of a live voice performance test and permission to proceed following an otologist's examination. Once an aid is chosen, there then follows a period during which little or no reassuring feedback is available and the most one can claim is that the choice of aid was not an unqualified disaster. More positively, however, having decided that an instrument must be chosen, a choice has to be made: is the hearing loss confined only to the high frequencies (upwards of 1000 Hz) or does the impairment affect the whole range of speech frequencies (say, 200 Hz to 4000 Hz in the context of aid selection)? If the low frequencies are intact, it is imperative that these be preserved and their potential exploited. This implies not impeding their reception by occluding the meatus with a standard earmould. Many children hear less of the frequencies they have learned from birth to depend on when wearing their aids, than when aidless. Either a vented earmould may be used that will allow free passage of unamplified low frequencies or an open earmould which fulfils the same purpose, though the latter will be effective only if very moderate gain is demanded in the high frequencies; otherwise, as the gain is increased, acoustic feedback will result. The crucial point is that the child must not be deprived of information-bearing sound that he has come to value at a time when new sounds (amplified high frequencies) are being fed to him, sounds which, as yet, may have little or no significance for him. If, on the other hand, the hearing impairment is not confined only to the high frequencies then the type of aid yielding most benefit would be an instrument having as wide a frequency range and as flat a frequency-response as possible. Even for frequency-response alone, a body-worn aid would be advised here, since low frequency handling capacity would be generally superior and if any extra emphasis were needed below 1000 Hz this would be furnished as a product of body-baffle (the enhancement of bass frequencies as a consequence of actually wearing the aid on the chest).

Acoustic considerations apart, a body-worn aid would be more practically manageable for a baby (ear-level aids tend to fall off unless taped in position), more easily attached to the infant's clothing and more easily accessible when in need of adjustment. Even more important, however, is that on the child's chest the aid is optimal for picking up the sound of his voice. This consideration cannot be emphasized too strongly. Even a normally-hearing adult with full command of language becomes insecure when deprived, even temporarily, of the sound of his own voice, and should the condition become permanent, as with the onset of total deafness, deviant features soon begin to creep into his speech patterns. With the infant language barrier the position is far more serious and it is important for this self monitoring medium to be available if voice quality and oral language structure are to approach normality.

The problem of setting hearing aid controls for the infant for whom pure-tone testing is still a distant goal cannot but be approximate. Firstly, once earmoulds have been made and the aid appears to be positioned sensibly, note the volume control setting at which the baby just detects the sound of a conversational voice, then measure the acoustic gain at this setting on a hearing aid test box. One now has a statement of the gain required to make the loudest of speech ingredients, stressed vowels, just audible. The second step is, with the help of the test box, to set the aid's volume control at a level that will furnish a further 30 dB of gain. The aim here is to attempt to make quiet consonants also audible to the child. Step three is extremely important and is a check on whether the theory underlying this 30 dB gain increase is actually practicable. The aid is replaced on the child and the same conversational level voice given whilst he is watched for startle response or any sign of discomfort or distress indicating that this volume setting is too high. If there are such signs there must be absolute silence until the volume control is turned down to a level where such evidence of discomfort is absent. If it now turns out that there is a low tolerance threshold, or that the intensity range between just hearing and discomfort is too narrow to accommodate the desired 30 dB dynamic range just referred to, then recourse must be made to an aid that will afford security and protection by incorporating output limiting circuitry (e.g. peak clipping) and perhaps compression.

For the hearing-impaired school age child the approach to aid selection can be more sophisticated. Much must be made of virtually normal low frequency hearing where this exists. It is from this range of speech that the child derives valuable information via intonation fluctuations and rhythmic patterns of speech. If normal vocal inflexions can be acquired and a sense of the correct grouping of words, with stressed elements in the right place, even though there may be grave errors and omissions elsewhere (e.g. in the articulation of high frequency consonants), then the goal of speech intelligibility is nearer. In an attempt to fit hearing aids to these children it is worth investigating the two or three ear-level aids that not only amplify high frequencies exclusively but also allow unamplified low frequencies to be leaked into the meatus and mixed with the enhanced high frequencies. Vented moulds are then not necessary.

Among congenitally deaf children the only positive feedback may be an indication that, when the aid is switched on, something can be heard. Nearly two generations of research effort has been exerted in improving and facilitating the selection of hearing aids, but as yet there is, unfortunately, no single infallible route to the right instrument. Levitt (1978) describes comprehenively four approaches to the task and discusses the controversies associated with each. The four approaches are:

1   Frequency-selective amplification

Earliest attempts at matching amplification systems to the needs of the hearing-impaired sought to restore the depressed pure-tone level to the normal position via differential amplification across the frequency range. It was a mirroring technique which proved unsatisfactory for sensori-neural loss patients, since whilst quieter speech sounds might well be brought within their audibility range, louder speech components became intolerably loud owing to the patients' restricted dynamic range.

Then came an attempt to offer the aid-wearer equally loud sounds across the speech spectrum, and another approach when the pure-tone configuration was mirrored by gain equal to only a fixed proportion of the hearing loss, usually around half (so that a 1000 Hz loss of 80 dB would be alleviated by 40 dB of gain). Yet another variant aims at delivering speech along a line half-way between the thresholds of detectability and discomfort—an attractive approach in its attempt to replicate normal experience.

No commercially produced aid has controls flexible enough to allow the fine adjustments prescribed. Also the time involved in deducing the individual's need, let alone seeking to fulfil it, is prohibitive in a clinical setting. Australian researchers, Byrne and Tonisson (1976) have revived this approach using predictions derived from their earlier data. Levitt (1978) maintains, however, that 'extensive experimental evaluations are still needed to establish the relative merit of this approach.'

2   Hearing aid selection

By contrast with what has been termed the 'speculative' or 'armchair' approach, described above, another method uses comparative testing of actual hearing aids on individuals. Results of speech tests are compared and a final selection made on this basis.

3   Fixed frequency-gain characteristics

The 1946–1947 Harvard research (Davis *et al.*, 1947) and the investigation carried out by the British Medical Research Council (Committee on Electro-Acoustics, 1947) led to advocacy of the 'uniform frequency characteristic', subsequently to be the basis of the specifications to which thousands of Medresco hearing aids were made in the UK. The electro-acoustic features of this design have satisfied the audiological needs of thousands of aid users for a whole generation and the rising frequency response blueprint approved at the time became the format adopted by many commercial hearing aid manufacturers. The Harvard report did, however, acknowledge the occurrence of 'unusual and difficult cases of hearing loss that require special attention' and certainly profoundly hearing impaired children with 'bottom left-hand corner' audiograms were not catered for by the first transistorized Medresco aids.

4   Adaptive fitting of a master hearing aid

This method involves the use of a master hearing aid, which can now be in wearable form, the controls of which are adjusted until the patient's needs are satisfied. An aid with similar characteristics is then sought.

None of these four methods is foolproof in locating the best aid for a very deaf child. Method 1 tends to be based on comfortable listening levels or preferred gain but, from our experience, listening levels required by children with the lowest linguistic attainments need to be more elevated than those selected by more sophisticated, linguistically competent aid users. Methods 2 and 4 depend too heavily on speech tests of hearing, involving language which the very deaf child may be wholly unable to cope with, and the protracted, fatiguing, listening sessions are quite unconducive to the furnishing of the reliable information needed for effective final selection.

Two brief final considerations are now examined. Firstly, although reference has been made to the hearing aid, in the singular, it is our very strong contention that, wherever possible, two aids should be fitted (Markides, 1977), and, providing that both electro-acoustic and ergonomic characteristics suit and there is no doubt whatsoever that the wearer receives good clear patterns of his *own* voice, the aids should be ear level rather than body-worn instruments.

At the beginning of this section three key words ('early', 'appropriate' and 'use') were extracted from a paper by Ross and Tomasetti (1980). The final intention is to emphasize another statement from the same paper concerning use of aids: 'early emphasis on amplification cannot take place in an habilitative vacuum'. In developing this concept the authors stress the need for having the aid worn consistently and for hearing adults in the child's environment, particularly his parents, being actively and understandingly involved in using the aid in helping language to develop. This has been a strong tenet of this University department in its long history of parent guidance practice, since without this back-up the world's most perfect method of aid selection will surely founder.

Early provision ... appropriate selection ... aids in constant use; one cannot better these ingredients if effective language development is the goal.

References

Benedict, H. (1978) 'Language comprehension in 9–15 month old children'. In *'Recent Advances in the Psychology of Language'* (eds R.N. Campbell and N.Y. Smith). Plenum Press, New York.

Bennett, M.J. & Wade, J.K. (1980) Automated newborn screening using the auditory response cradle. In *'Disorders of Auditory Function'* III. Academic Press, London.

Byers Brown, D.B., John, J.E., Owrid, H.L. & Taylor I.G. (1981) Linguistic Development. In *Foundations of Paediatrics* (eds J.A. Davis and J. Dobbing). Heinemann Medical Books, London.

Byrne, D. and Tonisson, W. (1976) Selecting the gain of hearing aids for persons with sensori-neural hearing impairments. *Scandinavian Audiology*, **5**, 51–59.

Chomsky, N. (1965) *Aspects of the Theory of Syntax*. M.I.T. Press, Cambridge, Mass.

Clare, M. (1981) Total communication. In *Ways and Means 3: Hearing Impairment* (ed. A. Jackson). Globe Education, Basingstoke.

Committee on Electro-Acoustics, *Hearing Aids and Audiometers* (1974) Medical Research Council, H.M.S.O., London.

Davis, H., Stevens, S.S. & Nichols, R.H. (1974) *Hearing Aids: An Experimental Study of Design Objectives*. Harvard University Press, Cambridge, M.A.

D'Souza, S.W., McCartney, E., Nolan, M. & Taylor, I.G. (1981) Hearing, speech and language in survivors of severe perinatal asphyxia. *Archives of Diseases in Childhood*, **56**, 245–252.

Fry, D.B. (1977) *Homo Loquens*. Cambridge University Press, Cambridge.

Fry, D.B. (1978) The role and primacy of the auditory channel in speech and development. In *Auditory Management of Hearing Impaired Children* (eds M. Ross & T.G. Giclas). University Park Press, Baltimore.

Gemmill, J.E. & John, J.E.J. (1977) A study of samples of spontaneous spoken language from hearing impaired children. *Journal of the British Association for Teachers of the Deaf*, **1** (6), 193–201.

Klima, E.S. & Bellugi, U. (1972) The signs of language in child and chimpanzee. In *Communication and Affect* (eds T. Alloway, L. Krames and P. Pliner). Academic Press, London.

Lenneberg, E.H. (1967) *Biological Foundations of Language*. John Wiley & Sons, Bristol.

Levitt, H. (1978) Methods for the evaluation of hearing aids. In *Sensori-neural hearing impairment and hearing aids* (eds C. Ludvigsen and J. Barfod). *Scandinavian Audiology Supplement* **6**.

Markides, A. (1977) *Binaural hearing aids*. Academic Press, London.

Nolan, M. & Tucker, I.G. (1977) A simple method of improving the acoustic seal of an ear mould. *The Teacher of the Deaf*, **1** (2), 74–77.

Nolan, M. & Tucker, I.G. (1981) *The Hearing Impaired Child and the Family*. Souvenir Press, London.

Notley, C. (1981) Paget Gorman Sign System. In *Ways and Means 3: Hearing Impairment* (ed. A. Jackson). Globe Education, Basingstoke.

Ross, M. & Tomassetti, C. (1980) Hearing aid selection for preverbal hearing-impaired children. In *Amplification for the Hearing Impaired* (ed. M.C. Pollack). Grune and Stratton, New York.

Simmonds, F.B. & Russ, F.N. (1974) Automated newborn hearing screening, the crib-o-gram. *Archives and Oto-Laryngology*, **100**, 1−7.

Sohmer, H., & Feinmesser, M. (1967) Cochlea action potentials recorded from the external ear in man. *Annals of Otology, Rhinology and Laryngology*, **76**, 427−435.

Snow, C.A. & Ferguson, C.E. (1977) *Talking to Children: Language Input and Acquisition*. Cambridge University Press, Cambridge.

Stark, R.E. (1979) Prespeech Segmental Feature Development. In *Language Acquisition* (eds P. Fletcher & M. Gorman). Cambridge University Press, Cambridge.

Taylor, I.G., Brasier, V.J., Hine, W.D., Morris, T. & Powell, C.A. (1973) Some aspects of the audiology of familial hearing loss. In *Disorders of Auditory Function, III*. Academic Press, London.

Taylor, I.G., Brasier, V.J., Hine, W.D., Chiveralls, K. & Morris, T. (1975) A study of the causes of hearing loss in a population of deaf children with special reference to genetic factors. *Journal of Laryngology and Otology*, **89**, (9), 899−914.

Tizard, B., Cooperman, O., Joseph, A. & Tizard, J. (1972) Environmental effects on language development: a study of young children in long stay residential nurseries. *Child Development*, **43**, 337−358.

Tough, J. (1977) *The Development of Meaning*. Unwin Education Books, London.

Wells, G. (1977) Language use and educational success: an empirical response to Joan Tough's 'The Development of Meaning'. *Research in Education*, **18**, (November 1977), 9−34.

Chapter 17
Children with Impaired Vision

Christopher Dodd

Children with impaired vision

Vision is a vital link between individuals and their environment. Bilateral visual impairment always retards general development. Unilateral visual loss restricts the development of binocular vision but does not markedly affect general development in a healthy child. However, a child handicapped by neurological disease needs maximum vision. Attention to the visual input from each eye and to the quality of binocular vision is therefore essential.

Most visual development is completed in the pre-school years. If remedial action is not taken to correct congenital defects then avoidable permanent visual loss occurs. Five examples are given:

1 Dense central bilateral congenital cataracts prevent retinal image formation. Deprivation amblyopia results.

2 Congenital glaucoma will lead to enlarged eyes with progressive anterior segment and optic nerve damage.

3 Suppresive amblyopia results from interrupted development of binocular reflexes. This may be caused by interference with the sensory input, e.g. anisometropia (unequal focussing), or the motor response e.g. oculo motor palsy (squint). Permanent reduction in central vision of the lazy eye, as well as loss of binocular vision results from late treatment.

4 Bilateral high refractive errors produce not only strain on accommodation and convergence but permanent reduction in central vision if optical correction is delayed.

5 The treatment of retinoblastoma is sight and life saving. The tumour may be in one or both eyes; it may be visible at birth or become apparent in childhood.

Amblyopia is a term used to denote visual loss without organic signs. Deprivation amblyopia from lack of visual stimulation will occur if vision is not restored within the 'critical period'. This means within the first three months of life, though there is plasticity for longer. Suppressive amblyopia is produced by cortical rejection of one of the two halves of the sensory visual input. This is reversible, if the duration is short, but irreversible damage occurs if treatment has not been started before school entry.

Acquired visual damage in the early years may lead to the additional defect of suppressive amblyopia. A corneal scar from infection or trauma may be sufficient to disrupt the dual sensory input, acquired cataract from trauma or Still's disease certainly will. Both the diagnosis of amblyopia and assessment of treatment is difficult in these situations because there is loss of vision from the original pathology. Usually the presence of a squint alerts the family or doctor. Treatment by patching must be discussed with the family. The child is asked to sacrifice the use of better sight to improve the vision in the damaged eye from bad to only fair. Occlusive therapy is therefore better outside school hours and for short periods. To avoid this secondary amblyopia a child with a corneal ulcer rarely has the eye covered if he is under the age of six.

Every child with neurological disease should have the special senses checked. Hearing and sight have a special interrelation since they bring all the information about surroundings outside the range of touch. Disease of either requires specialist assessment of both senses. What should an ophthalmic report provide? There are six basic aspects of vision, shown below.

Aspect of Vision	Comment
Light sense	Impairment in light or dark
Colour sense	Marked defects are clinically significant
Form sense	Visual acuity—distance and near including refraction and optical aids
Motility	Movement of eyes—lids
Visual fields	Monocular and binocular
Binocular vision	Stereopsis and muscle balance

They will be presented differently, since the medical examination of the visual system is arranged to concentrate on those aspects amenable to treatment by doctors. Diseases such as uveitis or glaucoma will affect all aspects of vision. The treatment of cataract involves form vision, binocular vision and visual fields. The ophthalmologist examines the visual pathways to diagnose disease treatable by the neurosurgeon or neurologist. Visual perception is tested as a part of the tests for acuity, fields and binocular vision. Higher visual functions are only tested in detail if there is a suspicion of abnormality.

Comprehensive examination of these basic aspects of vision requires a large amount of equipment. Light sense can only be measured objectively by dark adaptation tests using bulky, expensive apparatus. However, simple questions to the child and parents will usually allay or alert suspicion. The remaining aspects of vision can be tested with simpler equipment contained in two medical cases. One would contain diagnostic equipment and the other lenses. Examination of young handicapped children necessitates an additional box of test materials. A perimeter is needed for standardized visual field testing. A slit lamp microscope is essential for internal examination of the eyes, and intraocular tension measurement should be available. A binocular indirect ophthalmoscope is invaluable for examination of fundi after mydriasis. All this equipment should be available for use in routine examination of children with neurological disease. Since much of it is delicate and expensive it must be kept in a locked room. Electrodiagnostic equipment will cost more than all the preceeding apparatus and is only used in a minority of cases. It will only be available therefore in major centres and this means many families will have to travel long distances for it.

The area needed for patients, families, personnel and equipment is large. At least three examination rooms and a waiting area are needed. The doctor's room must have sufficient space for a child to have an area in which to crawl or walk around. This is additional to space for accompanying adults and siblings, equipment and students. Lack of a proper examination area may result in only a limited assessment of the child and a lost opportunity for the parents to learn about their child during the examination. It is essential to be able both to dim the lights and black out this room. Both the rooms for the orthoptist and refractionist need to be at least six metres long. Usual medical consulting rooms are unsuitable.

A large, warm, waiting area with a kitchen area, toys and adjacent toilet facilities are essential. Young children always need eye drops at their first examination to allow an accurate refraction and fundus examination. The drops temporarily paralyse accommodation (cycloplegia) and there is associated dilatation of the pupil (mydriasis). Half an hour is needed for the drops to work so there may well be two patients with accompanying relations in the waiting room.

To give the ophthalmologist more time with each child, a team which includes an orthoptist and refractionist should be chosen. Care with communication between team members and the families means that the many new faces are not too tiring for the child. A balance must be found between the amount of testing suitable for a particular child at one visit and the need for additional visits if testing is incomplete. Especially if long distances are involved, it is worth aiming for a comprehensive initial assessment. This may be facilitated by an interim break of say half and hour to allow the child to eat and express himself!

If the child is unco-operative and the examination a failure this should be regarded as an opportunity to gain the confidence of parents. Additional history can be taken and both the child and parents can see (hopefully) another child having similar tests happily. It may be suitable to show the parents a particular test to practice at home (e.g. single letter recognition test). This may give the child a sense of achievement and confidence at a second visit. Certainly, the more irritated a doctor may feel during an unsuccessful examination the more important it is to assuage the guilt feelings of parents. Several clinic visits may be necessary to gain the child's confidence. Examination under anaesthesia is occasionally necessary for ocular examination, special tests and refraction, but never replaces observation of the conscious child.

Internal examination of a child's eyes may often be achieved by using an indirect ophthalmoscope through dilated pupils. It has the following advantages:

1 Dim illumination only is needed which means the child is less likely to screw the eyes up.

2 The examiner is at arm's length and does not touch the child.

3 The disc and macula are in the same field of view. Both can be seen when the child looks straight at the examiner's light.

4 Eye movements become less important. The central fundi of a child with nystagmus can be seen quite adequately. The disadvantage is the reduced magnification so less detail is seen. Doubts about the disc, early papilloedema, and optic nerve hypoplasia require the magnified view of a direct ophthalmoscope.

An anaesthetic is often needed when the peripheral fundus must be seen: for instance for retinoblastoma, peripheral retinal degeneration in a high myope and in retinopathy of prematurity. Where there is a family history of congenital glaucoma the intraocular tensions must be measured and the drainage angles examined through a gonioscopic lens with an operating microscope. A child who has had congenital cataracts removed may need the initial refraction and contact lens fitting under anaesthetic if nystagmus is present. All such anaesthetics for examination purposes increase the waiting times for surgery.

The ophthalmic examination of the child has been considered at length because it is the initial occasion when the family and ophthalmologist meet. Not only is data being gathered but a relationship established. Rapport can be greatly helped by the way the child has been referred. Confidence in both the referring doctor and ophthalmologist will only decrease if the main source of information is the parents. Background medical information is essential, but family and personal information about attitudes or particular fears can alter ones approach. If some of this information is confidential then telephone contact prior to the consultation may well repay the time taken to get through!

Some children will only need one consultation when normal vision is found. Reassurance is given to the family and the information passed to the referring general practitioner, school health service and specialist (UK medical referral). Many retarded children will need several ophthalmic consultations spread over several years. They will be under more frequent care of a paediatrician and/or paediatric neurologist to whom information is passed and who will provide information for those who help the child. Some children will have primarily or solely a visual handicap. The child will see a paediatrician once for reassurance about general development but after that it is the ophthalmologist's responsibility to maintain liaison. This will be with the family, the general practitioner and the appropriate doctor who has contact with the educational service. Often direct contact with the school is helpful because educational decisions depend greatly on local arrangements so placement is an individual matter. Psychologists will usually be involved in assessing and helping the child; the earlier they are involved with the team work, the more worthwhile will be their contribution.

Since ophthalmology has a jargon of its own, it is important to translate it into terms the recipient of a report can comprehend. This is especially so for non-medical people and most of all for the family involved. When the family has only grasped part of the explanation it is helpful to record what they have been told. Repetition of the same explanation is often more helpful than varied ones, though particular aspects often need amplification. Questions that parents ask will be considered with examples.

Can the child see?

The child will have either an obvious visual difficulty or severe mental retardation for this question to be asked. The parents should be present while the ophthalmologist explains the test for fixation. The fixation reflex is the first basic step in development of vision and shows selection of some visual information from the mass of general visual information received by the eyes. It involves cortical function in giving priority to central retinal information over the peripheral, and maintenance of alignment of the eyes by commands to the mid brain centres that control eye movements. This reflex is partially innate and powerful with a normal brain; it is usually evident in the first few days of life and is well established by three months of age. The retinal image is initially out of focus since accommodation has not developed.

The parents will have decided whether the child can see their faces and probably tried toys to stimulate interest. If the response is negative then the most primitive stimulus of all is used, a moving light. To increase contrast, the background lighting is dimmed and if there is no response to a constant light then a flashing light is used; varying the colour makes little difference. If the child appears to fixate this must be confirmed by repositioning the target to see if refixation has developed or if the alignment was by chance. Occasionally, a globally retarded child will react by either increased or decreased body movements. This suggests light appreciation if the changes are repeatedly synchronous with the light.

Why can't he see?

There may be an obvious ocular defect but sometimes the eyes look normal. The pupil reactions and electrodiagnostic tests should provide an answer. Normal pupil reactions require a normal sensory visual input to the mid brain, intact central connections and a normal motor pathway to properly developed pupil muscles. The sensory input is generated by the retinal light receptors relaying information to the ganglion cells in the retina. The fibres from these cells form the optic nerves which pass several inches through the orbit and optic chiasm to the mid brain. Absent pupil reflexes mean there is either receptor and/or optic nerve damage. Generalized receptor damage may be associated with narrowed retinal arterioles; this sign is present long before optic atrophy appears. When atrophic optic discs are present it is necessary to discover if this is related to a retinal defect, primary neuronal disease or secondary to intra cranial disease.

An electroretinogram (ERG) should be arranged to help resolve this dilemma. A child may need to be referred specifically for this assessment.

These special arrangements and the aura of scientific equipment lead parents to expect much more information from the test that it can contribute. The ERG is an electrical record of the overall response of the retinal receptors to light. Part of the response is generated by the retinal pigment epithelium and bipolar cells but the ganglion cells do not contribute to it. Thus, a normal ERG is present both with ganglion cell disease from a neuronal degeneration such as Tay Sach's disease or ganglion nerve fibre damage from compression due to raised intracranial pressure. In an eye with tapeto-retinal degeneration where the primary defect is in the pigment epithelium and receptors the ERG is extinguished. The reduction in electrical response does not correlate with the loss of vision. Useful residual vision is often present although the ERG is absent. A contact lens is needed so it is necessary for a young child to have an anaesthetic for it. An averaged response from a lid electrode is under assessment.

If the pupil reactions are present then the defect in vision is due to damage in the optic radiation or occipital cortex. Cortical function is best assessed by simple psycho-physical tests. The only clinical use of the visual evoked response in this situation is to assess recovery of vision in a previously normal child. Thus, a child with head injury or meningitis showing little evidence of vision may show recovery of the evoked response before it is clinically apparent. Laterally placed occipital scalp electrodes may demonstrate a hemianopia. In each of these cases a flash stimulus is indicated rather than a structured stimulus used when steady fixation is present. An exception to this may be in the diagnosis of demyelinating disease.

How much can the child see?

This question must usually be answered imprecisely until the child can manage acuity tests based on the resolving power of the eye. It is important to remember certain aspects of form vision. The eyes are highly sensitive to moving objects. The cortex is firmly linked to ocular neuro-muscular control so that movement detected in the peripheral fields of vision results in movement of the eyes to line up the object of regard with binocular central vision. Any test dependent on a moving target is thus a poor indicator of resolution and will be insensitive to quite large changes in focus (e.g. rolled polystyrene balls). Initial movement of an object to obtain the interest of a child may well be needed but location of several static objects is much more informative about acuity. A test in which a single object is elicited from plain surroundings is less sensitive than one where one object is distinguished from several. The detection of a spot on the Catford Drum must be interpreted with caution on both these grounds. Small cake decorations are only roughly equivalent to a Snellen's 6/18. Both these tests are useful for young children who cannot manage a single letter recognition test, but are inaccurate. While emphasis is correctly placed on the comparison of monocular responses, it is apparent that the relative insensitivity of these tests may mask significant quality differences in vision between two eyes. Even the useful single letter recognition test (Sheriden-Gardener) may give equal results for two eyes which are shown to have a two line difference in acuity when tested with a Snellens chart. This test is made easier by screening of the rest of the chart from the line being read. This shows the importance of 'crowding' and of allowing cortical concentration on a small area of regard. Different tests thus have widely varying accuracy. Referral to the test a child can cope with gives some indication of the appropriate educational visual stimulus.

Mentally handicapped or severely visually handicapped children may never progress to letter recognition tests. Certainly they need to be conducted close to the child to obtain interest. A I metre test should be tried before abandoning the Sheriden-Gardener test. Edible test objects are most popular with the young or retarded child. Smarties for starters but quickly reducing to 'dolly mixtures' which can then be cut smaller will give a useful indication of vision. By using several sweets on a plain background a hemianopia can be excluded. The measured size of the stimulus used should be recorded for future comparison.

The handling of toys is the least sensitive way of assessing visual function but useful when other methods have failed. In attempting to gain a retarded child's interest the examiner usually finds he is moving the stimulus so the test is really one of establishing central fixation rather than testing acuity.

A child with very limited abilities or behaviour problems will take much longer to test. The tests should be made progressively simpler until a positive response is achieved and then this area of achievement is explored. When the child has confidence in succeeding, using both eyes, then the tests should be repeated using each eye separately. This is important to detect monocular defects. Latent nystagmus will produce individually poorer responses from either eye than with both eyes open. This applies even when a manifest squint is present and therefore binocular vision absent. It is the increased eye movement that decreases acuity.

Colour vision is always regarded with more interest by the parents and teachers than the ophthalmologist. The non-standard tests such as matching Lego blocks are useful but may disguise moderate defects. This is because there are other clues such as reflexisity which allow a correct match in the presence of a defect. The 'Guy's colour vision test' (a coloured S-G test) is useful, as is the 'City University test' for those with greater ability where children cannot manage an 'Ishihara' test. Testing for marked colour defect is not difficult and is of educational importance.

Visual field testing is an abnormal situation for a child. While an intelligent child will manage an 'adult' test as young as six years, the idea is foreign to him. To maintain fixation on a static dull target and ignore a moving one requires conscious inhibition of basic reflexes. Children therefore are best allowed to look at the peripheral object after initial distraction with a central one. Since anticipation is so much part of the response, two objects are best used coming from opposite sides. Lights or white balls on sticks in either hand work well, especially if the lights can be switched on or off with negligible finger movements. Since observation of the child's fixation is of paramount importance, the examiner should always face the child if he is single-handed. The lights or objects can be brought from behind if there is an assistant to maintain the child's interest and monitor fixation in front of him.

The question of how much a child can see has been answered by the parents being present during the tests and observing the child's abilities. If visual aids have been prescribed these should be used. If there is doubt about their usefulness it may be possible to demonstrate an improvement in skills with the aids. In some cases the aid will be worn for preventive purposes, i.e. to prevent loss of binocular vision. This should be explained at each visit. Difficulties with either glasses or other aids should be discussed and clear advice given.

Problems easily missed

Problems easily missed include scanning difficulties in reading. Nystagmus frequently increase in amplitude away from the primary positions. This leads to difficulties locating the start of a line or word. Crowding will be more of a problem for children with mental retardation. They need reading matter with a wide separation of words and lines more than increased magnification. Difficulties with visual concepts or memories need extra time for analysis. They are usually brought to light by teachers but suspicion may be aroused during routine tests. Difficulties with night vision and field defects sparing central vision usually remain silent until marked. Thus, retinitis pigmentosa may remain undiagnosed for years. A partial retinal detachment or juvenile glaucoma do not usually present until macular vision is affected.

What is the prognosis?

Although the answer is often that the prognosis is uncertain and several examinations will be needed to assess development, general comments can often helpfully be made.

A congenital defect is usually static. The vision will be reduced but it will improve as the child develops. Congenital nystagmus is a common example. Partial adaptation will develop so the child can learn to use his vision more usefully as he grows.

An acquired defect to vision resulting from say head injury, may be catastrophic in the short term but considerable long-term recovery is to be expected. If it occurs after the age of full development of vision, about eight, then there is an excellent fund of visual experience within the nervous system which is unlikely to be completely damaged. Even if total loss of sight occurs through ocular or optic nerve damage, the visual concepts previously gained will put that child in a much better learning position than one born blind. The psychological effects will be profound, however.

Both the above prognoses give hope for the future. Much the most difficult situation to share with the family is where progressive visual loss is expected. This may occur with metabolic disease such as Tay Sach's, with several specifically ocular diseases or as part of a generalized neurological degeneration. Accuracy of diagnosis is essential. Tests may well need repeating for the parents' sakes and a second opinion should be offered in all these cases. The doctor's understanding of the family's anxiety will help them accept what he says more easily. The parents will want to talk about the situation separately from the child and this will need to be done on several occasions. At some stage the child should join the discussion but not until the disease process is producing significant difficulty and the progressive nature is evident to the child. The news should be given by the doctor in charge of continuing care so it is both clear what has been said and to whom the patients return for further advice and information. Both retinitis pigmentosa and glaucoma will be considered later.

Will it happen again?

Genetic counselling should be offered to all parents and to children with significant risk at and just before school leaving age. The approach to this will be quite different in the two groups. Especially with immigrant families, the effects of consanguinity must be emphasized. Guidance may be given by the ophthalmologist or referral can be made to a geneticist.

Congenital cataracts can be dominantly inherited. New babies need to be examined within the first week of life. Congenital glaucoma can be familial; babies should be seen at, or as soon as possible after birth. Retinoblastoma is sporadic but occasionally it is familial. Children of such families need serial examinations under anaesthetic; peripheral tumours cannot be viewed otherwise. Retinal haemangioblastomas (Von Hippel's disease) are familial and may be bilateral. Large tumours are exceedingly difficult to treat but small asymptomatic ones often respond to laser treatment or cryotherapy. Retinitis pigmentosa may be inherited by dominant, recessive or sex-linked inheritance. It is important to explain the relevance to a particular family. Certain syndromes such as Stickler's or Marshall's syndrome are associated with high myopia and a retinal detachment risk as high as 50%. These are best treated by presentation with cryotherapy since the retinal tears that occur are often large and/or multiple with poor prognosis for vision.

When considering such high risk diseases it is necessary to create work by arranging to examine other family members. Taking a history of the other members is not sufficient, although an essential preliminary. An example is the examination for cataracts, not only in the child with dystrophia myotonica, but also among the relatives.

How soon will we know whether improvement is taking place?

It is useful to state that doctors are not prophets, but the family is entitled to some informed data. A range of examples from the literature can be discussed. If the disease is familial the advice is made more specific by considering the other members. In some families with retinitis pigmentosa some sight may be preserved throughout working life; in a few, sight is lost completely in childhood. Reference to the family pattern is therefore of general help but the individual variation needs to be emphasized.

Having said that the rate of improvement or deterioration can only be made after several examinations, it is useful to both the parents and doctor to record a time when a further prognosis will be attempted. This may well need changing but suggestion of a review period gives the family something to anticipate. This may well coincide with the period leading to nursery, primary or secondary school placement. Further review at school leaving is also important. The earlier the first assessment is made, the better will be the planning of educational and other assistance.

Pre-school assessment of the visually handicapped child is essential. By the age of five, a firm opinion about visual ability and the prognosis for binocular vision can be given. By the age of eight, a better idea of the effect of mental retardation on visual development can be gained. Development of binocular reflexes is then complete. The help that optical aids make to visual performance should be known so that educational recommendations on optional vision are made.

Educational placement
This can only be made if all the abilities of the child are considered and also the family support. Obtaining and correlating this information is difficult and this is one function of paediatric assessment units. The paediatrician will always be the co ordinator when the child is multiply handicapped. The ophthalmologist should be the leader when the child has a visual handicap only; that child should have had general development checked by a paediatrician.

Sometimes, the assessment is not complete in the preschool years because of failed hospital attendances, family mobility or instability. The assessment classes in nursery or primary schools are helpful in this situation. Close medical and educational liaison is best developed there. Evaluations by clinical and educational psychologists enhance communication between the professions. They need to have experience of the visually handicapped child and to know the local facilities and personalities. A big advantage of the assessment is that rapid changes in the child's abilities can be seen before a definite decision has been made.

There may well be medical factors which alter abilities, e.g., correction of undiagnosed high myopia will have a profound effect on the general, as well as, visual development. A child who has had congenital cataracts removed and given distance glasses only, may do much better with near vision tasks when supplied with reading correction.

The adverse effect of any handicap will be increased if the child is understimulated or emotionally disturbed. Marked changes in performance and happiness can be produced by sympathetic exploration of visual problems and a stable caring family. Advice by psychologists and child psychiatrists may be necessary. If this aspect of the child's development is neglected, serious errors can be made unintentionally. The general effect is for the child's potential to be underestimated. This makes the legal distinction of registration as partially sighted or blind unhelpful for children. Registration as a child with 'a visual handicap' is much more appropriate. Fortunately, the education of children by methods not involving the use of sight has not been carried out for a long time. The importance of using residual vision and its help in teaching non-visual skills is incorporated in teaching methods in all schools for the 'blind'. Mental power will govern the ability of the child to use visual skills. One dull child may develop better in a blind school when considerable residual vision is retained. Another more intelligent child will keep up with children in a partially sighted school though little vision is retained.

Special schools for the partially sighted are day schools. This causes problems to Education Authorities because of reducing numbers and travel costs, and to parents in travelling time. Schools for the blind are mainly residential. Disruption of family life has been reduced with emphasis on five-day residency and a four-term year. This produces stress on the Friday and Sunday evenings. This change puts more emphasis on the parents' handling of the child outside school hours and they need continuing support from the schools.

A clear distinction needs to be made between the educational needs of a child who has a static visual handicap and one who has a progressive one. In the latter case a child will adapt better in earlier placement at a special school rather than later. The natural transition periods may alter the timing to change. For instance, a child loosing sight from glaucoma may manage at an ordinary school with reducing visual fields during primary school, a direct move to a blind secondary school may well be the next step. If the sight is failing in secondary school years, consideration should be given to transfer to a blind school two years before school leaving. Minimal facility with non-visual skills can be learnt in one year. For the child's sake an earlier transfer should be suggested to the parents. The schools are always extremely understanding about such situations and welcome preliminary visits by parents. It is likely to be the ophthalmologist who is in the best situation to raise this problem and initiate discussion.

Can the child manage in a normal school?

This question will treble the output of adrenaline in certain parents and teachers! A decision must be made with consideration of the child's general and visual abilities, family situation and available educational facilities. Many visually handicapped children will manage in an ordinary school without markedly disrupting the running of the school. It is up to the family to show how little extra attention is needed. Explanation of the child's needs to the teacher is the first step. The child may need to sit near the front of the class on the side nearest the window. A demonstration of any aids used will help the teacher to know which ones are essential for which tasks. The biggest problem is usually speed of reading and writing, the child may well need to be in a slower stream and using spare intelligence to concentrate on minimizing the visual handicap. To some extent, the speed problem can be met by extra time spent both in and outside school hours. However, it is important that the child's need to be part of the children's community including play should not be sacrificed to academic educational ambitions of the parents.

Specific disorders of the nervous system
Hydrocephalus produces damage to the visual pathway. Raised intra-cranial pressure produces damage to both the visual cortex and the pre- and post-geniculate visual fibres. Some damage occurs before the pressure is controlled by one or more valves. The brain is much more tolerant of raised intracranial pressure before closure of the sutures than after fusion of the skull bones. A rise of intracranial pressure after closure of the sutures may be disastrous for vision, especially if there is already reduction in brain tissue. If there is a sustained block in outflow of cerebro-spinal fluid definite symptoms occur and papilloedema is often visible, though it may not be present if there has been only one intermittent increase of pressure. The valve will not empty when tested. The child needs urgent investigation and probably exploratory surgery if sepsis is excluded.

Intermittent blockage of the catheter may produce no symptoms, however, and the optic disc oedema is transitory. This gives no warning to either the family or doctor. The visual loss may thus be both sudden and unexpected. Kinking or alteration of position of the catheter from growth of the child may be relevant, but frequently no obstruction is demonstrated. Downward expansion of the third ventricles may produce the visual loss by pressure on the optic chiasm, nerves or tracts. Haemorrhage may have occurred within the visual cortex or optic radiations. Whatever the cause, it is unfortunately true that there is usually little recovery in vision. Serial brain scans allow ventricular size to be monitored but they often do not show a change in this situation. Serial visual fields allow optic atrophy to be monitored but the accuracy of this test depends on the co-operation and concentration of the child. Consistent results are rarely obtained so the use of this as a guide is limited.

Optic atrophy

Optic atrophy may result from many causes. It causes general reduction in quality of the vision and often a non-specific contraction of the visual field. Residual vision is helped by good lighting and magnification. It is more important for a child to be close to an object of interest than to wear glasses; visual aids are well tolerated by this group of children. If a unilateral central scotoma is present then binocular vision may be lost and a squint result. However, the squint may be due to a co-existing cranial nerve palsy and secondary amblyopia result. Such a child with bilateral optic atrophy may gain improvement in vision from part time occlusion. It is impossible to gauge the degree of acuity by visual inspection of the discs.

An occipital encephalocoele produces very variable visual loss. Often it is impossible to know how much visual cortex was present in the malformed tissue excised. There may be near normal vision but the defect is occasionally so severe that complete blindness occurs.

Prenatal infections

Prenatal infections produce damage to the developing eye in a serious degree only in the first two to three months of gestation. The eyes may be small and the most affected structures are the lens and retina. Rubella cataracts may be difficult to deal with surgically but the aim is to restore a focussed retinal image by the age of three months. Surgery restores a light path but the eye is grossly ametropic. Close liaison with a contact lens department is needed to keep a supply of powerful ($+15$ to $+30$ dioptres) lenses which usually have a life of only two months. The older child tolerates glasses well and will learn to use bifocals by school age.

Multiple retinal lesions are common from rubella and cytomegalic inclusion disease. Chorio-retinal foci are commoner with toxoplasmic infection. Usually the retinal periphery is involved and visual function may be little impaired. Loss of central vision will occur if the fovea is involved even if there is only one focus. Occasionally, significant reduction in peripheral vision occurs with disseminated foci; difficulty with night vision results.

Infection later in pregnancy may well lead to alterations in the retinal pigment epithelium. This is derived from the neural tissue of the optic vesicle and is essential for nutrition and maintenance of the receptors, the rods and cones. The pigment epithelium may show widespread alteration in pigmentation, especially at the posterior pole of the eye but usually the visual function is little impaired. In children with congenital rubella and nerve deafness this is a frequent incidental finding.

Tumours

Tumours affecting vision may be primary or secondary. Retinoblastoma is a highly radio sensitive tumour so small tumours may be destroyed with preservation of vision. Since the tumours may be multifocal and bilateral, careful follow-up is needed in a unit catering for children's needs. Both the lens and retina are at risk from repeated irradiation. Secondary deposits of neuroblastoma and primary optic nerve gliomas will produce proptosis. Neuroblastoma is treatable by chemotherapy and a glioma by surgical excision; the eye is usually preserved, although it is blind, for cosmetic reasons. Optic nerve gliomas may occur in association with Von Recklinghausen's disease. Intracranial tumours may affect ocular motility by causing cranial nerve palsies. This will produce a squint with amblyopia in a young child, but diplopia in a child who has established binocular vision. Posteria fossa tumours may produce nystagmus from cerebellar damage or raised intracranial pressure with papilloedema. The raised pressure may produce bilateral abducent palsy with convergence of the eyes.

The Sturge-Weber syndrome is a hamartoma with both intracranial and ophthalmic components. The skin and subcutaneous tissues may be largely replaced by vascular malformation. This should be left alone as long as the child can see out of the eye. The parents should be told that the lesion may grow for several years as the child grows but nature often produces autothrombosis. Laser treatment may be useful; excision and skin grafting is usually reserved for eyelids which cover the eye completely.

Internally, the eye may have a choroidal haemangioma associated with glaucoma. This is very difficult to control and progressive visual loss may occur in spite of both medical and surgical treatment.

Neurocutaneous syndromes may produce serious visual loss. Tuberose sclerosis (Bourneville's disease) is occasionally associated with a glioma of the optic nerve head. Von Recklinghausen's disease is much commoner; externally a mechanical ptosis may be produced by lid involvement. The optic nerve glioma has been mentioned but the chiasm and optic tract may also be affected. Involvement of the bones near the orbital apex may produce pulsating exophthalmos. The family should know that lesions may be multiple and that inheritance is dominant.

Demyelinating disease is uncommon in childhood. Rarely it affects the optic nerve in the second decade. At the same period, Leber's optic atrophy may manifest itself; this neuronal degeneration tragically affects one and then the second eye. No treatment is of proven benefit so general support is needed for younger siblings of a family when a child suddenly develops the typically acute visual loss in the first eye. Discussion about career prospects and further education is usually requested by the family for other members likely to become affected. Similar advice may be sought by those families with similar dominant optic atrophy that comes on much more gradually. The degree of residual vision is often fairly consistent within a family. Vision for mobility is usually retained but central vision is always lost in Leber's disease. Some central vision may be kept in dominantly inherited optic atrophy. Early provision of visual aids and mobility training is needed, and then retraining for alternative employment.

Retinitis pigmentosa (RP) may be an ocular disease present in an otherwise healthy individual. It may also be associated with other degenerative disorders affecting the nervous system. One of the most unfortunate associations is in Usher's syndrome where progressive hearing loss is associated with progressive visual loss. Since the onset of RP is slow and painless it may go undiagnosed for years. Clinically, it is only when the visual loss is falling below 30° that help is sought. Prior to that there is a peripheral island of vision outside a mid peripheral scotoma. Good central vision is retained for years in a 'tunnel' in most cases unless there is an associated macular degeneration. Cataracts develop late in the disease and very rarely produce sufficient opacity of the media to give significant visual improvement following extraction. The inheritance and variable clinical course in families has been mentioned. Visual aids are well used by this group and the new closed circuit television (CCTV) aids suit them well, even where there is a minimal field. None of the various 'visual field expanding glasses' have established themselves a place, though initial enthusiasm may be expressed.

Ocular myopathy

Ocular myopathy presents rarely in childhood. Congenital ptosis, often associated with a superior rectus weakness, is common. Surgery is essential when the frontalis overaction is causing headaches and an abnormal head posture is needed to maintain sight. Many other cases have cosmetic surgery. Myasthenia gravis occurs in childhood and a thymoma may be present; the disease responds well to medical treatment which may need reduction after removal of a thymus tumour. Ptosis and weakness of extra ocular muscles may occur late in the course of a systemic myopathy but they often are spared.

Trauma

Trauma is an important source of eye damage in childhood. Skull fractures or raised intracranial pressure often produce optic atrophy or cranial nerve palsies. Treatment for the latter is initially expectant and the visual prognosis for binocular vision depends on the age of the child, severity of brain damage and degree of palsy. Under the age of five, supressive amblyopia rapidly occurs if the visual axes are non aligned, and this is quite likely for a few years after that age. A small ocular deviation may be controlled by fresnel prisms. They will neutralize a fixed angle of deviation but control depends on the reserve of binocular vision. Since the angle of squint usually varies between distance and near vision, the development of binocular vision usually needs to be good for fresnel prisms to be helpful; a slight loss in acuity is associated with their wear. Severe concussion may produce loss of binocular vision with separation of visual axes without diplopia. Occasionally there is spontaneous recovery months later.

Direct eye damage is either concussive or penetrating. Both are serious and may lead to blindness. The most dreaded complication of penetrating ocular injuries is sympathetic ophthalmitis. This is most likely to occur if there is delay in diagnosis and repair. The inflammation is symmetrical and bilateral; it starts about three weeks after injury and tends to be progressive in spite of treatment. Removal of the injured 'exciting' eye is ineffective in stopping the inflammation once the bilateral process has begun. A decision about removal needs to be taken within two weeks of injury.

Other problems

Iatrogenic eye disease produces retrolental fibroplasia. Any drug may carry toxic side-effects and oxygen may inhibit the development of the premature retina of a baby of under 1 kg. Damage is infrequent in the 1−1.5 kg birth weight range. Monitoring arterial oxygen tensions has reduced the risk but some cases will occur unless lives are to be lost. Exposure to high oxygen tensions for as little as six hours may result in permanent retinal changes. Intermittent monitoring is safe but does not solve the problem of rapidly changing arterial oxygen tensions. This is frequently the situation in resolving hyaline membrane disease. Continuous monitoring carries risks; infection via the umbilical artery may cause necrotising enterocolitis and shunting of blood through a skin sensor may seriously affect the cardio-respiratory state of the baby. (see Chapter 2, Book 2).

Complete loss of sight from iatrogenic eye disease is rare but 'forme frustes' are not infrequent. Fibrous tissue in the temporal retinal periphery may drag the macula producing a pseudo-divergent squint. Distortion of central vision is then usually present. The late complication is retinal tear formation from continued tension on the retina; this leads to retinal detachment. However, minor changes in retinal architecture are compatible with continued good vision.

Psychogenic blindness or reduction in vision is related to stress. It is most commonly associated with problems at school. These are usually around exam times but may relate to difficult relations with a teacher or bullying by other children. Less commonly it results from severe emotional upset at home. Careful examination of the child and special investigations are quite therapeutic. Psychiatric and psychological help should be sought if the situation is not improving within a short period.

Squint surgery is either functional or cosmetic. When a squint is intermittent or only present is one direction of gaze then binocular vision is present some of the time. Surgical realignment of the eyes then allows the binocular reflexes to maintain control. This is a functional result. Most children with constant squints have lost binocular vision. If amblyopia is present requiring occlusion then achievement of alternating vision is usually a good visual result. Surgery may be done for cosmetic reasons and the repositioning is then approximate. When the vision is good in each eye the position is usually fairly stable, but when dense amblyopia is present that eye may well drift in later years.

An abnormal head posture may be adopted by some children with congenital nystagmus. The posture is used to minimize the amplitudes of the abnormal eye movements. Surgery to all four horizontal muscles can restore a normal head position. Vertical muscle surgery may be needed for congenital palsies such as a superior oblique weakness. The abnormal head posture is adopted to maintain binocular vision so the aim of surgery is to restore comfortable binocular viewing. Mechanical causes due to cervical spine abnormalities or muscular defects need to be excluded.

Further Reading

Black, P.D. (1980) Ocular defects in children with cerebral palsy. *British Medical Journal*, **ii**, 487–488.

Brant, J.C. & Nowotny, M. (1976) Testing of visual acuity in young children: an evaluation of some commonly used methods. *Developmental Medicine and Child Neurology*, **18**, 568–576.

Cole, G.F., Hungerford, J. & Jones, R.B. (1984) *Delayed visual maturation Archives of Disease in Childhood*, **59**, 107–110.

Dubowitz, L.M.S., Dubowitz, V., Morante, A. & Verghote, M. (1980) Visual function in the preterm and fullterm newborn infant. *Developmental Medicine and Child Neurology*, **22**, 465–475.

Fells, P. (1978) Recognition and management of squints. *Journal of Maternal and Child Health*, **40**, 8–14.

Gardiner, P.A. (1979) Cataracts. *British Medical Journal*, **i**, 36–38.

Gardiner, P.A. (1979) Blindness and partial sight. *British Medical Journal*, **i**, 180–181.

Gardiner, P.A. (1979) Evaluating common signs and symptoms. *British Medical Journal* **i**, 389–393.

Goble J.L. (1984) *Paediatric Habilitation Vol. 5 Visual Disorders in the Handicapped Child*. Marcel Decker.

Gordon, N. (1968) Visual agnosia in childhood. *Developmental Medicine and Child Neurology*, **10**, 377–379.

Gordon, N. (1969) Double vision. *Developmental Medicine and Child Neurology*, **11**, 242–245.

Hall, S.M., Pugh, A.G. & Hall, D.M.B. (1982) Vision screening in the under-5s. *British Medical Journal*, **ii**, 1095–1098.

Harcourt, B. (1976) Squint. *British Medical Journal*, **i**, 703–705.

Ingram, R.M. (1973) Role of the eye clinic in modern ophthalmology. *British Medical Journal*, **i**, 278–280.

Kennerley Bankes, J.L. (1974) Eye defects of mentally handicapped children. *British Medical Journal*, **i**, 533–535.

Kirkham, T.H. (1973) Preliminary testing of visual function. *British Journal of Hospital Medicine*, **10**, 299–306.

Mellor, D.H. & Fielder, R. (1980) Dissociated visual development: electrodiagnostic studies in infants who are 'slow to see'. *Developmental Medicine and Child Neurology*, **22**, 327–55.

Morante, A., Dubowitz, L.M.S., Levene, M. & Dubowitz, V. (1982) The development of visual function in normal and neurologically abnormal preterm and fullterm infants. *Developmental Medicine and Child Neurology*, **24**, 771–784.

Williams, H. (1976) Congenital cataracts. *Developmental Medicine and Child Neurology*, **18**, 806–808.

Wybar, K. (1979) Testing for squint. *Journal of Maternal and Child Health*, **4**, 38–40.

Chapter 18
Aids to Vision

George Marshall

Low vision aids

For those who have an impairment of vision, whether minor or serious, any aid that can assist in improving the quality of seeing must be given consideration. Improved visual acuity depends on producing a larger image at the retina by optical or non-optical means. In either case, the aim is to produce an image large enough for the person to recognize it and to give sufficient information to interpret the image correctly.

In many cases, the provision of some form of optical aid can be of value to those with less than normal vision. It is important, however, to pay careful attention to the psychological and training aspects of this provision. The person who is a recent victim of an accident or of an incapacitating eye disease or dysfunction is not prepared, at least initially, to accept the new visual status and is not at that stage a good subject for vision aids. At the other end of the scale, those who were born with a visual defect, and have had such a defect for a long time, have become psychologically adjusted to that state, and have usually become accustomed to a certain amount of pampering by their family, and to 'allowance' being made in school. Such persons usually lack the stimulus for adequate visual effort. Again, interpretation may be needed to overcome resentment of the short reading distance or restricted fields of vision required in order to see with high magnification, or of the nuisance of holding a lens, etc.

Although visual impairment does impose some restrictions on the life of the individual, many of these restrictions can be overcome. Visually handicapped people can often benefit greatly from the very many varieties of low vision aids which have been developed. This may well be accomplished with the aid of one type of low vision aid such as spectacles. At other times, and with other people, several aids may be required for different kinds of vision. One aid may be required for reading, and another for close work, and yet another different type of aid for long distance viewing. The use the individual makes of the low vision aid will depend upon the needs and upon the encouragement and training he or she has, in order to make the greatest use of those aids. Those who are partially sighted must be encouraged to make the full use of any low vision aid that is prescribed. The low vision aid may not enable the partially sighted person to see perfectly, but should it improve vision at all, then it is generally very well worth having. Many visually handicapped people may well refuse the help of any sort of low vision aid as they may be unwilling to admit, perhaps even to themselves, that the visual handicap is permanent. It may take a little time to accept the help, and to adjust to the necessity of it.

The handling of a child with less than normal vision is somewhat tedious at times, and always requires a great deal of patience and understanding. Low vision aids can be a help, but are not a 'cure-all' for restricted vision, or even the proper answer in many cases. From the point of view of education it is imperative that a child is trained carefully to use his residual vision to the fullest possible extent and efficiency. If an optical aid will assist, then it should be provided. If, however, when this training has been given, the child can then use his vision equally as effectively and with greater speed and accuracy without the aid, then he should be encouraged to do so.

An understanding of magnification is an essential if one is to understand how visual performance can be helped. If a person advances towards an object from say 20 feet to 10 feet, he will produce a magnification of two times. If he then moves to five feet from the object he will have produced a magnification of four times, and if then to two feet, the magnification will be ten. This might be termed the non-optical method of magnification and can have wide application. For instance, viewing television at one foot from the screen will produce a magnification of twenty times that when viewed at 20 feet. In other words, it is merely a question of moving closer. The fields of vision are not restricted. This non-optical method is just as valid for near vision as it is for distance vision. Thus, if one brings a book or card from 20 inches to four inches from the eyes, then there will be a magnification of five. Bearing in mind the value and direction of light therefore, it can be seen that many of those with only moderate degrees of near vision impairment can be helped by this non-optical method.

The higher the magnification of an optical aid, the smaller the field and the fewer the number of letters which can be encompassed in one eye span, the greater the peripheral distortion and the more difficult it is to get illumination between the magnifier and the page. The thicker the magnifying glass the more likely there are to be annoying light reflections on its outer surface.

It is difficult to tell which specific people will require, or will benefit from having a visual aid. In general, anyone who cannot perform ordinary school, work and home tasks with the best orthodox lens correction of spectacles, and who is not totally blind, may be considered a candidate for such help. It is then a matter of the amount of residual visual acuity, visual fields, and what the person is able to do with these, that is important. The exact cause of a visual impairment except when a progressive disorder needs to be diagnosed is usually of less importance than the amount of residual visual efficiency available and the effectiveness of the training of that vision. The appearance of the eyes is usually quite misleading but may have social implications.

It is very difficult for anyone with normal vision to understand how a person with limited vision sees. Anyone with normal vision will appreciate the difference in quality between well-made magnification systems that are expensive compared with cheaply made systems of similar power, and would choose the former. A person with a visual aberration may well choose the one of poorer quality, however, because the distortions actually help him to see better. The best in such circumstances, therefore, is not necessarily the most expensive.

There are a variety of low vision aids available. They may be held on the head, mounted so that they may be held in or on the hand, or rested on the reading material. Whether there is a minor or a severe vision loss, except for total blindness, one or more of such aids may be of value.

Low vision aids may be classified as either (A) for distance, or (B) for near.

(A)   Distance aids, always telescopic, may be monocular Fig. 18.1 or binocular. The binoculars normally used are always small enough to be easily carried in a pocket or handbag, but this smallness limits the magnification to 8×. The main disadvantage of distance aids is that generally they are too cumbersome to be mounted into spectacle frames, although this is done sometimes, especially for school children, but only produces magnifications up to 3×. Distance telescopes have a very small field of view so cannot be used for general moving around or driving.

(B)   Near aids can be sub-divided:

1   Spectacles/contact lenses.

2   Auxiliary magnifiers—Stand-mounted or hand-held giving up 25× magnification. Figs 18.2, 18.3, 18.4.

3   High binocular reading additions to spectacles with a prism to aid convergence where necessary, and giving up to 2× magnification. Fig. 18.5a.

4   Spectacle mounted monocular magnifiers (Fig. 18.5b), and simple or

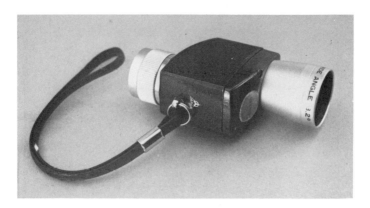

Fig. 18.1. Distance monocular.

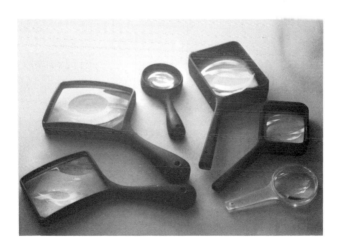

Fig. 18.2. Selection of hand magnifiers.

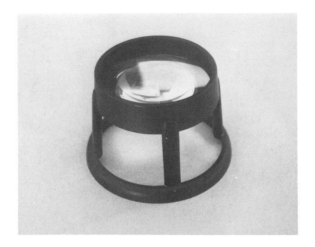

Fig. 18.3. Aspheric desk reader.

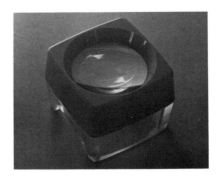

Fig. 18.4. Small field ×8 magnifier.

compound lenses, which may, in higher powers, be internally illuminated and/or hand held (Fig. 18.6). These can give up to 20× magnification.

5   Binocular telescopes, giving up to 5× magnification.

6   Monocular telescopes, giving up to 10× magnification.

7   Projection devices and instruments which give magnifications up to 25×—such as overhead projectors, closed circuit television systems, etc.

It is always advisable to determine the person's exact reading needs and then to fit with the weakest lens which will be satisfactory to that person.

Closed circuit television systems

Closed circuit television systems for the visually handicapped have been researched and developed in many countries, and many claims are made for them. The systems vary from moderately simple to quite advanced, and prices range accordingly.

Closed circuit television systems are electronic devices for use by those with severe visual limitations (i.e. for those with limited residual

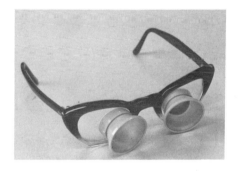

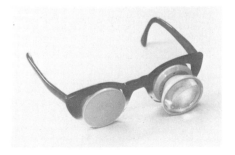

Fig. 18.5. (a) Binocular telescopic spectacles for near use. (b) These are also made as monoculars.

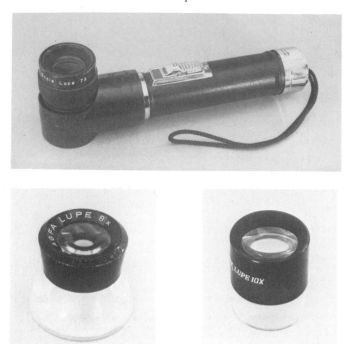

Fig. 18.6. Peak Light Lupe (×7) and Lupes (×8, ×10).

vision), which allow them to read and write. The systems can be used at home, at work, or at school. Although not readily portable—most are not portable at all—some manufacturers do produce small sets capable of being carried.

The systems are all based on an adaptation of closed-circuit television technology. Each system includes a television camera with zoom lens, a television monitor, which is a display screen in appearance similar to a home television receiver, and an X−Y platform. This latter is a platform on which material is placed for reading and writing and is capable of movement from left to right and backwards and forwards. Most systems have a reversal system incorporated, by which the user can view black letters, diagrams, etc., on a white background, or reverse to white letters, etc., on a black background. There are additional sophistications in some systems, such as electrical focussing ranges, typewriter viewing tables, and an extended range of magnifications from 2× to 200×.

Most low vision aids can be supplied through the hospital service in Britain. Referral is through the person's own General Practitioner, or by recommendation by Social Services, to an ophthalmologist. He will advise and make any necessary arrangements at the local hospital or nearest low vision clinic. There are low vision clinics at some hospitals and these are usually staffed by ophthalmic opticians. The best clinics hold a wide range of aids and have efficient follow-up services. Where a hospital does not have such a clinic, ophthalmic consultants may refer people to a private ophthalmic optician. This system, however, does not always provide a full range of aids nor a suitable follow-up system. In some cases, therefore, people may be referred by the consultant to another hospital for low vision services, whilst maintaining eye care and supervision himself.

Opticians may also supply aids privately. This is an expensive way, however. It is most advisable to consult an expert in the field of low vision aids before making purchases of what may well be useless equipment.

Light and vision

For the human eye to work efficiently and without undue strain, adequate light is needed. This is extremely important when doing close work, and for any vision aid to be of value, the problem presented by lighting when reading must be understood. Depending on the fineness of the work involved, the amount of light required will vary from an absolute minimum of 25 foot-candles up to as much as 100 foot-candles. A foot-candle is the amount of light emitted by a standard wax candle at a distance of one foot. Whether the light is natural or artificial it should be evenly distributed, free from glare and shadow and with any reflection away from the eyes. In daylight, of course, there should be no problem, since the illumination near a good window will vary from 100 to 200 foot-candles, depending on the brightness of the day and the size and exposure of the window. However, at some distance from the window, the daylight may very well need to be supplemented by artificial light.

Young children need some 60–70 foot-candles for continuous reading tasks, etc., whilst for studying, fine machine work, etc., for older children and adults at least 30–50 foot-candles are essential. In artificial light dependence should not be on ceiling lights alone. A table or reading lamp should be used also, some four feet or so from the working surface. The ceiling light should be kept on, however, to prevent sharp contrasts. The marked contrast between the bright light on the work and a dark background is annoying and fatiguing to the eye muscles. This is partly due to the constant changes made necessary in the size of the pupil to

compensate for the greatly varying amounts of light which enter the eyes
as the gaze alternates between the light on the work and the much darker
surroundings. The background therefore, should have a uniform illumination with non-glare light of less intensity than that used on the work,
but strong enough to prevent the sharp contrasts. This can be obtained by
natural light during daylight, and by ceiling or wall lights at night time.
White ceilings will improve the level of illumination, as will pastel-coloured
walls. It is most important to avoid glare, and it is quite surprising how
much glare we suffer without really being aware of the causes of it.
Furniture and floor surfaces, for instance, can produce quite uncomfortable glare, and they should, therefore, have a matt finish. Windows are
best situated so that the main light enters from one side. If there are
other windows in opposite or side walls then they should be more heavily
curtained or screened to prevent confusing cross lighting.

With sufficient non-glare light, proper background lighting and no
cross lighting, it is possible to study or work to close limits for hours
without any strain being imposed upon the eye and its muscles. Viewing
television under the proper conditions will not cause strain either. There
should be some other source of light in the room in addition to that
supplied by the television screen, to avoid annoying and fatiguing contrasts of light and dark.

For anyone who is visually impaired, the value of light is of tremendous importance. If a person with a visual impairment needs to read at a
distance of three inches, for instance, his head will obscure most of the
light. He needs to sit near a light source, therefore, and with the eye that
he uses nearer to that source. The light intensity required can be regu-
lated by the distance from the light source, and this will also diffuse the
light. It must be remembered that light can be a two-edged sword for
many who are visually handicapped. They need more light to see, but this
extra light often creates scatter because of aberrations in the eye. Light,
whether it be natural or artificial, should, therefore, be directed towards
the material being read so that it reflects away from the reader, and
scatter is thereby eliminated.

It is not enough just to give a visually handicapped person a vision
aid. For any vision aid to be of value, whether it be optical or non-
optical, the problems presented by lighting must be thoroughly understood also. In addition, the person must be helped to orientate himself
with it and be given careful training in how to adjust himself and his work
to the light.

Print, paper, books

Books are the most vital of educational tools and as such require special consideration for those with an impairment of vision. At one time it was considered necessary for books and reading material for visually handicapped children to be printed in large type. Much research with large groups of visually handicapped children and adults, with a very wide range of eye defects and over a considerable period of time, has taken place both in this country and in the United States of America. Very many type faces and type sizes were used, and varying spacings. As a result, the theory of large print materials for visually handicapped people has undergone considerable reappraisal. Properly prescribed and carefully used low vision aids make it possible for persons with vision sufficient to read large print also to read normal size print with such an aid equally as effectively. As the results of further technological advances become available, and as low vision aid services become more extensive, the range of reading materials suitable for visually handicapped people will become greatly expanded as they are able more easily to use generally produced materials. Only when low vision aids are widely available, however, will all visually handicapped readers have a true choice between large print material and ordinary print material. Large print books and materials do have their place, especially for older persons who have a visual impairment. The visually handicapped child should not be conditioned to accept the limitations that he can use only large print, thus restricting him to the limited number of titles available in that medium, compared to the much larger quantity in ordinary print.

The criteria of legibility are typeface, type size, inter-word and inter-line spacing, line length, quality of paper, page and illustration layout, margins and density of ink. These criteria apply to visually handicapped people as well as to the normally sighted. To be a fluent reader, word patterns rather than perception of individual letters must be immediately recognizable. In the reading learning process there has to be a period of word analysis and word formation, but this is a foundation period to help the child to acquire a large reading vocabulary which he can instantly recognize.

To understand the needs of the visually handicapped in the field of print and books, it is necessary to investigate the pattern of words. These are formed of outline, spaces enclosed by letters, spaces between letters and spaces between the words themselves. If the individual letters are printed in thick type then inevitably the spaces enclosed by each letter are reduced, and if great care is not taken, the ease of recognition can be reduced also. A suitable typeface is an essential, but there is no one single typeface which has proved to be universally correct. Since no two people perceive in exactly the same way, the development of a single set of standards for print and typeface is not simple nor is an ideal solution readily available. For some, type size may bear less relationship to re-adability than such factors as familiarity with the type style, illumination, contrast, focal distance, width of line and the spacing of letters, words and lines or combinations of them. What is of great importance, however, is the way in which the type is used. There are certain preferences in typography for visually handicapped children, but for the most part their needs in this field differ from those of the normal child. Generally speak-ing, the poorest sighted visually impaired children find good, slightly bolder than average typeface somewhat easier to read. Gill Sans and Plantin are good examples of these. At all times, however, one must bear in mind the problem of eye-span. In the normally sighted person the span at reading distance is about 10 cm. This allows the eyes to take in several words at once. Some visually impaired children, however, have a span of as little as 1.5 cm. Enlarging type, therefore, is defeatist. The child can only see one or two letters at any time in such a case. The whole word pattern is difficult and often impossible to see and the child in these circumstances will never become a fluent reader. Such children are slow and frequently inaccurate and invariably the child wearies of trying to read, becomes bored and frustrated with it, and often gives up.

There are other points to watch in choosing books for the visually handicapped. Unduly long lines make for poor follow-on, cramped margins are inhibiting and lines too close together cause visual confusion. To obtain reasonable spacing between words and lines will mean that the most suitable books are also more expensive. A much wider range of well printed material is now available which is suitable for visually handi-capped children. Illustrations can be a problem and there are one or two points on which care needs to be taken. It is essential, for instance, that illustrations should be adjacent to the relevant text. Those with a visual impairment can become confused visually if they are obliged to search for them. In some books, illustrations are allowed to sprawl unnecessarily across pages. Frequently, in such cases, the reading matter has been printed above, alongside and below the illustration, partly on white or partly on the coloured illustration. Obviously, in choosing for a visually handicapped person, such books should be avoided.

Where possible, the finish of the paper on which a book is printed should be prominent in the selection procedure. Art paper for instance, has too much reflection. The paper must have a dull, vellum, or non-glare finish. The colour of the paper should be white, but not bright white, and should be chosen to provide maximum contrast with the type, without glare. The paper should be durable, good to write upon and able to take duplicating and offset litho printing equally well.

Vision and child development

The development of a child may be affected by a physical disability, low intelligence or environmental deprivation. When a child suffers a loss in any one of these areas, his development will depend on his ability to utilize the other variables to compensate for the loss. When the child is unable to compensate adequately, there will be a lag in his development. Eighty per cent of learning experiences occur through vision, and there-fore much of the child's ability to discern relationships and to establish perceptual experiences necessary for normal development occur through vision. When a child has a visual loss, he must obtain information from his environment through other means. So spatial relationships and per-ceptual experiences necessary for normal development will suffer. The relationship between the degree of visual loss and development is not a straight forward one but will depend on the other variables and their interrelationship.

Since the visual sense has such a profound effect on a child's devel-opment, the child should be given every opportunity to learn through his vision, using aids if necessary. While prescribed lenses and low vision aids are important for improving visual acuity, they alone will not stop lags in the child's development. Developmental lags occur because of a variety of factors, and not solely because of a reduction of visual acuity. If this were so, then all children with 6/6 distance visual acuity and healthy eyes would show 'normal' development, and we know that this is not the case.

Low vision aids give the visual system the ability to function at a higher demand level. However, the discrimination and learning process is not a passive one. Learning involves the active process of probing, investigating and understanding relationships. If the child is able to see clearly but does not understand the relationships of what he sees, then there is no learning.

Low vision aids can cause perceptual distortions to the visual space world. Optical aids such as telescopes and microscopes improve visual acuity because they utilize concepts of optical magnification. The magnification enlarges the object and also makes it appear closer than it is. While magnification yields information about detail, it also causes a spatial distortion. For the normally sighted individual looking at an object across the room, the object gives information about size, distance, and detail. The visually handicapped individual using a telescopic aid sees a large magnified image of the object from which he can gain information about detail. However, the information about the actual size and distance of the object is false. The individual must look at the actual object to correctly interpret information about the latter.

If the individual can adapt quickly to changes in his visual world to gain the information he requires, he will have a greater probability of being successful with a low vision aid. The adaptation involves the ability quickly to screen and filter out certain information that is useless or erroneous. The child who is able to do this will be able to grasp 'the meaning of things' with greater efficiency than the child who cannot. For the child who cannot adapt readily, the aid can actually interfere with his ability to learn visually. It should not be inferred that optical aids should not be used because of this reason, but that support and help should be given to utilize motor movement and multi-sensory input to reinforce the visual perceptual inadequacies. The purpose is to enable the child to transfer information from one modality to another in order to establish the perceptual experience. As the child begins to understand what he is seeing through this approach, he will in turn have more trust and confidence to use his vision. Ultimately, the goal is to have the child gain the information predominately through a visual approach rather than a multi-sensory one and with motor reinforcement.

The visually handicapped child can also have functional vision problems that can interfere with his learning and development. This refers to difficulty in controlling pursuit tracking movements, difficulty in sustaining accommodation, problems in convergence of the eyes, or an inability to quickly redirect the eyes from one point to another point. Because vision is our dominant sense, energy will be expended to allow the individual to operate visually so long as the person derives some form of meaningful information from the visual process. Therefore, by only improving visual acuity and not analysing the visual process for possible causes of interference, the child may not function at his potential. In turn, visual interference may cause perceptual inadequacies leading to developmental lags.

The relationship of vision to development is profound. The science of optics has yielded great advances enabling the visually handicapped individual to function at high visual demand levels. However, the improvements in visual acuity alone do not enable the individual to operate with maximum efficiency. For the visually handicapped child, the learning experience is greatly influenced by his use of the visual process. Concern for helping the child visually should not end with a low vision prescription to improve his acuity, but should begin at this point. If we expect the child to function within our visual world, we must attempt to understand the interactive process between his physical abilities, psychological disposition and his environmental influences. When we understand this better, it may be possible to influence the learning process and so help the child to function to his potential.

Acquired visual handicap

If the onset of partial sight is sudden, as by accident, the individual may go through a period of great shock. It may well cause him to lose all motivation, to withdraw, and to become extremely depressed. This is a normal state of affairs, and precedes emotional recovery. It is during this period that the child needs great support, sympathy, and gradual encouragement towards becoming independent once again. Under no circumstances must he be offered a false hope of recovery. He needs to be helped to understand that although he has a handicap, he can learn to live with it, and move towards re-learning and adjustment of life. The quality of the help is absolutely vital. A realistic attitude is one which disregards stereotypes, and tries to understand each person as an individual. The child will always learn more easily to function with his visual handicap when he knows that others are interested in his well-being. He will need friendship and acceptance. He will take time to accept help from someone he does not know, and it may take time to develop a good relationship. He will need to be helped to trust others in their help, and patience is absolutely vital. He must be encouraged to respect himself, given a sense of his own worth and the assistance to look forward to the future.

Conclusions

It is important that the partially sighted person is helped to see as well as he possibly can with his less than normal vision. This may be accomplished with the aid of one type of low visual aid such as spectacles. At other times and with other people several aids may be required for different kinds of vision. One aid may be required for reading and other close-up work, and another different type of aid for long distance viewing. The use the individual makes of the low visual aid will depend upon his needs, and upon the encouragement and training he has to make the greatest use of those aids. The low visual aid may not enable the partially sighted person to see perfectly, but should it improve vision at all, then it is generally well worth having.

In acquired conditions, it is helpful to find out what the child's interests were before he became visually handicapped. Those who are not interested in reading books may well want a low visual aid to read letters, labels and tickets, or even television programmes. Some apparently minor activity might well provide the incentive to learn to use his low visual aid.

Besides the possibility of low visual aids, good lighting is imperative. It is so important for people with poor vision, that experiments should be made with various types of lighting. For many, the small, high intensity desk light, which can easily be carried around from one room to another, provides excellent lighting. Others find the excessive glare too much and may need to wear tinted glasses. Adjustable book stands may be helpful for reading and writing, and black felt-tipped marking pens are useful for larger writing. There are quite a number of books in large print, and many of them can be obtained from the local library.

Acknowledgement
The figures are published with the kind permission of Exhall Grange School (Headmaster, R.G. Bignell).

Index

Note:
Page references in italic indicate figures, those in bold indicate tables. Roman numerals refer to the Introduction.

399